PUBLIC HEALTH IN THE 21ST CENTURY

SPATIAL DISTRIBUTION OF HEALTH MANPOWER IN CHINA

EXPLORING ITS CHARACTERISTICS AND DETERMINANTS

PUBLIC HEALTH IN THE 21ST CENTURY

Additional books and e-books in this series can be found on Nova's website under the Series tab.

PUBLIC HEALTH IN THE 21ST CENTURY

SPATIAL DISTRIBUTION OF HEALTH MANPOWER IN CHINA

EXPLORING ITS CHARACTERISTICS AND DETERMINANTS

BIN ZHU, PhD
YING MAO, PhD
AND
CHIH-WEI HSIEH, PhD

nova science publishers
New York

Library of Congress Cataloging-in-Publication Data

Names: Zhu, Bin, 1957- author. | Mao, Ying (Public Health Scholar), author.
Hsieh, Chih-Wei, author.
Title: Spatial distribution of health manpower in China : exploring its characteristics and determinants / Bin Zhu, Ying Mao, Chih-wei Hsieh.
Description: New York : Nova Science Publishers, Inc., [2020] | Series: Public health in the 21st century | Includes bibliographical references and index.
Identifiers: LCCN 2020006806 (print) | LCCN 2020006807 (ebook)
ISBN 9781536175721 (paperback) | ISBN 9781536175738 (adobe pdf)
Subjects: LCSH: Medical personnel--Supply and demand--China--Statistics. Medical personnel--Supply and demand--Research--China. | Medical offices--Location--China. | Medicine--Practice--China. | China--Statistics, Medical.
Classification: LCC RA410.9.C6 Z48 2020 (print) | LCC RA410.9.C6 (ebook) DDC 338.4/761069--dc23
LC record available at https://lccn.loc.gov/2020006806
LC ebook record available at https://lccn.loc.gov/2020006807

Published by Nova Science Publishers, Inc. † New York

CONTENTS

List of Figures		**vii**
List of Tables		**xiii**
Preface		**xix**
Abbreviations		**xxi**
Chapter 1	Introduction	**1**
Chapter 2	Literature Review and Research Framework	**13**
Chapter 3	Research Methodologies	**31**
Chapter 4	Characteristics of the Health Manpower Distribution in China	**51**
Chapter 5	Determinants of the Health Manpower Distribution in China	**95**
Chapter 6	Discussion	**113**
Chapter 7	Conclusion	**127**
References		**137**
Appendices		**153**

About the Authors **221**

Index **223**

LIST OF FIGURES

Figure 1.1. Classification of health manpower in China (National Health and Family Planning Commission of the PRC 2018) 2

Figure 1.2. The Classification of eastern, central and western China 6

Figure 2.1. The Lorenz curve of equity in health manpower distribution 15

Figure 2.2. Research model for the characteristics of the health manpower distribution in China 21

Figure 2.3. Health workforce planning model 24

Figure 2.4. Research model of the determinants of health manpower distribution (B. Zhu, Fu, Liu, and Mao 2018) 25

Figure 2.5. The health manpower distribution (a) between countries and (b) within countries (B. Zhu, Fu, Liu, and Mao 2018) 28

Figure 3.1. Research procedures and related methods 32

Figure 3.2. Two types of spatial clusters detected by Kulldorff's space-time scan statistics 36

Figure 3.3. Four types of spatial clusters (HH, HL, LH, LL) detected by local Moran's I 39

Figure 3.4. Model selection procedures of the spatial panel econometric models (J. P. Elhorst 2010) 48

Figure 4.1. Average densities of different subtypes of health manpower during 2012–2016 52

Figure 4.2. Average densities of different subtypes of licensed doctors during 2012–2016 54

Figure 4.3. Average densities of different types of urban health manpower during 2012—2016 55

Figure 4.4. Average densities of different types of rural health manpower during 2012–2016 56

Figure 4.5. Boxplots of the density of total health manpower during 2012–2016 58

Figure 4.6. Boxplots of the density of urban health manpower during 2012–2016 59

Figure 4.7. Boxplots of the density of rural health manpower density during 2012–2016 59

Figure 4.8. Space-time clusters of higher rates of change of the densities of different subtypes of health technicians 61

Figure 4.9. Space-time clusters of lower rates of change of densities of different subtypes of health technicians 63

Figure 4.10. Space-time clusters of higher rates of change of densities of different subtypes of licensed doctors 66

Figure 4.11. Space-time clusters of lower rates of change of densities of different subtypes of licensed doctors 67

Figure 4.12. Space-time clusters of higher rates of change of densities of different subtypes of urban health technicians 69

Figure 4.13. Space-time clusters of lower rates of change of densities of different subtypes of urban health technicians 70

Figure 4.14. Space-time clusters of higher rates of change of densities of different subtypes of urban health technicians 74

Figure 4.15. Space-time clusters of lower rates of change of densities of different subtypes of urban health technicians 75

Figure 4.16. Hierarchical maps and univariate LISA cluster maps of the densities of health technicians 77

Figure 4.17. Hierarchical maps of the densities of different subtypes of health technicians 79

Figure 4.18. Univariate LISA cluster maps of the densities of different subtypes of health technicians 80

Figure 4.19. Hierarchical maps of the densities of different subtypes of licensed doctors 82

Figure 4.20. Univariate LISA cluster maps of the densities of different subtypes of licensed doctors 83

Figure 4.21. Hierarchical maps and univariate LISA cluster maps of the densities of urban health technicians 84

Figure 4.22. Hierarchical maps of the densities of different subtypes of urban health technicians 86

Figure 4.23. Univariate LISA cluster maps of the densities of different subtypes of urban health technicians 87

Figure 4.24. Hierarchical maps and univariate LISA cluster maps of the densities of rural health technicians in 2012, 2014, and 2016 89

Figure 4.25. Hierarchical maps of the densities of different subtypes of health technicians 90

Figure 4.26. Univariate LISA cluster maps of the densities of different subtypes of health technicians 91

Figure 5.1. Summary of direct and spillover effects of outpatient health services demand on the densities of different subtypes of health manpower 107

Figure 5.2. Summary of direct and spillover effects of inpatient health services demand on the densities of different subtypes of health manpower 108

Figure 5.3. Summary of direct and spillover effects of medical graduate density on the densities of different subtypes of health manpower 109

Figure 5.4. Summary of direct and spillover effects of government health expenditure on the densities of different subtypes of health manpower 110

Figure 5.5. Summary of direct and spillover effects of social health expenditure on the densities of different subtypes of health manpower 111

Figure 6.1. Summary of locations and manpower types that display low-low cluster feature in 2016 116

Figure 6.2. Summary of locations and manpower types that display low-high cluster feature in 2016 117

Figure 7.1. Research scales in geography 135

Figure B1. Boxplots of the density of total health manpower during 2007–2016 178

Figure B2. Boxplots of the density of urban health manpower during 2007–2016 179

Figure B3. Boxplots of the density of rural health manpower during 2007–2016 185

Figure B4. Space–scan for units with higher change rates of health technician density during 2007–2016 186

Figure B5. Space–scan for units with lower change rates of health technician density during 2007–2016 187

Figure B6. Space–scan for units with higher change rates of urban health technician density during 2007–2016 188

Figure B7. Space–scan for units with lower change rates of urban health technician density during 2007–2016 189

Figure B8. Space–scan for units with higher change rates of rural health technician density during 2007–2016 190

Figure B9. Space–scan for units with lower change rates of rural health technician density during 2007–2016 191

Figure B10. Hierarchical maps and univariate LISA cluster maps of the density of health technicians in 2007, 2010, 2013, and 2016 192

Figure B11. Hierarchical maps and univariate LISA cluster maps of the density of licensed doctors in 2007, 2010, 2013, and 2016 193

Figure B12. Hierarchical maps and univariate LISA cluster maps of the density of registered nurses in 2007, 2010, 2013, and 2016 194

Figure B13. Hierarchical maps and univariate LISA cluster maps of the density of pharmacists in 2007, 2010, 2013, and 2016 195

Figure B14. Hierarchical maps and univariate LISA cluster maps of the density of technologists in 2007, 2010, 2013, and 2016 196

Figure B15. Hierarchical maps and univariate LISA cluster maps of the density of interns in 2007, 2010, 2013, and 2016 197

Figure B16. Hierarchical maps and univariate LISA cluster maps of the density of urban health technicians in 2007, 2010, 2013, and 2016 198

Figure B18. Hierarchical maps and univariate LISA cluster maps of the density of urban registered nurses in 2007, 2010, 2013, and 2016 200

Figure B19. Hierarchical maps and univariate LISA cluster maps of the density of urban pharmacists in 2007, 2010, 2013, and 2016 201

Figure B20. Hierarchical maps and univariate LISA cluster maps of the density of urban technologists in 2007, 2010, 2013, and 2016 202

Figure B21. Hierarchical maps and univariate LISA cluster maps of the density of urban interns in 2007, 2010, 2013, and 2016 203

Figure B22. Hierarchical maps and univariate LISA cluster maps of the density of rural health technicians in 2007, 2010, 2013, and 2016 204

Figure B23. Hierarchical maps and univariate LISA cluster maps of the density of rural licensed doctors in 2007, 2010, 2013, and 2016 205

Figure B24. Hierarchical maps and univariate LISA cluster maps of the density of rural registered nurses in 2007, 2010, 2013, and 2016 206

Figure B25. Hierarchical maps and univariate LISA cluster maps of the density of rural pharmacists in 2007, 2010, 2013, and 2016 207

Figure B26. Hierarchical maps and univariate LISA cluster maps of the density of rural technologists in 2007, 2010, 2013, and 2016 208

Figure B27. Hierarchical maps and univariate LISA cluster maps of the density of rural interns in 2007, 2010, 2013, and 2016 209

LIST OF TABLES

Table 1.1. Health manpower classification and definition in China (National Health and Family Planning Commission of the PRC 2018) 3

Table 2.1. Comparison of main methods for measuring equity in health manpower distribution 17

Table 3.1. Indicators included in the study of characteristics 34

Table 3.2. Variable measurements, codes, and descriptions 43

Table 4.1. Space-time clusters of higher and lower rates of change of densities of different subtypes of health technicians during 2012–2016 64

Table 4.2. Space-time clusters of higher and lower rates of change of densities of different subtypes of licensed doctors during 2012–2016 72

Table 4.3. Space-time clusters of higher and lower rates of change of densities of different subtypes of urban health technicians during 2012–2016 73

Table 4.4. Space-time clusters of higher and lower rates of change of densities of different subtypes of rural health technicians during 2012–2016 76

Table 5.1. Descriptive statistics of the variables 96

Table 5.2. Estimation results of spatial panel econometric models for health technician density 97

Table 5.3. Direct effects of independent variables on the densities of different subtypes of health technicians and their sum 99

Table 5.4. Spillover effects of independent variables on the densities of different subtypes of health technicians and their sum 101

Table 5.5. Total effects of independent variables on the densities of different subtypes of health technicians and their sum 103

Table 5.6. Direct effects of independent variables on the densities of different subtypes of licensed doctors 104

Table 5.7. Spillover effects of independent variables on the densities of different subtypes of licensed doctors 105

Table 5.8. Total effects of independent variables on the density of different types of licensed doctors 106

Table A1. Health technicians stock in each provincial unit during 2007–2016 155

Table A2. Licensed doctors stock in each provincial unit during 2007–2016 156

Table A3. Clinicians stock in each provincial unit during 2007–2016 156

Table A4. TCM doctor stock in each provincial unit during 2007–2016 157

Table A5. Dentists stock in each provincial unit during 2007–2016 158

Table A6. Public health doctors stock in each provincial unit during 2007–2016 158

Table A7. General Practitioners stock in each provincial unit during 2007–2016 159

Table A8. Registered nurses stock in each provincial unit during 2007–2016 160

Table A9. Pharmacists stock in each provincial unit during 2007–2016 160

Table A10. Technologists stock in each provincial unit during 2007–2016 161

Table A11. Interns stock in each provincial unit during 2007–2016 162

Table A12. Number of population in each provincial unit during 2007–2016 162

Table A13. Urban health technicians stock in each provincial unit during 2007–2016 163

Table A14. Urban licensed doctors stock in each provincial unit during 2007–2016 164

Table A15. Urban registered nurses stock in each provincial unit during 2007–2016 164

Table A16. Urban pharmacists stock in each provincial unit during 2007-2016 165

Table A17. Urban technologists stock in each provincial unit during 2007–2016 166

Table A18. Urban interns stock in each provincial unit during 2007–2016 166

Table A19. Urban population in each provincial unit during 2007–2016 167

Table A20. Rural health technicians stock in each provincial unit during 2007–2016 168

Table A21. Rural licensed doctors stock in each provincial unit during 2007–2016 169

Table A22. Rural registered nurses stock in each provincial unit during 2007–2016 169

Table A23. Rural pharmacists stock in each provincial unit during 2007–2016 170

Table A24. Rural technologists stock in each provincial unit during 2007–2016 171

Table A25. Rural interns stock in each provincial unit of China during 2007–2016 172

Table A26. Rural population in each provincial unit during 2007–2016 172

Table A27. Government and social health expenditure in each provincial unit during 2012–2016 173

Table A28. Outpatient and inpatient visits in each provincial unit during 2012–2016 174

Table A29. The number of medical graduates in each provincial unit during 2012–2016 175

Table B1. Detailed information of space–time clusters of higher and lower rate of health technicians from 2007 to 2016 180

Table C1. Estimation results of spatial panel econometric models for licensed doctor density 210

Table C2. Estimation results of spatial panel econometric models for clinician density 211

Table C3. Estimation results of spatial panel econometric models for traditional Chinese medicine doctor density 212

Table C4. Estimation results of spatial panel econometric models for dentist density 213

Table C5. Estimation results of spatial panel econometric models for public health doctor density 214

Table C6. Estimation results of spatial panel econometric models for general practitioner density 215

Table C7. Estimation results of spatial panel econometric models for registered nurse density 216

Table C8. Estimation results of spatial panel econometric models for pharmacist density 217

Table C9. Estimation results of spatial panel econometric models for technologist density 218

Table C10. Estimation results of spatial panel econometric models for intern density 219

PREFACE

The misdistribution of health manpower is one of the major challenges faced by the Chinese health sector hindering people's access to healthcare. However, this subject remains underexplored, as spatial distribution characteristics have not been fully mapped out, nor have its causes been determined at the macro regional level. To fill this research void, this study aims to conduct sophisticated spatial analyses to examine the characteristics of health manpower distribution and test various determinants of health manpower densities. By introducing spatial techniques, this study sheds light on the distribution of health manpower in China, thus offering invaluable evidence for making national and regional policies to facilitate a more effective distribution of health manpower in China.

On the one hand, this study used spatial statistics (space-time scan statistics and Moran's I statistics) to reveal, visualize, and compare the temporal trends, spatio-temporal dynamics, and spatial clustering patterns of different subtypes of health manpower (clinicians, doctors of traditional Chinese medicine, dentists, public health doctors, general practitioners, registered nurses, pharmacists, technologists, and interns) and their total. The results reveal that regional disparities and huge urban-rural imbalances exist in China's health manpower distribution, indicating that some provincial units have been left behind. In addition, spatial distribution characteristics varied across different subtypes of health manpower, which still held with respect to either the urban or rural health manpower distribution.

On the other hand, this study theoretically modeled and empirically measured various determinants of health manpower distribution from both the supply and demand sides while taking the spillover effect between adjacent geographical units into consideration. Based on the results of the estimation, the health service demand was, as expected, found to forcefully drive the health manpower distribution across the nation. In light of this, the increase in health services demands in a province could significantly help one unit attract licensed doctors and registered nurses from adjacent units. Unexpectedly but intriguingly, the power of medical education capacity was relatively limited in increasing the health manpower density in local units compared to its spillover effect on neighboring units. In addition, government and social health expenditure played different roles in the health labor market, the former being more effective in increasing the stock of licensed doctors and registered nurses, the latter doing better in attracting dentists and general practitioners.

This study has the potential to make profound contributions to the theory and practice of health manpower distribution in China. First, this study advances our understanding of characteristics of health manpower distribution by introducing spatial statistics. By doing so, this study visualizes the detailed spatial distribution characteristics with maps and identifies the priority areas for health manpower allocation in China. Second, this study provides a comprehensive research framework to understand the potential drivers of health manpower distribution, and more importantly, takes spillover effects into consideration and measures them for the first time. Third, this study systematically explores and compares the distribution characteristics and determinants of different subtypes of health manpower, which differ greatly. By exploring both the characteristics and determinants, this study gives a full picture of the health manpower distribution and provides new evidence for making health manpower allocation policies in China.

ABBREVIATIONS

ASEAN	Association of Southeast Asian Nations
ASGC-RA	Australian geographical classifications — Remoteness Areas
GDP	Gross Domestic Product
GNI	Gross National Income
HH	High-High
HL	High-Low
HMD	Health Manpower Density
HT	Health Technicians
IQR	Interquartile Range
LD	Licensed Doctors
LISA	Local Indicators of Spatial Association
LH	Low-High
LL	Low-Low
MAUP	Modifiable Areal Unit Problem
MDGs	Millennium Development Goals
OLS	Ordinary Least Squares
PH	Pharmacists
PRC	People's Republic of China
RMES	Rural-oriented Medical Education Scheme
RN	Registered Nurses

SDGs	Sustainable Development Goals
SDPM	Spatial Durbin Panel Model
SEPM	Spatial Error Panel Model
SLPM	Spatial Lag Panel Model
TCM	Traditional Chinese Medicine
TE	Technologists
WHO	World Health Organization
5+3	5 year undergraduate and 3 year standardized residency training

Chapter 1

INTRODUCTION

1.1. RESEARCH BACKGROUND

In December 2015, the United Nations General Assembly adopted 17 Sustainable Development Goals (SDGs) to provoke worldwide efforts to address global development issues for the coming 15 years (United Nations 2015). In consonance with the United Nations' Millennium Development Goals (MDGs), which were introduced in 2000 and have since contributed to improved human wellbeing around the globe, the SDGs also position health as a key feature of continuing human development but take the further step of establishing the goal of health improvement with 13 specific targets (WHO 2015). More effective human resource management in healthcare is one of the 13 targets, which is made exclusively for developing countries and is now drawing attention from countries with transitional health systems, including China.

Health manpower (also referred as health workers, health personnel, healthcare workforce, health workforce, human resources for health, and health human resources) refers to people who deliver healthcare services (WHO 2006b). As one of the major resource inputs, human resources are crucial for the proper functioning of any national healthcare system (Doull and Campbell 2008). Many studies have shown a significant relationship between the density of health manpower and health outcomes. For instance, in an analysis of the global workforce, Chen and colleagues (L. Chen et al. 2004) reported that the increased density of healthcare workers in a population is associated with the improvement of population-based health and human survival. By examining 192 countries around the world, the World Health Organization (WHO) (2006a) also found that the density of health manpower is negatively correlated with maternal mortality rates. Additionally, Anand and Bärnighausen (Anand and Bärnighausen 2004) reported that health manpower density is negatively related to the infant and under-five mortality rate. WHO (2013) has therefore used the density of skilled health professionals per 1000 population as an important indicator to assess the performance of a healthcare system. There is no doubt that wider and more effective coverage of health manpower makes a positive contribution to achieving the health-related SDGs.

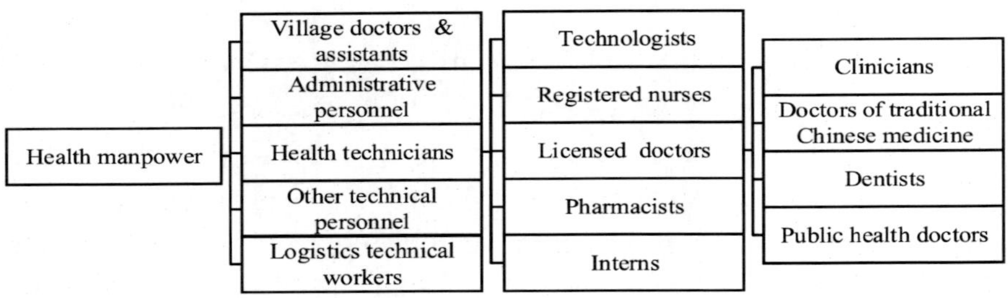

Figure 1.1. Classification of health manpower in China (National Health and Family Planning Commission of the PRC 2018).

Broadly speaking, health manpower in China includes all the people working in the healthcare system. They comprise health technicians (licensed doctors, registered nurses, pharmacists, technologists, and interns), village doctors and assistants, other technical personnel, administrative personnel, and logistics technical workers (National Health and Family Planning Commission of the PRC 2018). Different subtypes of health manpower have their respective roles to play in the operation of the healthcare system. The detailed classification of health manpower in China as adopted by the National Health Commission of the PRC is shown in Figure 1.1. The definition of each subtype of health manpower is given in Table 1.1.

Table 1.1. Health manpower classification and definition in China (National Health and Family Planning Commission of the PRC 2018)

Category		Definition
Health technicians	Licensed doctors (LD)	Doctors with the certificate of (assistant) medical practitioner who are engaged in medical practice, exclusive of those in managerial positions. Licensed doctors can be further divided into clinicians, traditional Chinese medicine (TCM) doctors, dentists, and public health doctors.
	Registered nurses (RN)	Nurses with a registered nurse license who are engaged in nursing practice, exclusive of those in managerial positions.
	Pharmacists (PH)	Health professionals who practice in pharmacy and focus on safe and effective medication use.
	Technologists (TE)	Technologist includes different levels of medical laboratory technicians and diagnostic imaging technicians.
	Interns	Interns include various interns for medical practice (licensed doctor interns, registered nurse interns, technologist interns etc.).
Village doctors & assistants		Those doctors who serve in the village clinics with the "village doctor" certification are listed as the village doctors while those serving at the same places without the certification are listed as assistants.
Other technical personnel		Professionals who are responsible for technical, research, health education and promotion.
Administrative personnel		Professionals who are responsible for the management duties and daily operation of the hospitals and clinics.
Logistics technical workers		Personnel who are responsible for repair and logistic services.

In a narrow sense, health manpower in China only refers to the health technicians, who make up the most important component of health manpower and account for three-fourths of the total number of health workers. This study adopts the narrow definition of health manpower due to the direct, significant role of health technicians in healthcare delivery.

During the past decades, the problem of health manpower in China, like many developing countries, was deemed a "crisis" due to the severe shortage of qualified health professionals (Chen et al., 2004; Mandeville, Lagarde, Hanson, & Mills, 2016). With the concerted efforts of WHO, many countries have made several global, regional, and national investments, most of which center on addressing concerns about the number of skilled healthcare workers (Shamian et al. 2015). In order to cope with the issue of health manpower shortage, China launched a major expansion campaign of tertiary education combined with a growing number of medical and nursing schools in 1998 (Anand et al. 2008). In 2009, the Chinese government undertook new healthcare reforms, which also placed health manpower as one of the priorities (Yip et al. 2012). As a result of continuous efforts, significant changes in the quantity of health manpower have begun in China and the shortage of health manpower has gradually eased. According to the *China Health Statistical Yearbook 2007* (National Ministry of Health of the PRC 2007) and the *China Health and Family Planning Statistical Yearbook 2017* (National Health and Family Planning Commission of the PRC 2018), the number of health technicians in China has increased from 4,624,140 in 2006 to 8,444,403 in 2016, almost doubling in 10 years. In addition, the proportion of health technicians educated at the college level or above increased from 46.4% in 2005 to 71.5% in 2016 (64.7% to 81.1% for licensed doctors, 31.7% to 65.1% for registered nurses) (National Health and Family Planning Commission of the PRC 2018), which means that the quality of health manpower in China has increased dramatically.

However, the increase in health manpower quantity and quality at the national level tends to obscure the misdistribution of health manpower (Kanchanachitra et al. 2011). The shortage of health manpower in the past has drawn attention to the total number of health workers, making an equal distribution of health manpower between regions difficult. Additionally, in recent decades, China's booming economy has compelled millions of Chinese villagers to move into cities and facilitated the development of provincial units for a better living. Accordingly, health resources have increasingly been poured into densely populated cities at the expense of those who live in rural and remote areas (B. Zhu, Fu, Liu, He, et al. 2018). As the inappropriate allocation of resources contributes greatly to inequities in healthcare services (Asante, Zwi, and Ho 2006), manpower misdistribution has become one of the major challenges faced by the Chinese health sector.

As the largest developing country in the world, the problem of health manpower misdistribution is exacerbated due to China's vast territory. There are 32 administrative units in mainland China, which consist of 21 provinces, 4 municipalities, 5 autonomous regions, and 2 special administrative regions at the province level[1] (Figure 1.1). They are directly under the central government but differ in a number of ways. First, in terms of economic strength, the difference in the gross domestic product (GDP) per capita between the richest and the most underdeveloped provinces can be as much as a factor of four, with the eastern region being relatively high in GDP per capita. Second, as for population, the density decreases gradually from the eastern region to the western region, with most people living in the eastern and central regions. Third, differences also exist in geographical features among these administrative units, as the western region has a much vaster territory. The differences in economy, population, and geography aggravate the imbalance in the distribution of health manpower. The natural geographical advantages of the coastal region and policy support make eastern China dominant in the recruitment and retention of health workers. In contrast, central and western China are disadvantaged in various aspects because of their underdeveloped economy and unfavorable geographic position.

In the relevant literature, initial efforts have already been made to explore and explain the misdistribution of health manpower in China. Anand and colleagues (2008) calculated three measures of inequity across provinces (Gini coefficient, Theil-T, Theil-L) using the density of health workers weighted by population and concluded that the misdistribution of health manpower occurs along various gradients, including the urban-rural, regional, and national levels. Chen et al. (2014) also estimated the inequity in the distribution of community health manpower by considering population size and geographical area (i.e., the Lorenz curve and Gini coefficient). In addition, Liu et al. (2016) disaggregated data into three regions (west, central, and east) by geographical location and used the Theil index to measure the trend of equity in health manpower distribution after the New Medical Reform launched in 2009. Li et al. (2018) analyzed the distribution inequality of doctors and nurses with a concentration index

---

[1] Please see *the Constitution of the People's Republic of China*. http://www.npc.gov.cn/englishnpc/Law/2007-12/05/content_1381903.htm.

and concluded that there was an inequality in the distribution of health human resources in mainland China in 2014.

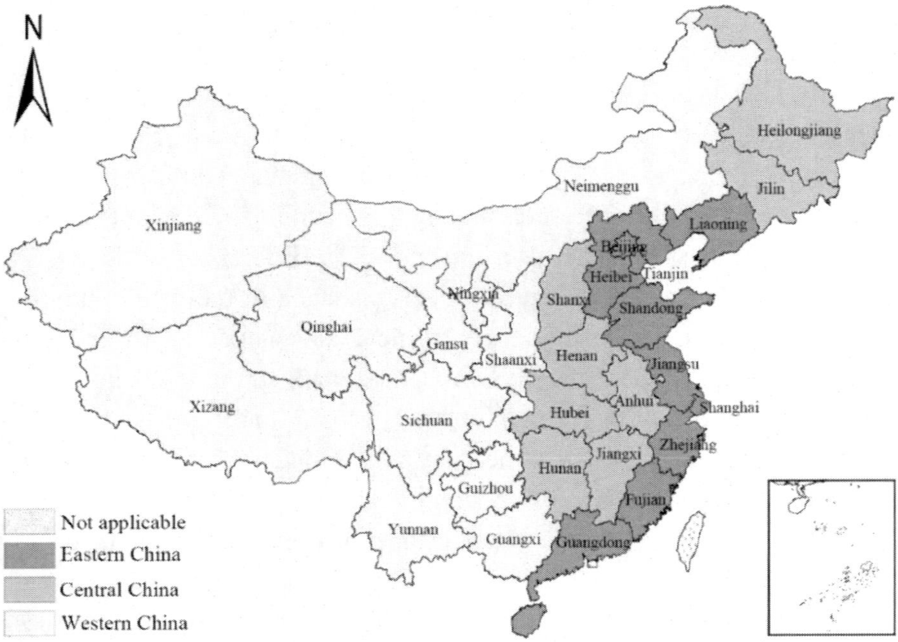

Figure 1.2. The Classification of eastern, central and western China.

Despite the fact that knowledge has accumulated, existing research is by and large based on traditional economic methods, which have significant defects. For example, to measure the degree of equity in health manpower distribution at the provincial level, the first step is often to sort provincial units on the basis of health manpower density. However, space position information is lost in the process of sorting. As a result, detailed spatial distribution characteristics and spatio-temporal dynamics of health manpower distribution have not been explored in existing studies. More importantly, few studies have tried to explore the underlying causes of health manpower misdistribution in China due to the absence of a widely acknowledged theoretical framework.

1.2. RESEARCH QUESTIONS AND OBJECTIVES

To fill the research void, this study proposed to reveal distributional characteristics of health manpower in China and to understand the determinants of its density with spatial analysis methods. Unlike existing literature, this study applied spatial statistics and spatial econometrics so that the spatial characteristics and determinants of health manpower distribution can be fully analyzed. This study selected administrative units at the provincial level (including provinces, municipalities, and autonomous regions) as the research subjects. I hope that findings of this study can provide a basis for planning more effective regional-oriented health manpower allocation policies.

To attain its goal of determining the spatial distribution of health manpower in China, this study introduces spatial statistics and spatial econometrics to explore the distributional characteristics of different subtypes of health manpower at the provincial level, and also its determinants from the regional perspective.

To be more specific, this study aims to answer the following questions:

(1) How is health manpower distributed in China?
(2) What factors may contribute to regional differences in the health manpower distribution in China?

The first question concerns the characteristics of the distribution and examines how health manpower is distributed and clustered at the province level. The second question regards the determinants of distribution and examines how the determinants from the supply and demand sides in each provincial unit influence the health manpower density and their spillover effects to adjacent units. Because characteristics and determinants are relatively independent and reflect different aspects of the health manpower distribution, research activities in this study can be generally divided into two parts, namely the study of characteristics and the study of determinants. Accordingly, the objective of the present research is twofold:

The Study of Distribution Characteristics Aims

(1) to reveal, visualize, and compare the temporal trends of the densities of different subtypes of health manpower in each provincial unit,
(2) to discover, visualize, and compare the spatio-temporal dynamics of different subtypes of health manpower distribution, and
(3) to identify the spatial cluster areas of different subtypes of health manpower.

The Study of Distribution Determinants Aims

(1) to test and compare the effect of supply-side factors on the distribution of different subtypes of health manpower,
(2) to test and compare the effect of demand-side factors on the distribution of different subtypes of health manpower, and
(3) to showcase and compare the spillover effects of supply-side and demand-side factors to adjacent units on the distribution of different subtypes of health manpower.

1.3. Significance of This Study

This study is the first to apply spatial analysis methods to comprehensively investigate the characteristics of the health manpower distribution in China and build a research framework to understand its determinants. The introduction of spatial statistics and spatial econometrics will provide an innovative perspective to understand the health manpower distribution in China, either the current status or its causes. This study contributes to the health manpower literature in three ways as follows.

First, this study advances the understanding of the characteristics of health manpower distribution, as previous studies mainly used traditional economic methods, which have significant defects. Traditional economic methods (Gini coefficient, Theil index, etc.) can only reveal the overall equity level for an entire region but ignore the detailed local spatial distribution characteristics due to a neglect of spatial location information. In this study, two complementary spatial statistics are introduced to display the detailed spatial distribution characteristics of health manpower, thus not only providing more evidence for understanding the health manpower distribution in China but also serving as a methodological reference for future studies of equity in the distribution of health manpower. In addition, this study further tracks the changes in spatial distribution characteristics of health manpower distribution over time. The panel dataset provides an opportunity to conduct a spatial analysis from two different analytical angles. The cross-sectional analysis explores the comparative features of health manpower distribution at the provincial level, while the longitudinal analysis reveals the spatial-temporal dynamics of health manpower distribution during the research period.

Second, this study represents one of the first attempts to interpret the health manpower distribution with supply and demand theory. Supply and demand theory has been widely employed to elucidate the dynamics of the labor market but has rarely been applied to the health field (Lee and Wolpin 2010; Hawkins et al. 2000). This study builds a research framework on supply and demand theory so as to explain the imbalances of health manpower distribution. This research framework also has the merit of explaining the health manpower distribution in other contexts similar to China's. More importantly, this study refines supply and demand theory when applied to explain the health manpower distribution within countries. As Anselin (1988) pointed out, a given area would be more or less affected by its neighbors, but spatial spillovers between administrative units have been overlooked by existing studies on health manpower distribution. Considering the increasingly close connections of Chinese provinces, this study reasonably suspects that spatial spillovers could exist in the distribution of health manpower at the provincial level. Thus, spillover effects between adjacent units are incorporated into the research model, providing a theoretical reference for further in-depth studies. In other words, the health manpower density in one provincial unit is not only explained by the direct effects of within-province factors but also by the spillover effects of the factors in adjacent provincial units. Moreover, both direct effects and spillover effects are empirically measured with the spatial panel econometric models, which verify the rationality and validity of the proposed research model.

Third, the majority of existing studies have only focused on limited subtypes of health manpower, which substantially limits our understanding of the health manpower distribution in China. This study aims to expand the scope of current research by systematically exploring and comparing the characteristics and determinants of all subtypes of health technicians (clinicians, dentists, TCM doctors, public health doctors, registered nurses, pharmacists, technologists, and interns), as these are the most important components of health manpower in China. Results generated by the present research can reveal the relatively different spatio-temporal dynamics and potential drivers of the distribution of different subtypes of health manpower. Thus, it would be beneficial for scholars to understand the differences between different subtypes of health manpower.

The study also has profound policy implications. The results can strengthen the knowledge of policy makers in the central and provincial governments on the health manpower distribution in China, as the study of both characteristics and determinants can serve as a basis for promoting a balanced distribution of health manpower in China. First, spatial statistics can identify distinctive regions or administrative units displaying spatial cluster features, which tend to be the priority areas for health manpower allocation. Accordingly, based on the spatial distribution characteristics of each subtype of health manpower, policy makers can easily find these areas and formulate different policies for different subtypes of health manpower. Second, as this study theoretically models and empirically measures the underlying causes of health manpower misdistribution, the results enable policy makers to fulfill their appointed roles. These include a series of measures to boost the health manpower stock in disadvantaged areas, such as the increase of government or social health expenditures, more quotas for medical universities, and the prevention of a brain drain of health manpower. Third, as the results show the changing spatial patterns of the health manpower distribution, this study allows policy makers to evaluate policy effectiveness in the past decade and thus serves as a reference for making more effective policies in the future.

1.4. STRUCTURE OF THE THESIS

Including this chapter, this thesis comprises seven chapters. So as not to repeat what has been introduced above, I will explain the content of Chapters 2 to 7 as follows:

Chapter 2 reviews the existing literature concerning the characteristics and determinants of health manpower distribution. The research frameworks of the characteristics and determinants of health manpower distribution are then introduced. Regarding the study of characteristics, spatial statistics are used to explore the detailed spatial distribution characteristics of health manpower; as for the study of determinants, a "supply-demand-spillover" research model is constructed to explain the driving factors of health manpower distribution in China based on supply and demand theory.

Chapter 3 outlines the methods employed in studies of characteristics and determinants. The first section explains the data, indicators, spatial statistics (space-time statistics, Moran's I statistics), and corresponding map tools for exploring the characteristics (temporal trends, spatial-temporal dynamics, and spatial clustering patterns). The second section explains the data, variables, and spatial panel econometric models for exploring the determinants of health manpower distribution in China. The model selection principle is also discussed in this section.

Chapter 4 presents the analytical results of health manpower distribution characteristics during 2012–2016. It first displays the temporal trends of the densities of different subtypes of health manpower with boxplots and tables and identifies the provincial units that displayed higher or lower rates of increase with space-time scan statistics and then visualizes the spatio-temporal dynamics and spatial clustering patterns of each subtype of health manpower with maps. The urban-rural differences in the characteristics of health manpower distribution are also revealed.

Chapter 5 presents the estimation results and model selection of spatial panel econometric models by each subtype of health manpower based on China's panel dataset during 2012–2016. Direct and spillover effects of each independent variable (government health expenditure, social health expenditure, outpatient services, inpatient services, and the number of medical graduates) on the densities of different subtypes of health manpower are estimated and compared.

Chapter 6 presents an in-depth discussion of the characteristics and determinants of health manpower distribution based on the findings presented in Chapters 4 and 5. Special attention is paid to lessons drawn from the characteristics and determinants of health manpower distribution for improving the overall health manpower distribution in China.

Chapter 7 concludes the thesis by summarizing the major findings and lessons drawn from the presented study. This chapter also discusses policy and theoretical implications of this study, followed by the acknowledgement of research limitations and suggested directions for future research.

Chapter 2

LITERATURE REVIEW AND RESEARCH FRAMEWORK

This chapter first reviews the related literature and then builds a research framework based on existing studies. The structure of the literature review is arranged as follows: The first section summarizes the studies and methods for characteristics of health manpower distribution and builds a research model to explain the characteristics of health manpower distribution in China. Likewise, the second section reviews existing studies and models of the determinants of health manpower distribution and builds a research model to test the determinants of health manpower distribution.

2.1 CHARACTERISTICS OF THE HEALTH MANPOWER DISTRIBUTION

2.1.1. Existing Studies

2.1.1.1. Health Equity and the Health Manpower Distribution

Health equity has long been a primary concern for policy makers (Waters 2000; WHO 2008a; Shadmi et al. 2014; Sheldon and Smith 2000).

WHO (1996) defined health equity as a situation in which people's needs rather than social privileges guide the distribution of opportunities for well-being. It involves many aspects (health financing, health services, health resources, etc.) in the health field, and intense discussions are generated when health needs are confronted by resource constraints (Sheldon and Smith 2000; B. Zhu, Hsieh, and Zhang 2018).

As one major health resource, health manpower is always limited and even rare in the rural and remote areas of most countries (Chen, 2010; Serneels, Lindelow, Garcia-Montalvo, & Barr, 2005). Therefore, the distribution of health manpower among health care departments or regions reflects the degree of health equity (Culyer & Wagstaff, 1993). The necessity of promoting the equitable distribution of health manpower has gained the interest of international communities. WHO (2004) also put forward equity as one of the basic principles of health manpower allocation.

Nonetheless, the principle that clearly defines the equitable distribution of health manpower remains controversial (Campbell et al. 2013). One major reason for the lack of consensus on this issue is that there are various interpretations of the term "equity." To be specific, expenditure, input, access, utilization, and health status can all indicate health equity under different circumstances (Asante, Zwi, and Ho 2006). However, it is widely recognized that health equity is commonly divided along the horizontal and vertical dimensions, where the former refers to equal treatments for people with equal needs and the latter emphasizes different levels of treatment for people with unequal needs (Braveman 2006). Almost all theoretical or empirical studies, as well as the equitable health manpower distribution, have advocated the horizontal rather than the vertical dimension (Kreng and Yang 2011; X. Zhang et al. 2015).

2.1.1.2. Methodology for Measuring Equity in Health Manpower Distribution

The measurement of equity in health manpower distribution is inevitable when scrutinizing the health manpower distribution in one health system (Kreng and Yang 2011). With respect to the operationalization and measurement of equity in health manpower distribution, equal access to health workers is advocated by numerous researchers and WHO. For instance, Kreng and Yang (2011) interpreted an ideal distribution of health manpower as a condition where most people have equal access to health services despite geographical and/or economic differences. WHO (2016) also proposed to accelerate progress toward sustainable development goals by ensuring equitable access to health manpower. The main methods for measuring equity in health manpower distribution are summarized as follows.

Gini Coefficient and Lorenz Curve

The Gini coefficient (Catalano, Leise, and Pfaff 2009) is the primary measure of income inequality, which is always combined with the Lorenz curve (Figure 2.1). The degree of equity in health manpower distribution as indicated by one-dimensional number can also be calculated from Gini coefficient and Lorenz curve. The Gini coefficient can be calculated as follows:

$$\text{Gini coefficient} = \text{Area A}/(\text{Area A}+\text{Area B}) = 2 \times \text{Area A} \quad (2.1)$$

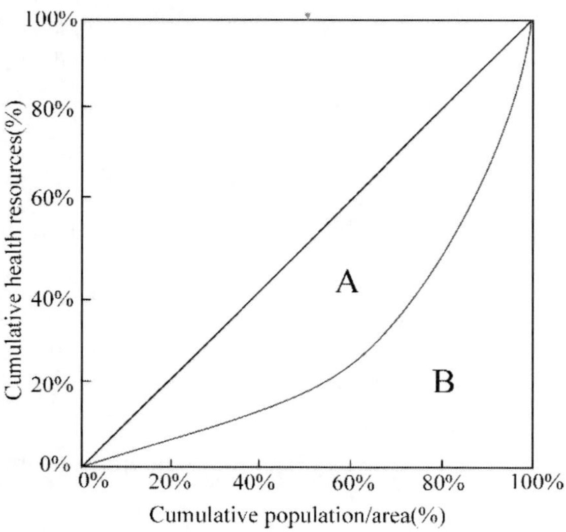

Figure 2.1. The Lorenz curve of equity in health manpower distribution.

The Gini coefficient ranges from 0 to 1. The standards of the Gini coefficient in health manpower distribution are taken from the corresponding standards in economics: 0–0.3 indicates a perfect equity condition; 0.3−0.4 a normal condition; 0.4–0.6 an alert condition; and 0.6−1.0 a highly inequitable, perilous condition (Tao et al. 2014).

Theil index

The Theil index also ranges from 0 to 1, where a smaller value means a more equitable health manpower distribution. It is a tool mainly used for the measurement of income equity, but scholars have increasingly adopted this method to measure equity in the health manpower distribution. It can be calculated as follows:

$$Theil\ index = \sum_{i=1}^{n} P_i \ln \frac{P_i}{Y_i} \tag{2.2}$$

P_i: Proportion of population in one area out of the total population;

Y_i: Proportion of health manpower in one area out of the total health manpower.

If the areas are divided into several groups, i.e., k groups in the formula, the Theil index can also be decomposed into the $T_{\text{intra-class}}$ and $T_{\text{inter-class}}$ (Tao et al. 2014). The contributions within and between groups can be calculated by dividing the Theil index into $T_{\text{intra-class}}$ and $T_{\text{inter-class}}$ as follows.

$$\begin{aligned} Theil\ index &= T_{intra-class} + T_{inter-class} \\ T_{intra-class} &= \sum_{g=1}^{k} P_g T_g \\ T_{inter-class} &= \sum_{g=1}^{k} P_g ln \frac{P_g}{Y_g} \end{aligned} \tag{2.3}$$

$T_{intra-class}$: Degree of equity in health manpower distribution within the group.

$T_{inter-class}$: Degree of equity in health manpower distribution between the groups.

T_g: Theil index of health manpower distribution in subgroups.

P_g: Proportion of population in one group out of the total population.

Y_g: Proportion of health manpower in one group out of the total health manpower.

Concentration Index

The concentration index is similar to the Gini coefficient, but the population along the *x*-axis is ranked by social-economic indicators (income). The concentration index ranges from −1 to 1, where a positive value indicates the concentration of health manpower among low-income people and a negative value among high-income people. The higher the absolute value, the greater the degree of inequity. It is defined as

$$C = \frac{2}{\mu} cov(h, r) \tag{2.4}$$

where *h* is the health manpower, *r* is the fractional rank in terms of household economic status, and μ is the mean health manpower (X. Zhang et al. 2015).

Table 2.1. Comparison of main methods for measuring equity in health manpower distribution

Measure	Advantages	Disadvantages
Gini coefficient and Lorenz curve	• Easily to interpret and compare when combined.	• Only shows the overall equity level. • Overlook of space location information
Theil index	• Shows the contributions to inequity within the subgroup and among subgroups. • Sensitivity to the efficiency of health manpower distribution.	• Poor visualization • Overlook of space location information
Concentration index and Contentration curve	• Social-economic factors are taken into considerations • Reflects the social class allocated more resources.	• Only shows the overall equity level. • Overlook of space location information

To summarize, different methods have different advantages as shown in Table 2.1. Different indicators have their respective advantages and disadvantages in measuring equity in health manpower distribution. However, they both ignored the space location information of the research subjects, which limits the understanding of equity in health manpower distribution.

2.1.1.3. Equity in the Health Manpower Distribution

Internationally, health manpower distribution has been the concern of all the countries. In some cases, the academic word explored this topic just by comparing the health manpower availability indicators in different regions. Tokuhata et al. (1975) analyzed the distribution of physicians and other licensed health personnel in the state of Pennsylvania by comparing the their densities in different counties. Ahmed et al. (2011) compared the physician and nurse density in urban and rural Bangladesh by using national sample survey data. Gupta (2003) compared and mapped the geographical variations in health manpower distribution in Kenya, Mexico and Viet Nam and concluded the strong inequalities in health workforce distribution in these three countries. In other cases, the economic indicators were adopted to empirically measure the equity in health manpower distribution. For instance, Hazarika (2013) investigated the inequalities in the distribution of doctors, dentists, nurses and midwives by calculating the Gini coefficient. Theodorakis et al. (2006) measured the health inequalities in general practitioner distribution in Albania by plotting Lorenz curves and calculating Gini coefficients. Honarmand et al. (2017) calculated the Gini coefficient and Robin Hood index to investigate the equity in general practitioners, midwives, pediatricians, and gynecologists distribution in Iran. Wiseman (2017) adopted Lorenz Curve/Gini Coefficient and Theil Index to explore the inequality in health manpower distribution in Fiji for doctors, nurses, and all health manpower (doctors, nurses, dentists and health support staff).

Thus far, while there have been some empirical studies of the health manpower distribution in China, almost all existing studies tried to understand the status quo of the health manpower distribution through the lens of health equity. Zhang et al. (2015) adopted the concentration index and Gini coefficient to evaluate the equity in the distribution of health technicians in 2011. Chen et al. (2014) analyzed the inequity in the distribution of health manpower by population size and geographical area based on survey data from 190 community health service centers in China. Zhou et al. (2015) computed the Gini coefficient and Theil index from 1985 to 2011 to investigate changes in inequalities in the distributions of health manpower in the different stages of health reform. Song and associates (2016) analyzed the equity in the distribution of pediatricians and pediatric nurses using the Gini coefficient and Theil index. Severe inequity was found in the distribution of the pediatric workforce across the nation, especially in western and eastern China. Jin, Wang, Ma, Wang, and Li (2015) used the Gini coefficient to measure the equity of the distribution of medical personnel in 2013 and concluded that China's demographically assessed distribution of health manpower is greater than that of its geographically measured distribution. Sun and Luo (2017) employed the Gini coefficient to measure the equity in the distribution of total health manpower and concluded that distinct regional disparities exist in the distribution of health manpower. Liu et al. (2016) used the Theil index to measure the trends of the equity in the distribution of health technicians in western, central, and eastern China from 2009 to 2013.

2.1.2. Limitations of Previous Research

Despite the accumulation of knowledge, there are limitations to existing research due to the shortcomings of research methods, i.e., the neglect of spatial location information. These methods for measuring the equity of the health manpower distribution have something in common: They were all initially designed to describe income inequality and then transferred to measure the equity of the health manpower distribution (Zhu, Hsieh, and Zhang 2018). Nevertheless, income equality is slightly different from the equity of a health manpower distribution. Income equality is represented by the distribution of socio-economic resources within a population, whereas equity in health manpower distribution involves the distribution of health manpower not only within a population but also across geographical units. Simply put, the spatial distributions of the same values within different administrative units are of little relevance to the former but of great importance to the health manpower distribution. For instance, an equal Gini coefficient value may correspond to hundreds of different kinds of spatial distribution patterns indicating different types of local characteristics. Accordingly, such existing studies could only focus on the "what" rather than the "how," which means that these studies can only explore whether health manpower is distributed equally rather than where the inequitable areas are (Tao et al. 2014). Due to the evident limitations of existing studies, further studies are needed in order to understand the detailed characteristics of the health manpower distribution in China.

2.1.3. Proposed Research Framework

Health equity is a widely used proxy for understanding the characteristics of health manpower distribution, but it bears limitations due to the shortcomings of traditional economic methods. How to make up for the shortcomings of existing methods? By definition, the inequity in health manpower distribution depends on the spatial concentration of health manpower—excessive in some areas and insufficient in others (Gilles Dussault and Franceschini 2006). Therefore, methods that can explore the concrete details of spatial distribution can also be applied by health scholars to understand the health manpower distribution more effectively (Zhu, Hsieh, and Zhang 2018).

As an emerging technology, spatial statistics focuses on the distribution details and features excellent visualization by means of maps. It has been widely used in revealing the regional inequalities of societal resources, like education resources, agricultural resources and infrastructures (Haddad and Nedović-Budić 2007; Travnikar and Juvancic 2015) and identify the priority areas for corresponding policies (Thongdara et al. 2012). In recent years, the spatial distribution of air pollutants or carbon emissions have also been explored with the help of spatial statistics (Chuai et al. 2012; Y. Liu et al. 2014; Kang, Zhao, and Wu 2016; Hao and Liu 2016). In the public health field, a variety of spatial statistics have been introduced to explore the infectious diseases epidemiology, visualizing the spatial distribution patterns and highlighting the hotspots of disease cases (Abbas, Younus, and Muhammad 2015; Abdullayev et al. 2012; Wu et al. 2017).

The introduction of spatial statistics as aids can provide two distinct benefits in understanding the characteristics of health manpower distributions. First, spatial statistics can identify those distinctive regions or administrative units that tend to have priority for promoting an equitable health manpower distribution. Second, spatial statistics can reveal the spatial-temporal dynamics of the health manpower distribution, providing more evidence for evaluating the effectiveness of past policies and directing future policies to achieve a better health manpower distribution.

Therefore, the present study will employ spatial statistics to reveal the characteristics of the health manpower distribution in China. This study will specifically explore the spatial-temporal dynamics and spatial clustering patterns of the health manpower distribution. The proposed research model is outlined in Figure 2.2.

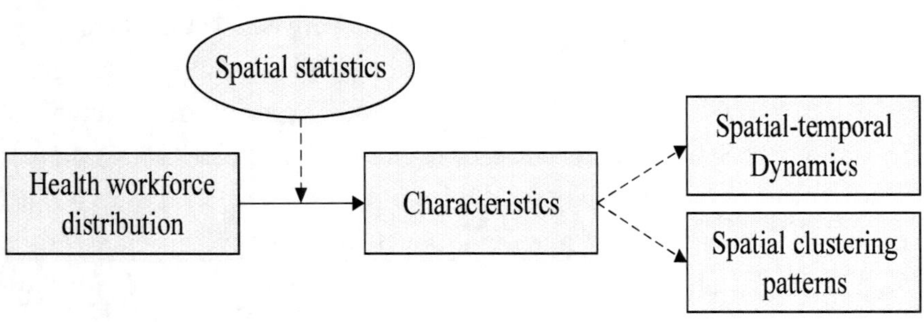

Figure 2.2. Research model for the characteristics of the health manpower distribution in China.

2.2. Determinants of the Health Manpower Distribution

2.2.1. Exiting Studies

Existing studies of the determinants of the health manpower distribution can be categorized into two complementary lines of research: 1) studies for understanding the determinants of health manpower distribution between countries; and 2) studies for understanding the determinants of health manpower distribution within countries.

2.2.1.1. Studies of the Determinants of the Health Manpower Distribution between Countries

Health manpower is essential for the operation of health systems, but what determines the size of different types of health manpower in a given country? The World Bank (2008) stated that it is a complex issue, as a nation's history, culture, politics, social structures, and economy may all play a role. Dussault and Franceschini (2006) categorized the determinants of geographical imbalances into five categories: individual; organizational; health care and educational systems; institutional structures; and the broader sociocultural environment. On the empirical level, Kanchanachitra et al. (2011) determined a significant relation between health manpower densities (the number of health workers per 1000 population) and gross national income (GNI) in ten countries from the Association of Southeast Asian Nations (ASEAN) region. Freed, Nahra, and Wheeler (2004) plotted the relationship between inflation-adjusted gross domestic product (GDP) per capita and the number of all active physicians and pediatricians in the United States for all available years and showed the linear relationship. Zaman, Gemmell, and Lievens (2014) performed a cross-country analysis of 183 United Nations member countries and grouped the predictors for health manpower density into three categories: demographic factors, economic factors, and political factors. In Zaman et al.'s study, literacy rate, total health expenditure, and social stability stand out as the most important explanatory factors when all the variables are entered into the model. In conclusion, except for the effects of economic factors (economic strength or health investment), there was no other consistent conclusion reached by these empirical studies.

2.2.1.2. Studies of the Determinants of the Health Manpower Distribution within Countries

Health manpower is always unequally distributed within countries, with the shortage being much more serious in rural and remote areas. Many studies have tried to study health manpower misdistribution within countries from an individual perspective (B. Zhu, Fu, Liu, and Mao 2018). For example, studies of job satisfaction, burnout, and motivation help explain the turnover behavior of health workers in rural and remote areas (Bonenberger et al. 2014; Y. Zhang and Feng 2011), while studies of medical students have shown how socio-economic characteristics and rural early exposure programs affect medical students' intentions to choose rural medical work after graduation (J. Liu, Zhu, and Mao 2018; King et al. 2016; Somers, Strasser, and Jolly 2007). These studies explain how individual choices contribute to the health manpower misdistribution.

At the macro-regional level, there is no widely used model for understanding the health manpower availability in a certain area. As the health manpower planning also needs to model the dynamics of the health labor market, therefore the health manpower planning models own implications for us to explore the determinants of health manpower distribution. A typical model of health manpower planning is shown in Figure 2.3. It follows a path to match supply and demand in one certain area (Parsons 2010). On the supply side, the supply of health manpower at a point in time is measured by *Current Stock+Increments–Migration–Exits*, which is proposed by the WHO (2006b). On the demand side, the demand for health manpower is calculated based on the population needs, which are driven from three aspects: population, health status and level of services. Based on the planning model, the health manpower availability in one certain area is influenced by both the supply chain of health manpower and health services required.

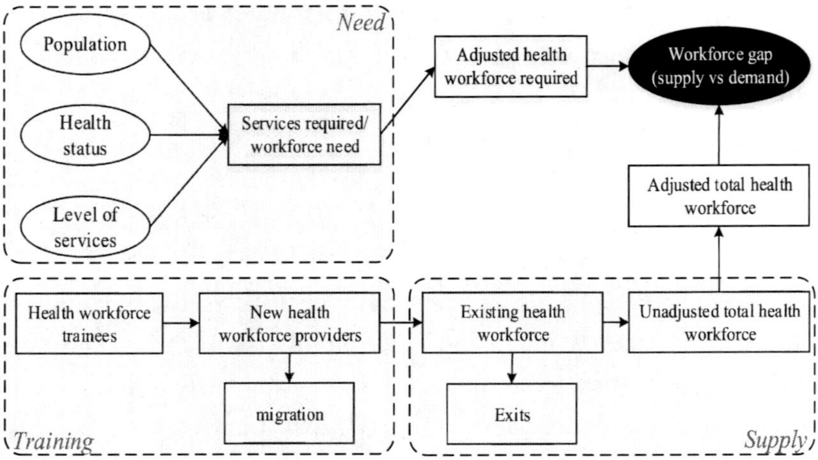

Figure 2.3. Health workforce planning model.

Based on the health manpower planning model, some studies have been conducted to explore the influence of health manpower supply and demand in ceterin regions. Scholz, Graf von der Schulenburg, and Greiner (2015) found significant effects of demand/need factors (population morbidity/financial incentives) on health manpower in Germany. Laurence and Karnon (2016) modeled the inflence of population size, health needs, and service utilisation rates on the health manpower supply in Australia. Murphy et al. (2014) simulated how various factors affect the supply of health manpower in different scenarios in Jamaica. However, the generalizability of their findings to other countries is limited.

2.2.2. Limitations of Previous Research

It is quite clear that why regional disparities exist in the distribution of health manpower is largely unanswered in existing studies. As an important part of the labor market, the distribution of health manpower is a function of not only health workers' self-determination but also a "product" of macro-regional factors. More studies are needed to theoretically model and empirically measure the determinants of the health manpower distribution within countries.

2.2.3. Proposed Research Framework

"The observed differences in the availability of health workers, both within countries and between countries, can be explained by differences in the demand for and supply of health workers" (World Bank, 2008, p77).

-Dussault and Vujicic

The theory of supply and demand has served as an important basis to understand the dynamics of the labor market. According to Dussault and Vujicic (2008), the differences in supply and demand help us to understand the health manpower distribution both within and between countries. The demand of health manpower can be defined as the number of health workers that the health facilities are willing to hire, the supply as the number of health workers who want to work in health facilities (World Bank, 2008). "In a perfect health labor market, supply would equal demand and there would be no imbalances" (World Bank, 2008, p. 83). However, in reality, the stock of health manpower is neither just the supply nor demand of health manpower, but is determined by the interactions of supply and demand (McRae and Butler 2014).

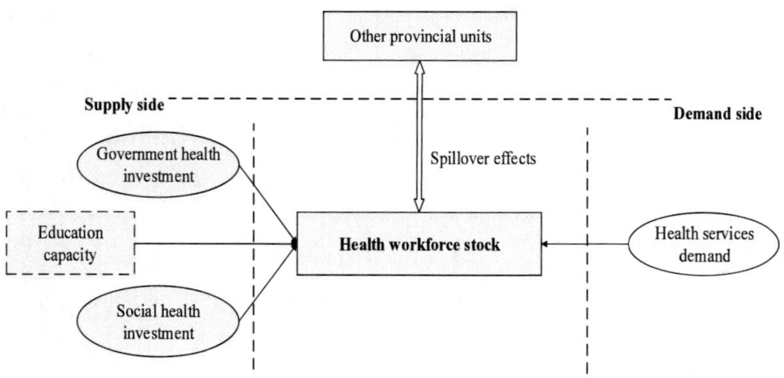

Figure 2.4. Research model of the determinants of health manpower distribution (B. Zhu, Fu, Liu, and Mao 2018).

Figure 2.4 shows the research framework built to explain the determinants of the health manpower distribution in China, which can generally be divided into three parts: supply-side factors, demand-side factors, and the spillover effects of other geographical units.

2.2.3.1. Demand Side

The population's medical needs provide the fundamental impetus to hire health workers. If there are no medical needs, health manpower would have no value (Murphy et al. 2014). However, it is important to differentiate the concepts of demand and need. The concept of need is normative—what ought to be, i.e., how many health workers we should have (G Dussault and Vujicic 2008). It is determined by the population health status and demographic situation (Parsons, 2010). The concept of demand refers to how many workers the health system wants; it is only driven by people's demand for health services. In general, there is not much difference between the demand and need for health manpower. The demand is invariably lower than the need for health workers as there are always some unmet medical needs that are not reflected in the demand for health services on account of multiple social and individual factors (B. Zhu, Fu, Liu, and Mao 2018). In other words, even though a large number of people have medical needs, the unmet needs cannot translate into the motivation of health facilities to recruit health workers if they do not go to the hospitals or other health institutions. That is, the determination of health manpower demand is driven by the people's demand for health services rather than people's medical needs (O'Brien-Pallas et al. 2001). The higher the health services demand, the more health manpower is needed. Therefore, I hypothesize the relationship between health services demand and health manpower stock as follows:

> *Hypothesis 1:* The demand for health services is positively related to the health manpower stock.

2.2.3.2. Supply Side

In an ideal market, the health manpower stock is totally driven by the demand side, as there is no imbalance between supply and demand. In reality, the health manpower supply has normally failed to keep up with rising demand. Owing to the relatively undeveloped education system and growing medical needs, I reasonably believe that health manpower availability in China is restricted, even to a large degree, by the supply side (B. Zhu, Fu, Liu, and Mao 2018). The supply chain of health manpower can be divided into two steps: training and recruitment.

As the first stage, the education system serves as a pipeline from inexperienced students to skillful health workers. Given that health technicians need to acquire professional job-related skills in order to provide quality services, medical education plays a crucial role in the supply of health manpower. More concretely, the education capacity determines the size of the pool of potential health workers. Thus, this study hypothesizes that there is a positive relationship between education capacity and health manpower stock as follows:

Hypothesis 2: Education capacity is positively related to the health manpower stock.

Next, following the graduation of medical students, the recruitment of health workers relies on the attraction and retention of health facilities. In China, medical institutions are classified into two groups, public health institutions (not-for-profit) and private health institutions (for-profit).

In public health institutions, the number of employees is mainly determined by the budget allocated, as a significant portion of government health expenditures are assigned to health workers (Ranson et al. 2010). Therefore, those provincial units with greater financial resource allocations by the government are better positioned to recruit, retain, and compensate healthcare workers. For this reason, I postulate:

Hypothesis 3: Government health investment is positively related to the health manpower stock.

In private health institutions, the workforce enrollment is mainly determined by the investment of social capital. As far as province units are concerned, greater social health investment indicates an influx of more health workers, as it brings more employment opportunities in private health facilities in its train. In addition, the competition of public and private hospitals tends to offer better working conditions, thus attracting more health workers working in the area. Therefore, this study proposes the following hypothesis about the relationship between social health investment and health manpower stock:

Hypothesis 4: Social health investment is positively related to the health manpower stock.

2.2.3.3. Spillover Effects

In addition to the intra-regional factors, it is important to note that the spillover effects (the effects of within-province factors on adjacent provinces) (Yang and Wong 2012) cannot be ignored when studying the health manpower distribution in China.

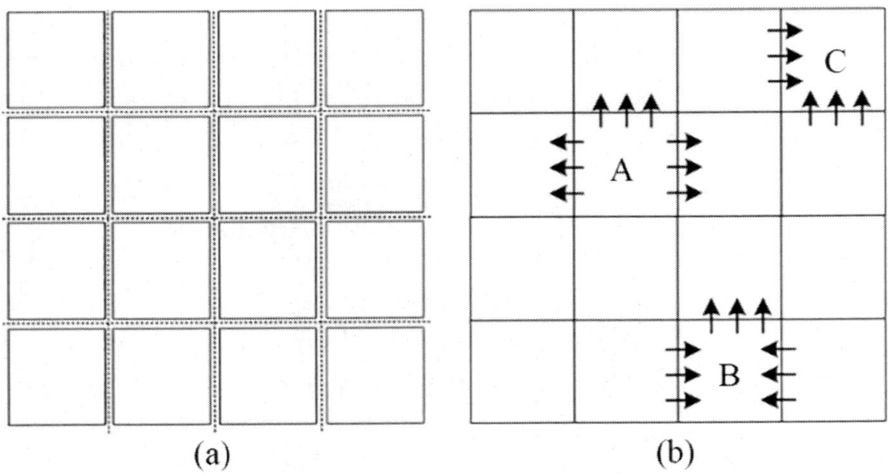

Figure 2.5. The health manpower distribution (a) between countries and (b) within countries (B. Zhu, Fu, Liu, and Mao 2018).

Figure 2.5 displays two circumstances impacting the health manpower distribution. In Figure 2.5 (a), each square represents a country; the health manpower in different countries are relatively independent because of the existence of borders and customs. In Figure 2.5 (b), each square represents one provincial unit or state, where innumerable links exist between provincial units, resulting in the spillover effects of intra-regional factors to other units. For instance, the immigration of health manpower that results from wage differentials is the embodiment of the spillover effects between different geographical units.

Therefore, the health manpower stock in one provincial unit calls for explanation not only by the supply-side factors and demand-side factors in the local unit but also through its interactions with other provincial units. The stronger the supply-side and demand-side factors in one area, the more health workers in other areas are likely to be affected, and vice versa. For instance, if the government health investment in one unit is higher than in other units, health workers from adjacent units are more likely to be attracted to it. Therefore, this study suggests the following hypothesis:

> *Hypothesis 5:* The health service demand, education capacity, government, and social health investment in one provincial unit may have spillover effects on the health manpower stock in adjacent units.

Chapter 3

RESEARCH METHODOLOGIES

This research aims to study the spatial distribution characteristics of health manpower in China and identify its causes at the province level. Overall, the research methodology can be divided into two phases. In the first phase (the study of characteristics), spatial statistics are used to explore the characteristics (temporal trends, spatial-temporal dynamics, spatial clustering patterns) of health manpower distribution in China. In the second phase (the study of determinants), spatial panel econometric models are introduced to explore the determinants of health manpower distribution at the provincial level. Due to the specificity of these techniques, this chapter explains each in depth in the following section in order to make the analyses and findings more comprehensible.

3.1. METHODOLOGY FOR CHARACTERISTICS OF HEALTH MANPOWER DISTRIBUTION

3.1.1. Data Resources

The study of the characteristics of the distribution uses the provincial-level year-end data collected in China during 2012–2016. Only the provincial administrative units in mainland China are included in this study; Hong Kong and Macau are excluded because of data accessibility. The data in this part are obtained from China's *Health Statistical Yearbook* and *Health and Family Planning Statistical Yearbook*,[2] both published by the National Health Commission of China under its own data authority. All the original data adopted in the study of characteristics can be found in Appendix A. This study also displays the spatial-temporal dynamics and spatial changing patterns of different subtypes of health manpower during 2007–2016 for reference; please see the Appendix B for more details.

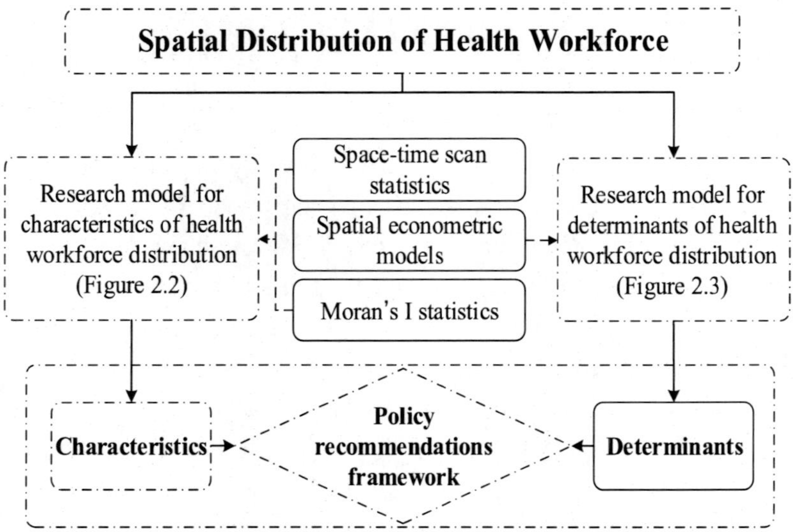

Figure 3.1. Research procedures and related methods.

3.1.2. Measurement of the Indicators

The total number of health manpower workers is an important indicator to evaluate the health manpower availability in one

[2] China's Health Statistical Yearbook is the predecessor of the latter but was renamed after the National Ministry of Health merged with the Population and Family Planning Commission in 2013.

region/country. However, as regions differ in population, the total health manpower cannot be used for comparison across different regions or nations. To exclude the effect of population, the health manpower density is widely used as an indicator for regional comparison (WHO 2008b). It is defined as the ratio of health manpower quantity to population size and conventionally calculated as the total health manpower per 1000 population (Formula 3.1). It is widely used in WHO reports, government statistical files, and academic research to evaluate the performance of a health system (Altman & Ph, 1961; Bigbee & DeMeyer, 2007; Dal Poz et al., 2010; Shetty & Shetty, 2014), and is also the only quantitative target indicator in the *Long-Term Medical Personnel Development Plan of China (2011–2020)* (National Health and Family Planning Commission of the PRC 2011).

$$Health\ manpower\ density = \frac{(Urban/rural) Health\ manpower\ number}{(Urban/rural)\ Population} \times 1000 \qquad (3.1)$$

This study adopts the narrow concept of health manpower and only focuses on health technicians due to their direct, significant role in healthcare delivery. This study seeks to give a full picture of the health manpower distribution by examining the spatial distribution characteristics for different subtypes of health manpower. Overall, the total, urban, and rural densities of health technicians and their five subtypes (licensed doctors, registered nurses, pharmacists, technologists, interns) are included in this study. As for the subtypes of licensed doctors (clinicians, TCM doctors, dentists, public health doctors, and general practitioners), this study can only explore their total densities due to data accessibility. In total there are 23 indicators of health manpower included in the study of characteristics (Table 3.1).

Table 3.1. Indicators included in the study of characteristics

Manpower type	Indicators*	Calculation
Health technician	Health technician density (HTD)	$\frac{health\ technician\ number}{population} * 1000$
	Urban health technician density (UHTD)	$\frac{urban\ health\ technician\ number}{urban\ population} * 1000$
	Rural health technician density (RHTD)	$\frac{rural\ health\ technician\ number}{rural\ population} * 1000$
Licensed doctor	Licensed doctor density (LDD)	$\frac{licensed\ doctor\ number}{population} * 1000$
	Urban licensed doctor density (ULDD)	$\frac{urban\ licensed\ doctor\ number}{urban\ population} * 1000$
	Rural licensed doctor density (RLDD)	$\frac{rural\ licensed\ doctor\ number}{rural\ population} * 1000$
	Clinician density (CD)	$\frac{clinician\ number}{population} * 1000$
	Traditional Chinese medicine (TCM) doctor density (TCMDD)	$\frac{TCM\ doctor\ number}{population} * 1000$
	Dentist density (DD)	$\frac{dentist\ number}{population} * 1000$
	Public health doctor density (PHDD)	$\frac{public\ health\ doctor\ number}{population} * 1000$
	General practitioner density (GPD)	$\frac{general\ practitioner\ number}{population} * 1000$
Registered nurse	Registered nurse density (RND)	$\frac{registered\ nurse\ number}{population} * 1000$
	Urban registered nurse density (URND)	$\frac{urban\ registered\ nurse\ number}{urban\ population} * 1000$
	Rural registered nurse density (RRND)	$\frac{rural\ registered\ nurse\ number}{rural\ population} * 1000$
Pharmacist	Pharmacist density (PD)	$\frac{pharmacist\ number}{population} * 1000$
	Urban Pharmacist density (UPD)	$\frac{urban\ pharmacist\ number}{urban\ population} * 1000$
	Rural Pharmacist density (RPD)	$\frac{rural\ pharmacist\ number}{rural\ population} * 1000$
Technologist	Technologist density (TD)	$\frac{technologist\ number}{population} * 1000$
	Urban technologist density (UTD)	$\frac{urban\ technologist\ number}{urban\ population} * 1000$
	Rural technologist density (RTD)	$\frac{rural\ technologist\ number}{rural\ population} * 1000$
Intern	Intern density (ID)	$\frac{intern\ number}{population} * 1000$
	Urban intern density (UID)	$\frac{urban\ intern\ number}{urban\ population} * 1000$
	Rural intern density (RID)	$\frac{rural\ intern\ number}{rural\ population} * 1000$

* HTD = LDD+RND+PHD+TED+IND.
UHTD = ULDD+URND+UPHD+UTED+UIND.
RHTD = RLDD+RRND+RPHD+RTED+RIND.
LDD = CD+TCMD+DD+PHDD.

3.1.3. Analytical Tools

This study adopts two complementary spatial statistics (space-time scan statistic and Moran's I statistics) to explore the spatio-temporal dynamics and spatial clustering patterns of health manpower in China. The former is used to explore the spatial variations in the temporal trends of health manpower density during 2012–2016, the latter to explore the spatial changing patterns of health manpower distribution during the same period.

3.1.3.1. Space-Time Scan Statistics

Kulldorff's space-time scan statistic explores the spatial variations in temporal trends of health manpower densities. More specifically, it identifies those units in which the rates of change of health manpower density are significantly higher or lower than the others. Kulldorff's space-time scan statistic is defined by a circular window with a geographic base (L. Huang et al. 2017). The first step of space-time scan analysis is to impose the window on the map that is then moved in space and time. The window visits each possible geographical position with each possible window size. The null hypothesis is that the trends of geographical units in different windows are the same, while the alternative hypothesis is that the trends are different. On the basis of the hypotheses, the difference in the rates of change inside and outside the windows is evaluated by the Log Likelihood Ratio (LLR, Formula 3.2) (B. Zhu, Liu, et al. 2018), which is lower the more likely it is that the trend difference is due to chance.

$$\mathrm{LLR} = \log\{(C/n)^{c}[(C-c)/(C-n)]^{(C-c)}\} \tag{3.2}$$

C: Total rate of change of health manpower density.

c: Observed rate of change of health manpower density inside the space-scan window.

n: Expected rate of change of health manpower density inside the space-scan window.

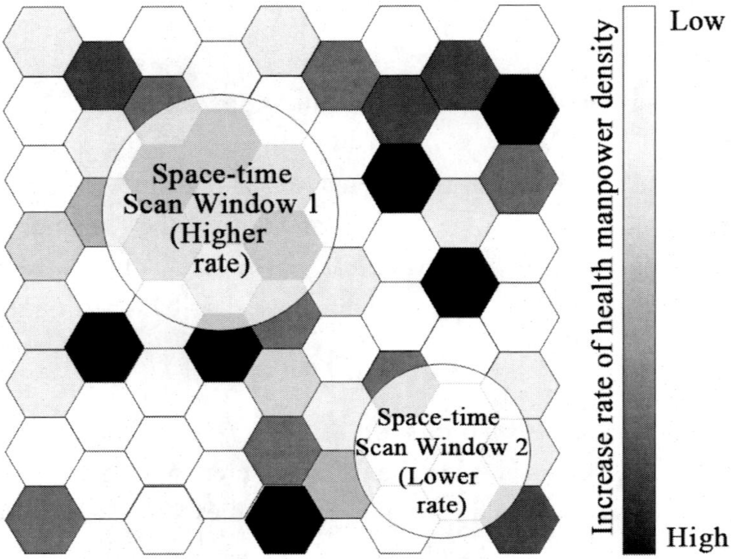

Figure 3.2. Two types of spatial clusters detected by Kulldorff's space-time scan statistics.

Based on the values of the LLR, the space-time scan statistic can identify both the higher and lower-rate clusters (the rate of change of the health manpower density within the geographical units inside the window is higher or lower, respectively, than that of units outside of the window). For either higher-rate or lower-rate clusters, the window with the largest LLR is referred to as the most likely cluster for which the trend inside the window is most unlikely to be the same as the units outside the window, while others (if any) are known as secondary clusters. For this analysis, a Poisson-based model was used and Monte Carlo randomization (999 permutations) was employed to compute the significance of the Kulldorff's space-time scan statistics.

3.1.1.2. Moran's I Statistic

Spatial autocorrelation, which means the correlation among values of a single variable resulting from the proximity of those values in geographical space (Fischer and Griffith 2008), particularly targets the spatial disparities resulting from the geographical location. Moran's I is one of the most common spatial autocorrelation indicators (L Anselin 1995; Hajizadeh,

Campbell, and Sarma 2016; Long, Shao, and Chen 2016), which has the unique advantage of describing and visualizing geographical distributions and identifying units or subset of units that are unusual. There are two forms of Moran's I—global Moran's I and local Moran's I.

Global Moran's I is a measure describing the overall spatial distribution characteristic of the whole area (Cheng et al. 2014; Long, Shao, and Chen 2016). Therefore, only one value is calculated for the entire sample. It is defined as

$$\text{Global Moran's I} = \frac{n\sum_{i=1}^{n}\sum_{j=1}^{n} W_{ij}(x_i-\bar{x})(x_j-\bar{x})}{\left(\sum_{i=1}^{n}\sum_{j=1}^{n} W_{ij}\right)\sum_{i=1}^{n}(x_i-\bar{x})^2} \tag{3.3}$$

Spatial locations are represented by a spatial-weighted $n \times n$ matrix (W), which represents neighboring relations between geographical units, where n is the total number of those units (L Anselin 1988). Contingent upon the definition of the neighboring criterion, there are several options for constructing a spatial weight matrix (Luc Anselin 2002). This study adopts the widely used strategy of constructing the spatial weight (Q. Li et al. 2014), a binary contiguity matrix (formula 3.4) with the rook criterion, i.e., a spatial neighboring criterion based on border sharing. If administrative unit i borders unit j, then the matrix element $W_{ij} = 1$, and $W_{ij} = 0$ otherwise. To control the effect of the number of neighbors, the matrix is row-standardized so that the sum of each row is constant.

$$W_{ij} = \begin{bmatrix} W_{11} & W_{12} & \cdots & W_{1,30} & W_{1,31} \\ W_{21} & W_{22} & & W_{2,30} & W_{2,31} \\ \vdots & & W_{ij} = \begin{cases} 1 \text{ adjacent} \\ 0 \text{ otherwise} \end{cases} & & \vdots \\ W_{30,1} & W_{30,2} & & W_{30,30} & W_{30,29} \\ W_{31,1} & W_{31,2} & \cdots & W_{31,30} & W_{31,31} \end{bmatrix} \tag{3.4}$$

If y is the health manpower density, the difference between the average of y ($\bar{y}$) and y values of adjacent units (i.e., y_i and y_j) plays an important role in determining whether Moran's I is positive or negative. With $\bar{y}$ as the point of reference, all the values of y are classified into two categories, high and low. Global Moran's I, similar to the Pearson Correlation Coefficient, ranges from −1 to 1. Zero refers to a random spatial distribution, which means high and low values are scattered randomly on the map. When the global Moran's I is greater than zero, it means that geographical units with a similar value (e.g., high with high or low with low) tend to cluster together in space. In contrast, when the global Moran's I is negative, it means that geographical units are surrounded by neighbors with dissimilar values (Luc Anselin and Bera 1998). However, the global Moran's I only has limited significance in this study, as the spatial cluster features of health manpower vary across space in China (B. Zhu, Hsieh, and Zhang 2018). To examine the characteristics of health manpower distribution at smaller scales, the local Moran's I statistic needs to be investigated.

Local Moran's I, which is also referred to as the local indicator of spatial association (LISA), is an indicator for a particular area. It can be regarded as the result of the decomposition of Global Moran's I (L Anselin 1995). It is defined as

$$\text{Local Moran's I} = \frac{(y_i - \bar{y})}{m_0} \sum_j W_{ij}(y_j - \bar{y}) \quad m_0 = \sum_j (y_i - \bar{y})/n \qquad (3.5)$$

The operation of summing over unit j is limited to the neighbors of unit i (Q. Li et al. 2014). Akin to global Moran's I, a positive value of local Moran's I indicates a resemblance between one geographical unit and its adjacent areas, whereas a negative value implies a dissimilarity between units (Q. Li et al. 2014). Normally it is used to identify outliers and leverage points, i.e., units with statistical significance. Based on its value and significance, the local Moran's I can detect four types of clusters (Figure 3.3), reflecting the high-low (HL, geographical units with high values surrounded by geographical units with low values), high-high (HH, geographical units with high values surrounded by geographical units with high value), low-low (LL, geographical units with low values surrounded by geographical units with low values) and low-high (LH, geographical units with low values surrounded by geographical units with high values) clustering patterns. As the spatial cluster features of health manpower vary across space, the outliers and leverage points that display fairly unique characteristics have relatively abundant or inadequate health manpower, and thus should be precisely the places on which to focus to promote an equitable distribution.

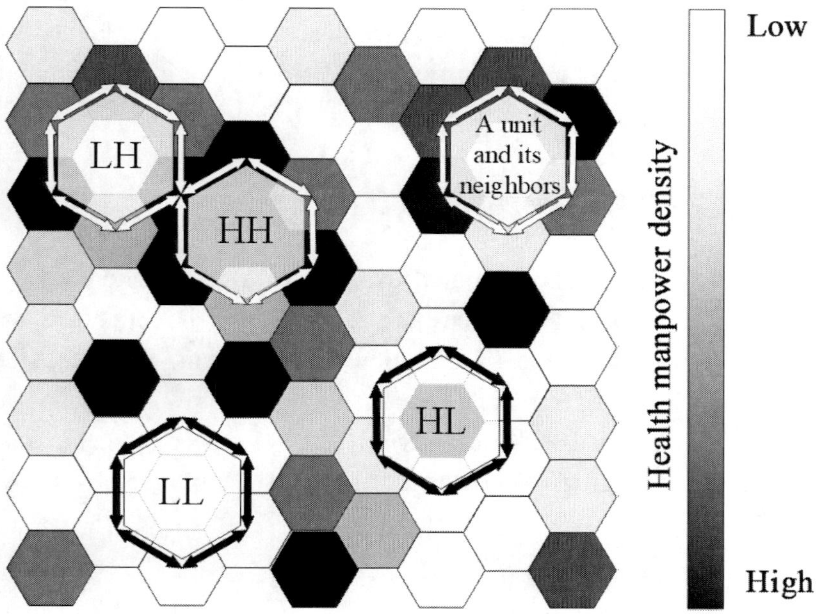

Figure 3.3. Four types of spatial clusters (HH, HL, LH, LL) detected by local Moran's I.

To illustrate statistically significant spatial autocorrelations (also known as spatial clusters) on China's geographical map, a graph which displays those units whose Local Moran's I passes the significance level (i.e., $\alpha = 0.05$) will be presented. As marked areas highlight positive or negative spatial autocorrelations, this graph is known as the univariate LISA cluster map. In order to visualize the dynamics of health manpower distribution more effectively and concisely, three equidistant time points 2012, 2014, 2016 are selected to display the univariate LISA cluster map. Besides, the hierarchical maps of the corresponding indicator are also be displayed alongside the cluster map for reference. In the hierarchical maps, the density of one certain type of health manpower is classified into five classes, which are displayed in different colors. The class breakdown in the hierarchical maps is based on the maximum and minimum of health manpower density during 2012, 2014 and 2016. The differences between these two values are divided evenly into five categories. For instance, if the maximum and minimum are 20 and 0 respectively, then the five classes are 0–4, 4–8, 8–12, 12–16, and 16–20. After that, the data were loaded into China's administrative map with provincial boundaries indicated.

3.1.4. Software

The local Moran's I is computed using GeoDa 1.12.1 (Luc Anselin, Syabri, and Kho 2006). The space-time scan analysis is conducted with SatScan 9.5 (Kulldorff and Information Management Services, Inc., Boston, MA, USA). Hierarchical maps and univariate LISA maps are developed with ArcGIS 10.0. The descriptive functional boxplots are made with Microsoft Excel 2016 (Microsoft Corporation, Redmond, WA, USA).

3.2. Methodology for the Determinants of the Health Manpower Distribution

3.2.1. Data Resources

The study of determinants, like that of characteristics, uses the provincial level year-end data in China from the period 2012–2016. As with the study of characteristics, only the provincial administrative units in China mainland are included in this study. The data in this part were obtained from the *China Statistical Yearbook*, *China Health Statistical Yearbook*, *China Health and Family Planning Statistical Yearbook*, and

China Education Statistical Yearbook. All the original data adopted in the study of determinants can be found in Appendix A.

3.2.2. Measurement of the Variables

3.2.2.1. Health Manpower Stock: Health Manpower Density

To ensure consistency with the study of characteristics, the study of determinants also uses the health manpower density as the dependent variable. As different subtypes of health manpower play different roles in the operation of the healthcare system, different subtypes of health manpower will be discussed separately. Moreover, this study only adopts the total health manpower density and excludes the urban/rural health manpower density as the dependent variable because the urban-rural health manpower distribution differs greatly at the provincial level due to the differentiated allocation policies in the units. That is, the urban-rural health manpower allocation is more like the self-determined business of the provincial units rather than stemming from inter-regional imbalances.

3.2.2.2. Health Service Demand: Outpatient Visits per Capita and Inpatient Visits per Capita

Health services are defined as a certain quantity or a combination of different services, such as diagnosis, observation, treatment, and intervention services, that are delivered by health institutions (Vujicic and Zurn 2006). Health services can be roughly divided into outpatient services and inpatient services (Lv et al. 2016). An outpatient means a patient who visits health institutions (hospital, clinic, etc.) but is not hospitalized overnight, while inpatients receive lodging in health institutions. As patients are only hospitalized overnight when they are extremely ill or have severe physical trauma, the outpatient and inpatients visits therefore reflect different aspects of health services demand. This study adopts the ratios of both outpatient and inpatients visits and population, i.e., outpatient visits per capita and inpatient visits per capita, to measure the health services demand, as higher per capita inpatient and outpatient visits reflect stronger health service demand.

3.2.2.3. Education Capacity: Medical Graduate Density

Medical schools serve health institutions by pipelining trained medical graduates into the health manpower pool. Even though the number of medical graduates does not fully represent the medical education capacity in one unit, it directly determines the number of potential health workers. The more students the medical education system trains, the larger the potential labor force for the health industry. To maintain consistency with the dependent variable, this study adopts the medical graduate density, i.e., the ratio of the number of medical graduates to the population size, to represent the education capacity in a unit.

3.2.2.4. Government and Social Health Investment: Government Health Expenditure per Capita and Social Health Expenditure per Capita

In a previous study, Zaman et al. (2014) used the total health expenditure to represent the government and social investment in one country. In the Chinese context, the health expenditure is divided into three parts: government, social, and personal health expenditure. Government and social health expenditure correspond exactly to the government and social health investment. The government health expenditure represents the investment in the health care industry by all branches of governments, while the social health expenditure refers to the investment in the health care industry by all sectors of society other than the government (National Health and Family Planning Commission of the PRC 2018). Likewise, this study also adopts the ratio of health expenditure to the population, that is, the government health expenditure per capita and social health expenditure per capita, to represent the investment level of government and society, respectively.

A summary of all the variables and their codes and descriptions is shown in Table 3.2.

Table 3.2. Variable measurements, codes, and descriptions

Variable	Measurement	Code	Description
Health manpower density (HMD)	Health technician density	HTD	Number of the health technicians divided by the population and multiplied by 1000
	Licensed doctor density	LDD	Number of the licensed doctors divided by the population and multiplied by 1000
	Clinician density	CD	Number of the clinicians divided by the population and multiplied by 1000
	TCM doctor density	TCMDD	Number of the TCM doctors divided by the population and multiplied by 1000
	Dentist density	DD	Number of the dentists divided by the population and multiplied by 1000
	Public health doctor density	PHDD	Number of the public health doctors divided by the population and multiplied by 1000
	General practitioner density	GPD	Number of the general practitioners divided by the population and multiplied by 1000
	Registered nurse density	RND	Number of the registered nurses divided by the population and multiplied by 1000
	Pharmacist density	PD	Number of the pharmacists divided by the population and multiplied by 1000
	Technologist density	TD	Number of the technologists divided by the population and multiplied by 1000
	Intern density	ID	Number of the interns divided by the population and multiplied by 1000
Health services demand	Outpatient visits per capita	OV	Number of the outpatient visits divided by the population
	Inpatient visits per capita	IV	Number of the inpatient visits divided by the population
Government health investment	Government health expenditure per capita	GHE	Government health expenditure divided by the population
Social health Investment	Social health expenditure per capita	SHE	Social health expenditure divided by the population
Education capacity	Medical graduate density	MGD	Number of medical graduates divided by the population and multiplied by 1000

3.2.3. Analytical Tools

The study of the determinants is based on the following model (Formula 3.5) derived from the theoretical model in Section 2.2.3 and the measurement of the variables.

$$
\begin{aligned}
Ln(HMD)_{it} = \alpha + \beta_1 ln(OV)_{it} + \beta_2 ln(IV)_{it} + \beta_3 ln(GHE)_{it} \\
+ \beta_4 ln(SHE)_{it} + \beta_5 ln(MGD)_{it} + \epsilon_{it} \\
i = 1,2 \ldots 31; t = 2012, 2013, 2014, 2015, 2016 \qquad (3.5)
\end{aligned}
$$

where the subscript i represents 31 province units (i = 1, 2, …, 31) and t denotes time (t = 2012, 2013, 2014, 2015, 2016). α stands for the constant term and ϵ for the error term. It is important to note that this study uses the logarithmic transformation in the regression models to minimize the effect of heteroskedasticity. This implies that the coefficients reflect the percentage change of dependent variables with changes in the independent variables.

The spillover effects of within-province factors to other units should be considered, but the traditional regression models fail to measure the spillover effects between adjacent geographical units. This study therefore adopts spatial panel econometric models so as to produce a more accurate estimation of model coefficients and spillover effects (Y. Liu et al. 2014). Spatial panel econometric models can be regarded as the extension of conventional regression models by adding information of adjacent units (Hao and Liu 2016). They have been widely used to model the spillovers between geographical units, such as the education spillovers (Yajuan 2010), education expenditure spillovers (Qi 2016), economic development spillovers (X. Jiang et al. 2016), economic incentives spillovers (Amin 2016), transport infrastructure spillovers (Belt 2017), human capital spillovers (Fu and Gabriel 2009) and spillovers in tourism flows (Yang and Wong 2012).

In general, the spatial panel econometric model includes three basic models: the Spatial Lag Panel Model (SLPM), the Spatial Error Panel Model (SEPM), and the Spatial Durbin Panel Model (SDPM) (L. Jiang and Ji 2016; Z. Zhou, Ye, and Ge 2017). In order to avoid estimation bias caused by Ordinary Least Squares (OLS) estimation when spatial effects exist (L Anselin 1988), the maximum likelihood method is adopted to estimate the coefficients of the spatial panel econometric models.

3.2.3.1. Spatial Lag Panel Model

$$Ln(HMD)_{it} = \rho \sum_{j=1}^{n} W_{ij} ln(HMD)_{it} + \beta_1 ln(OV)_{it} + \beta_2 ln(IV)_{it} + \beta_3 ln(GHE)_{it} + \beta_4 ln(SHE)_{it} + \beta_5 ln(MGD)_{it} + \alpha + \mu_i + \gamma_t + \varepsilon_{it} \quad (3.6)$$

The SLPM (Formula 3.6) is mostly employed to analyze the spatial autocorrelation of the dependent variable, that is, whether the value of a unit is influenced by values of its neighboring regions (Cheng et al. 2014). In the SLPM, W_{ij} is a spatial weight matrix (row-standardized) for the 31 geographical units in China, which is the same as the spatial weight matrix in the study of characteristics (Formula 3.4). $W_{ij}ln(HMD)_{it}$ is a vector of the spatial lag (average of the neighbors) of health manpower density; β are the regression coefficients, which are the same as the coefficients in non-spatial models; ρ is a spatial regression coefficient; and μ_i and γ_t indicate the spatial fixed effects (space-specific, time-invariant) and time-period fixed effects (time-specific, space-invariant), respectively (Fischer and Getis 2010).

3.2.3.2. Spatial Error Panel Model

The SEPM (Formula 3.7), however, is used most often to address the circumstance where the dependent variable is related to a group of variables as well as to the spatially autocorrelated error term. The parameter λ is the spatial autoregressive coefficient, reflecting the influence of the residuals of neighbors on the residuals of a certain area; ε is the spatially autoregressive error term; and the other parameters are as for the SLPM.

$$\begin{aligned} ln(\mathrm{HMD})_{it} &= \beta_1 ln(OV)_{it} + \beta_2 ln(IV)_{it} + \beta_3 ln(GHE)_{it} \\ &\quad + \beta_4 ln(SHE)_{it} + \beta_5 ln(MGD)_{it} + \alpha + \mu_i + \gamma_t + \varepsilon_{it} \\ \varepsilon_{it} &= \lambda \textstyle\sum_{j=1}^{n} W_{ij}\, \varepsilon_{it} + v_{it} \qquad (3.7) \end{aligned}$$

3.2.3.3. Spatial Durbin Panel Model

SDPM (Formula 3.8) is most useful when the dependent variable should be explained by the independent variables in both the local unit and adjacent geographical units (J. Huang and Xia 2016). In the SDPM, $\theta_1, \theta_2, \theta_3, \theta_4$ in Formula 3.8, as spatial parameters, indicate the impacts of the independent variables in adjacent units on the health manpower density of the target area. The other parameters are the same as for the SLPM and SEPM.

$$Ln(HMD)_{it} = \rho \sum_{j=1}^{n} W_{ij} Ln(HMD)_{it} + \beta_1 ln(OV)_{it} + \beta_2 ln(IV)_{it} + \beta_3 ln(GHE)_{it} + \beta_4 ln(SHE)_{it} + \beta_5 ln(MGD)_{it} + \theta_1 \sum_{j=1}^{n} W_{ij}\, ln(OV)_{it} + \theta_2 \sum_{j=1}^{n} W_{ij}\, ln(IV)_{it} + \theta_3 \sum_{j=1}^{n} W_{ij}\, ln(GHE)_{it} + \theta_4 \sum_{j=1}^{n} W_{ij}\, ln(SHE)_{it} + \theta_5 \sum_{j=1}^{n} W_{ij}\, ln(MGD)_{it} + \alpha + \mu_i + \gamma_t + \varepsilon_{it}) \tag{3.8}$$

Since SDPM exploits the complicated dependence structure between units, the effect of an explanatory variable change for a specific unit will affect the unit itself and potentially affect all adjacent units indirectly. The changes of variables in the neighboring units can further affect the specific unit via feedback. Hence, the coefficients in the SDPM cannot be explained as the percentage change of dependent variables with respect to the independent variables, as the derivative of y with respect to x usually does not equal to β_k. To better interpret the coefficients of the SDPM models, the effects of independent variables on the dependent variable in SDPM models can be further decomposed into direct and spillover effects.

"By definition, the direct effects refer to the influence of a unit change in an independent variable x in geographical unit i on the health manpower density in geographical unit i averaged across all the geographical units. In comparison, the spillover effects (indirect effects) refer to the influence of a unit changes in the independent variable x in all the geographical units excluding unit i on the health manpower density in geographical unit i, averaged across all the geographical units. The total effects equal the sum of the average direct and average spillover effects and measure the impact of a unit change in independent variable x in all the units on health manpower density in geographical unit i, again averaged across all the geographical units" (Belotti & Hughes, 2017, p. 28).

The SDPM (Equation 3.8) can be rewritten in the following vector form (formula 3.9) (Lesage and Pace 2009):

$$Y_{it} = (1-\rho W)^{-1}(X_{it}\beta + WX_{it}\theta) + (1-\rho W)^{-1}\mu_i + (1-\rho W)^{-1}\gamma_t + (1-\rho W)^{-1}\varepsilon_{it} \quad (3.9)$$

The matrix of partial derivatives of Y_{it} with respect to the kth exogenous variable of X from unit 1 to unit n is represented as follows (formula 3.10) (Z. Zhou, Ye, and Ge 2017). Based on the matrix of partical derivatives, the direct effect can be calculated as "the sum of the diagonal elements of the matrix at the bottom of [Formula 3.10] (Lesage & Pace, 2009, p. 36), and the indirect effect can be calculated as the average of either the row sums or column sums of the non-diagonal elements of the matrix" (Lesage & Pace, 2009, p. 36).

$$\left[\frac{\partial Y}{\partial X_{1k}} \cdots \frac{\partial Y}{\partial X_{Nk}}\right] = \begin{bmatrix} \frac{\partial y_1}{\partial X_{ik}} & \cdots & \frac{\partial y_1}{\partial X_{ik}} \\ \vdots & \cdots & \vdots \\ \frac{\partial y_n}{\partial X_{ik}} & \cdots & \frac{\partial y_n}{\partial X_{ik}} \end{bmatrix}$$
$$= (1-\rho W)^{-1} \begin{bmatrix} \beta_k & W_{12}\theta_k & \cdots & W_{1N}\theta_k \\ W_{21}\theta_k & \beta_k & \cdots & W_{2N}\theta_k \\ \vdots & \vdots & \cdots & \vdots \\ W_{N1}\theta_k & W_{N2}\theta_k & \cdots & \beta_k \end{bmatrix} \quad (3.10)$$

3.2.3.4. Model Selection

The procedures for the specification of spatial panel econometric models are shown in Figure 4. Following the strategy proposed by Elhorst and colleagues (P. Elhorst, Piras, and Arbia 2010), researchers should start with the SDPM and test for alternatives. That is, we estimate the SDPM but would like to know if it is the best model for the specific data. However, as this study uses the panel data, the first task is to make a judgment between all the SDPM sub-models. Therefore, the model selection can be divided into two phases. First, we estimate all the SDPMs to test which is the best. Second, we run two tests to judge whether the best SDPM can be simplified into SLPM or SEPM (B. Zhu, Fu, Liu, and Mao 2018).

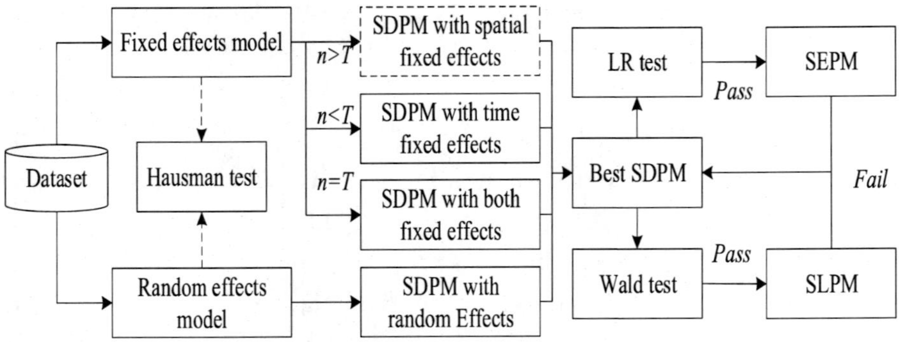

Figure 3.4. Model selection procedures of the spatial panel econometric models (J. P. Elhorst 2010).

In the first phase, the SDPM can be divided into a model with spatial-fixed effects (controlling the "space-specific, time-invariant" variables, which are excluded from the model), a model with time fixed effects (controlling "all time-specific, space-invariant variables," which are excluded from the model), a model with spatial and time fixed effects (controlling the above two), and a random effects model based on different assumptions (L. Jiang and Ji 2016). According to Greene (2012), we should choose one-way fixed models (spatial-fixed or time-fixed) if the sample size n does not equal T compared with the two-way fixed model. More specifically, a model with spatial fixed effects for short panels (n > T) and a model with time fixed effects for long panels (n < T). Furthermore, the choice between models with fixed and random effects should be made based on the Hausman test (Hausman 1976).

In the second phase, the Wald test (H_0: $\theta = 0$) and LR (Likelihood Ratio) test (H_0: $\theta = -\rho\beta$) are successively used to test the alternatives of SDPM. It is easily shown that if $\theta = 0$ and $\rho \neq 0$, the SLPM is a better one, while if $\theta = -\rho\beta$, the model is SEPM where errors are spatially correlated. But if the conditions $\theta = 0$ and $\theta + \rho\beta = 0$ are both rejected, the most fit one would be SDPM (Kang, Zhao, and Wu 2016). To fully capture the possible spatial correlations between adjacent units, both these spatial panel econometrics models will be estimated and compared in order to choose the model that can best illustrate the relationship between the dependent and independent variables.

3.2.4. Software

GeoDa 1.8.16 (Version 1.8.6116, the University of Chicago, Chicago, IL, USA) is employed to constitute the spatial weight matrix. The spatial panel econometric models are computed with the STATA 12.0 (Version 12.0, College Station TX, STATA Corporation, 1996.) (Belotti and Hughes 2017).

Chapter 4

CHARACTERISTICS OF THE HEALTH MANPOWER DISTRIBUTION IN CHINA

This chapter presents the analytical results on the characteristics of the health manpower distribution in China. First, this chapter presents the descriptive statistics of different subtypes of health manpower densities and then displays the temporal trends with boxplots. Second, the spatial variations in the temporal trends of the health manpower densities are displayed. That is, the units that displayed relatively higher or lower rates of change in health manpower density during 2012–2016 are identified and visualized with maps; the detailed parameters are shown in tables. Third, the changing spatial patterns of health manpower distribution are visualized through hierarchical maps and univariate LISA cluster maps in 2012, 2014, and 2016 for different subtypes of health manpower.

4.1. Descriptive Statistics

Figure 4.1 displays the average health manpower densities of all subtypes of health technicians in each provincial unit during 2012–2016 and the original data are appended below the figure.

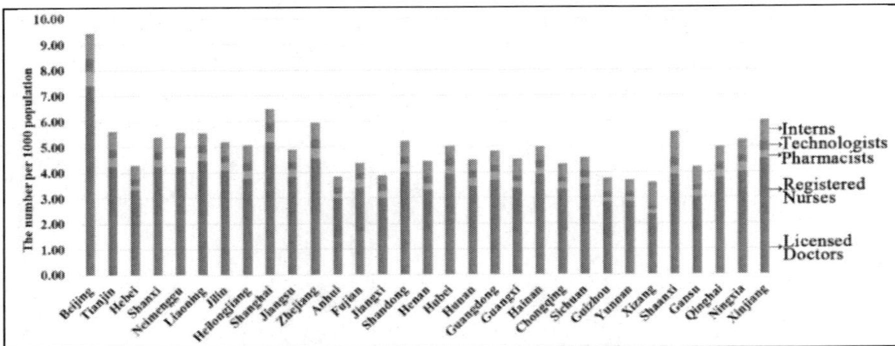

Region	HT	LD	RN	PH	TE	Interns
Beijing	10.035	3.799	4.159	0.593	0.525	0.960
Tianjin	5.701	2.257	2.110	0.347	0.314	0.672
Hebei	4.781	2.153	1.656	0.205	0.246	0.522
Shanxi	5.770	2.453	2.191	0.275	0.300	0.551
Neimenggu	6.189	2.510	2.263	0.394	0.325	0.697
Liaoning	5.927	2.373	2.451	0.304	0.331	0.468
Jilin	5.583	2.355	2.094	0.288	0.292	0.555
Heilongjiang	5.534	2.133	2.031	0.298	0.328	0.743
Shanghai	6.777	2.515	2.968	0.378	0.394	0.522
Jiangsu	5.746	2.261	2.370	0.320	0.290	0.506
Zhejiang	6.863	2.679	2.655	0.441	0.350	0.738
Anhui	4.373	1.690	1.823	0.211	0.259	0.389
Fujian	5.314	1.955	2.218	0.352	0.272	0.517
Jiangxi	4.412	1.619	1.845	0.301	0.293	0.354
Shandong	6.101	2.336	2.447	0.324	0.311	0.683
Henan	5.200	1.994	2.011	0.252	0.307	0.636
Hubei	5.784	2.162	2.496	0.308	0.302	0.517
Hunan	5.118	2.043	2.034	0.300	0.281	0.459
Guangdong	5.455	2.039	2.206	0.340	0.278	0.594
Guangxi	5.396	1.832	2.183	0.302	0.283	0.796
Hainan	5.667	1.964	2.520	0.295	0.303	0.584
Chongqing	5.165	1.942	2.103	0.257	0.245	0.618
Sichuan	5.479	2.165	2.136	0.274	0.271	0.633
Guizhou	4.817	1.679	1.912	0.196	0.275	0.755
Yunnan	4.435	1.629	1.763	0.187	0.239	0.617
Xizang	3.944	1.726	0.865	0.178	0.183	0.991
Shaanxi	6.674	2.039	2.577	0.357	0.418	1.283
Gansu	4.784	1.835	1.712	0.230	0.247	0.761
Qinghai	5.762	2.249	2.118	0.296	0.340	0.760
Ningxia	5.968	2.275	2.289	0.364	0.327	0.714
Xinjiang	6.646	2.386	2.595	0.315	0.389	0.96

Figure 4.1. Average densities of different subtypes of health manpower during 2012−2016.

In terms of the total number of health technicians, Beijing, the capital, far outweighed all the other provincial units, with an average density of 10.035 health technicians among 1000 population during 2012−2016, while that of Xizang (the Tibetan Autonomous Region) was only 3.616, which was less than that half of Beijing. In addition, Shanghai and Zhejiang also had relatively high average densities of health technicians (6.777 and 6.843, respectively), while those in most of the other units were less than 6. This indicates the great gap and unevenness in the distribution of health manpower at the provincial level in China.

Examining the five specific categories shows that the blue and red bars, which represent licensed doctors and registered nurses, respectively, usually had the largest shares of the manpower in most of the provincial units, while the proportions of pharmacists and technologists were often the smallest. Beijing ranked first in the average densities of four subtypes of health manpower (LD, RN, PH, and TE), all except interns. Regarding licensed doctors, the value for Beijing was 3.799 per 1000 population, whereas the minimum value was 1.690 in Anhui, which was less than half of the former. This situation was even more dramatic for the density of registered nurses: The density of Beijing was 4.159 per 1000 population, yet in some provincial units, Xizang for instance, registered nurses (0.865) were relatively scant in all the subtypes, at approximately one-fifth that of the capital city. In contrast, the average density of interns in Shaanxi (1.283) ranked first, higher than in Beijing (0.960).

Figure 4.2 shows the average health manpower densities of all subtypes of licensed doctors in each provincial unit in China; the original data are appended below the figure. Among its four components, clinicians accounted for the largest proportion of health technicians in all the provincial units, while the density of public health doctors in a provincial unit was usually smaller than that of dentists and TCM doctors. Beijing had the highest density of all subtypes of licensed doctors, while the lowest average densities of clinicians, TCM doctors, dentists, and public health doctors were located in Xizang, Anhui, Xizang, and Hebei, respectively. As general practitioner was the second identity of some of the licensed doctors, the density of general practitioners was not displayed in the histogram. In general, only a small proportion (usually less than 10%) of licensed doctors registered as general practitioners at the same time.

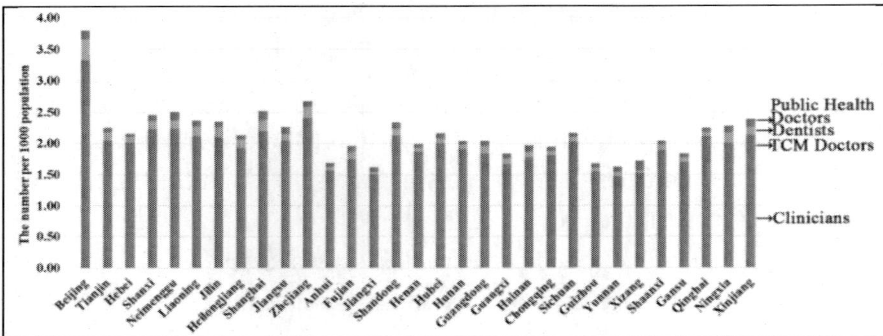

Region	Clinicians	TCM doctors	Dentists	Public health doctors	GP
Beijing	2.625	0.700	0.332	0.143	0.389
Tianjin	1.638	0.414	0.130	0.076	0.115
Hebei	1.703	0.314	0.090	0.046	0.101
Shanxi	1.849	0.383	0.130	0.091	0.095
Neimenggu	1.766	0.476	0.131	0.137	0.106
Liaoning	1.844	0.272	0.157	0.099	0.084
Jilin	1.782	0.315	0.164	0.094	0.084
Heilongjiang	1.675	0.254	0.134	0.070	0.091
Shanghai	1.904	0.290	0.181	0.141	0.278
Jiangsu	1.790	0.257	0.106	0.108	0.247
Zhejiang	2.040	0.373	0.175	0.091	0.337
Anhui	1.385	0.186	0.054	0.066	0.099
Fujian	1.431	0.323	0.117	0.084	0.112
Jiangxi	1.272	0.230	0.047	0.070	0.064
Shandong	1.832	0.289	0.119	0.096	0.091
Henan	1.575	0.291	0.067	0.060	0.089
Hubei	1.741	0.255	0.089	0.077	0.099
Hunan	1.634	0.285	0.053	0.071	0.072
Guangdong	1.542	0.293	0.119	0.084	0.125
Guangxi	1.415	0.252	0.089	0.076	0.090
Hainan	1.578	0.189	0.104	0.093	0.079
Chongqing	1.393	0.409	0.082	0.058	0.082
Sichuan	1.510	0.512	0.080	0.063	0.108
Guizhou	1.328	0.219	0.057	0.075	0.067
Yunnan	1.271	0.204	0.070	0.084	0.087
Xizang	1.180	0.350	0.041	0.154	0.036
Shaanxi	1.592	0.297	0.094	0.056	0.060
Gansu	1.264	0.437	0.069	0.065	0.102
Qinghai	1.708	0.396	0.068	0.076	0.139
Ningxia	1.714	0.288	0.161	0.112	0.071
Xinjiang	1.854	0.280	0.120	0.133	0.135

Figure 4.2. Average densities of different subtypes of licensed doctors during 2012−2016.

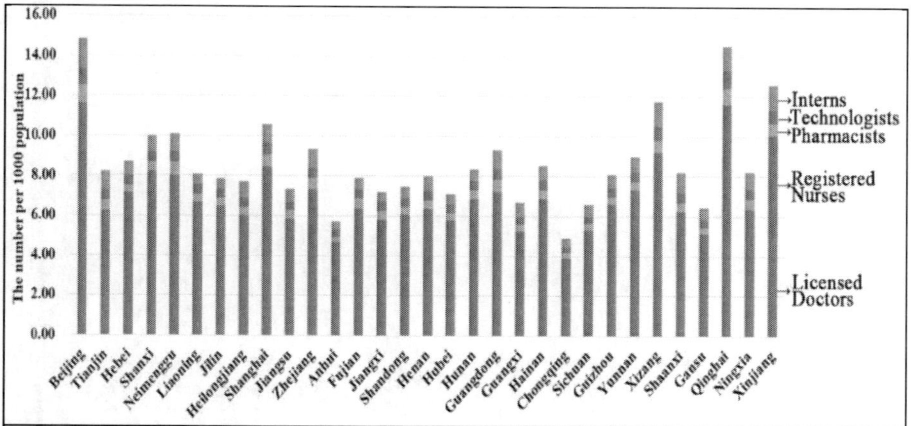

Region	HT	LD	RN	PH	TE	Interns
Beijing	16.394	6.186	6.828	0.96	0.855	1.577
Tianjin	8.898	3.404	3.432	0.551	0.505	1.024
Hebei	10.228	4.144	4.42	0.429	0.537	0.696
Shanxi	11.44	4.522	5.032	0.507	0.604	0.782
Neimenggu	11.692	4.408	4.974	0.742	0.618	0.944
Liaoning	9.078	3.478	4.066	0.447	0.516	0.554
Jilin	9.594	4.032	4.012	0.452	0.53	0.576
Heilongjiang	8.978	3.272	3.844	0.418	0.509	0.93
Shanghai	11.542	4.214	5.11	0.646	0.675	0.9
Jiangsu	9.116	3.31	4.098	0.488	0.483	0.756
Zhejiang	11.366	4.218	4.75	0.691	0.623	1.062
Anhui	6.452	2.274	3.082	0.288	0.365	0.433
Fujian	9.94	3.652	4.396	0.624	0.524	0.732
Jiangxi	8.714	2.976	4.17	0.496	0.548	0.526
Shandong	9.188	3.482	4.094	0.463	0.464	0.688
Henan	9.872	3.412	4.63	0.45	0.54	0.847
Hubei	8.81	3.122	4.2	0.431	0.472	0.58
Hunan	10.192	3.638	4.89	0.485	0.544	0.626
Guangdong	11.262	4.038	4.82	0.693	0.605	1.105
Guangxi	7.92	2.716	3.556	0.417	0.408	0.806
Hainan	10.834	3.684	5.18	0.549	0.623	0.805
Chongqing	5.804	2.076	2.602	0.297	0.297	0.529
Sichuan	7.866	2.858	3.534	0.379	0.413	0.655
Guizhou	10.31	3.778	4.686	0.422	0.559	0.878
Yunnan	11.08	4.244	4.816	0.501	0.608	0.931
Xizang	12.41	5.456	4.146	0.62	0.69	1.483
Shaanxi	9.642	3.118	4.254	0.472	0.57	1.231
Gansu	7.2	2.784	3.024	0.355	0.408	0.609
Qinghai	17.362	6.252	7.814	0.876	1.024	1.381
Ningxia	9.362	3.408	3.912	0.523	0.5	0.997
Xinjiang	15.082	5.69	6.44	0.711	0.764	1.456

Figure 4.3. Average densities of different types of urban health manpower during 2012—2016.

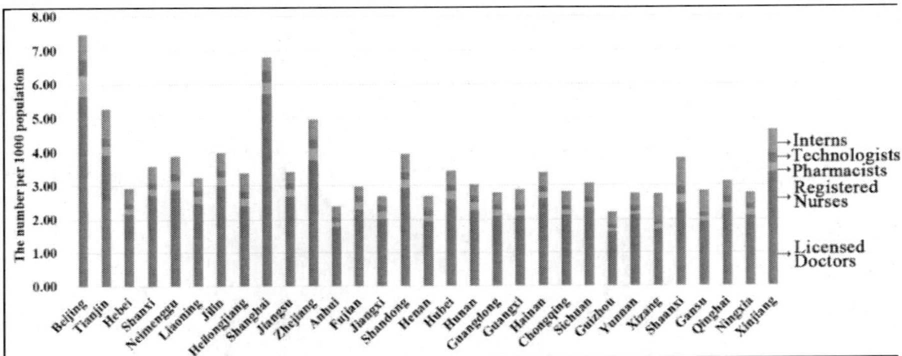

Region	HT	LD	RN	PH	TE	Interns
Beijing	8.16	3.72	2.68	0.669	0.487	0.562
Tianjin	6.024	3.028	1.57	0.316	0.255	0.73
Hebei	3.298	1.614	0.932	0.143	0.167	0.388
Shanxi	3.866	1.77	1.196	0.199	0.197	0.424
Neimenggu	4.364	1.884	1.346	0.28	0.227	0.529
Liaoning	3.594	1.568	1.216	0.2	0.193	0.368
Jilin	4.344	1.844	1.458	0.241	0.218	0.495
Heilongjiang	3.828	1.59	1.114	0.244	0.24	0.565
Shanghai	7.622	4.16	2.34	0.37	0.354	0.375
Jiangsu	4.22	1.84	1.55	0.245	0.201	0.342
Zhejiang	5.93	2.422	2.096	0.401	0.281	0.619
Anhui	2.764	1.142	0.992	0.143	0.171	0.264
Fujian	3.772	1.368	1.466	0.263	0.188	0.388
Jiangxi	3.018	1.162	1.148	0.229	0.208	0.255
Shandong	4.786	1.836	1.754	0.265	0.246	0.584
Henan	3.166	1.298	1.038	0.16	0.196	0.397
Hubei	4.05	1.588	1.578	0.231	0.206	0.389
Hunan	3.532	1.512	1.204	0.233	0.198	0.328
Guangdong	3.29	1.352	1.142	0.212	0.145	0.37
Guangxi	3.51	1.188	1.296	0.205	0.187	0.539
Hainan	3.9	1.38	1.604	0.209	0.194	0.43
Chongqing	3.434	1.396	1.172	0.162	0.141	0.482
Sichuan	3.744	1.568	1.28	0.193	0.176	0.451
Guizhou	2.952	0.994	1.066	0.119	0.173	0.476
Yunnan	3.476	1.244	1.32	0.141	0.185	0.484
Xizang	2.992	1.288	0.484	0.133	0.122	0.762
Shaanxi	4.716	1.348	1.544	0.276	0.313	1.014
Gansu	3.392	1.274	1.008	0.159	0.159	0.627
Qinghai	3.588	1.51	1.038	0.187	0.212	0.538
Ningxia	3.346	1.396	1.028	0.24	0.194	0.415
Xinjiang	5.708	2.012	2.144	0.271	0.351	0.782

Figure 4.4. Average densities of different types of rural health manpower during 2012–2016.

Figures 4.3 and 4.4 present the urban-rural divide of different subtypes of health manpower for the period 2012–2016. In general, the comparison between urban and rural areas was more revealing due to the significant urban-rural differences in health manpower distribution in China. The average urban heath technician density could be twice the average rural health technician density. Beijing also ranked first for the average densities of almost all subtypes of urban and rural health manpower. Apart from Beijing, Qinghai, Xinjiang, and Xizang were three units with a higher density of urban licensed doctors than the other units. However, the densities of rural licensed doctors in these units were much lower. The urban-rural imbalances were more dramatic in the case of registered nurses. The density of urban registered nurses was extremely high in Beijing, Qinghai, and Xizang, while the lowest density was found in the provincial unit of Chongqing. In contrast, Xizang had the lowest density of rural registered nurses, with only 0.484 registered nurses per 1000 population. Similar urban-rural discrepancies were found in the distribution of these subtypes of health manpower.

4.2. Temporal Trends

Figure 4.5 displays the temporal trends of the densities of different subtypes of health manpower during 2012–2016. Generally speaking, China experienced a rapid increase in the density of almost all subtypes of health manpower, as evidenced by the rising trend lines. The maximum, upper quartile, median, lower quartile, and minimum of the density of health technicians have all increased dramatically since 2012. In spite of rapid growth nationwide, the health manpower distribution was relatively unbalanced, with the range (the difference between the maximum and minimum) of the densities of each type of health technicians being relatively huge. This finding could apply just as well to the subtypes of health technicians.

Figures 4.6 and 4.7 show the temporal trends of the densities of each subtype of urban and rural health manpower during 2012–2016, respectively. Evidently, the density of urban health manpower had more rapid growth than rural health manpower. For instance, the median density of rural licensed doctors remained almost unchanged during the research period, while that of urban licensed doctors increased by about 1 unit.

Moreover, the range of densities of rural health manpower was much larger in terms of the IQR.

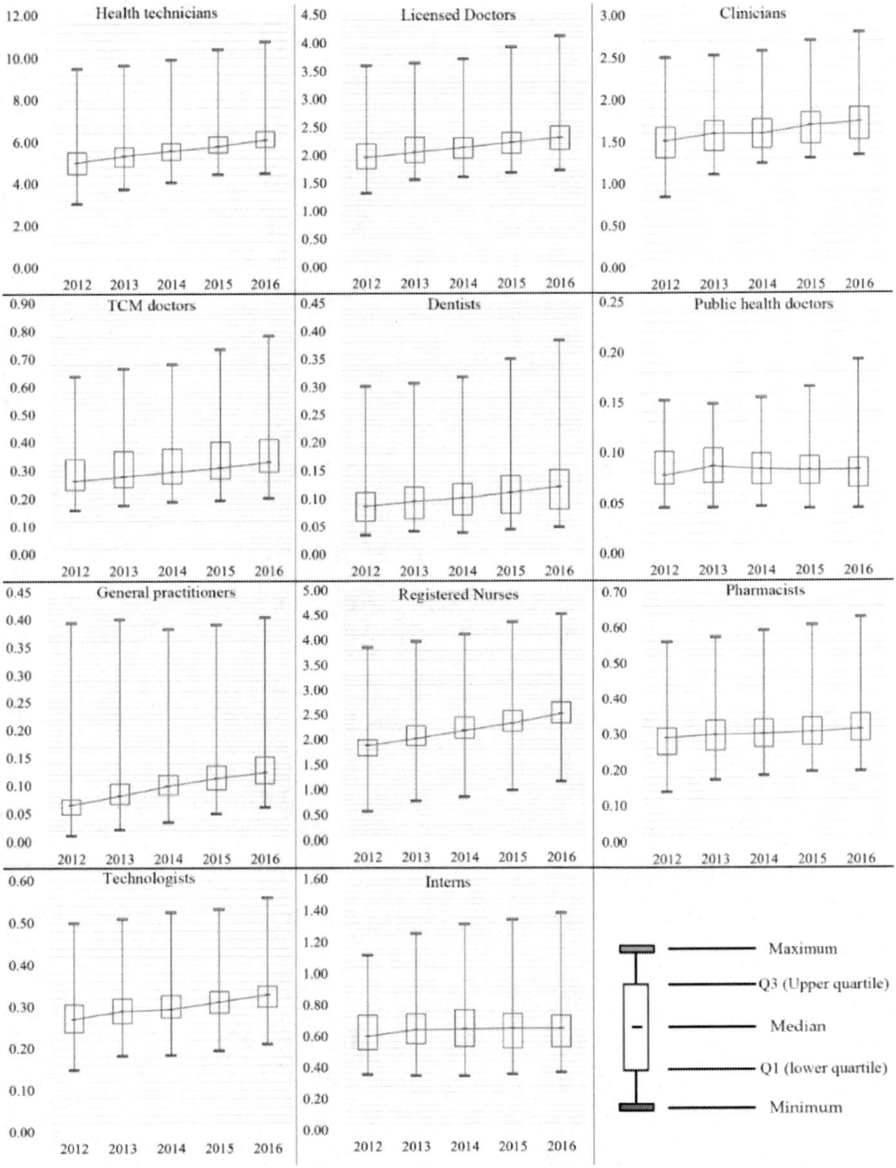

Figure 4.5. Boxplots of the density of total health manpower during 2012–2016.

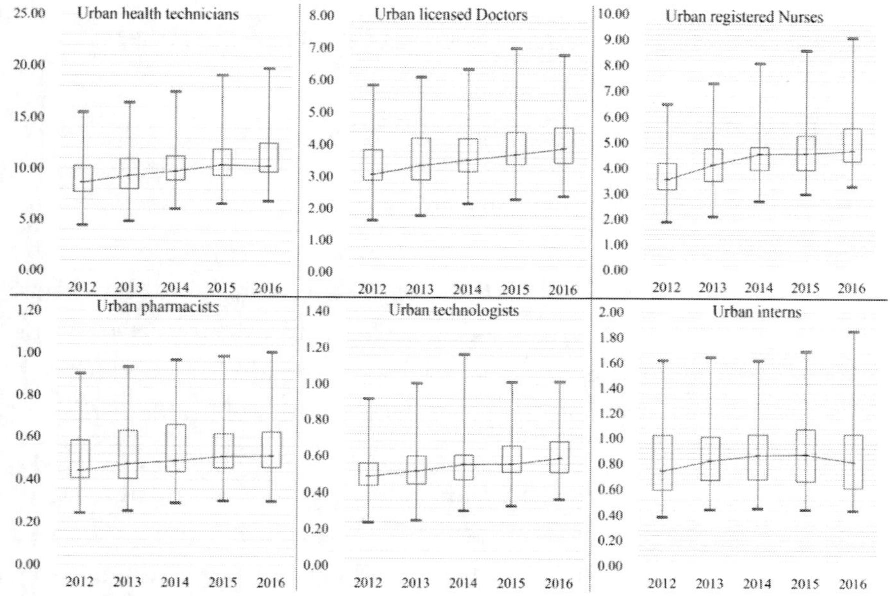

Figure 4.6. Boxplots of the density of urban health manpower during 2012–2016.

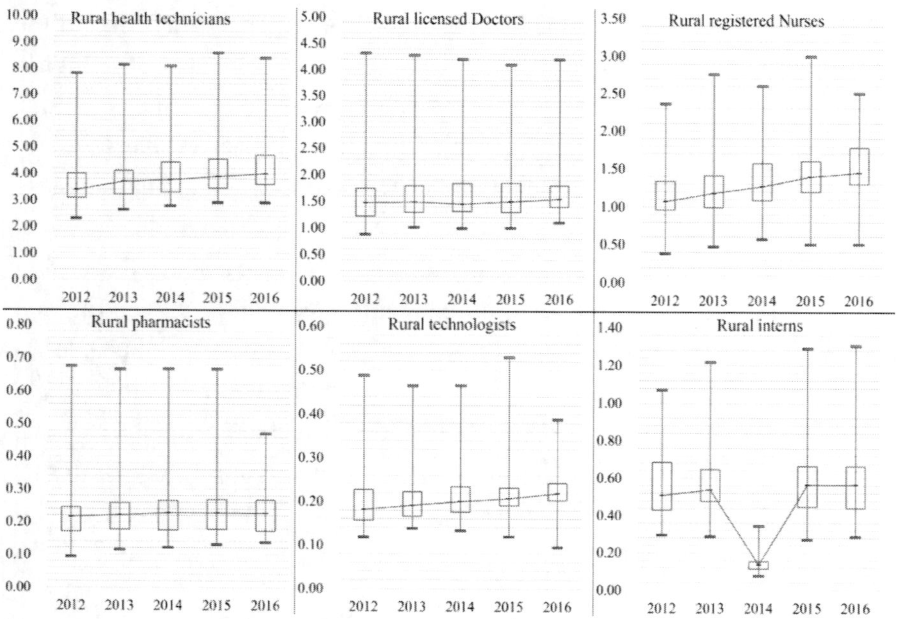

Figure 4.7. Boxplots of the density of rural health manpower density during 2012–2016.

4.3. Spatial Variation in Temporal Trends

4.3.1. Total Health Manpower Distribution

As shown in Section 4.2, the densities of almost all subtypes of health technicians, especially the urban group, maintained rapid growth during 2012–2016, whereas spatial variations may exist in the temporal trends. This section employs the space-time scan statistics to detect those provincial units that displayed higher or lower rates of change, which will help us to fully understand the temporal characteristics of health manpower distribution in China.

Figure 4.8 visualizes the space-time clusters of higher change rate of densities of different subtypes of health technicians. Regarding the total health technicians, two significant clusters of higher rates of change during 2012–2016 were detected, the most likely cluster being identified in two provincial units, with Yunnan the cluster center. The mean annual increase rate for these two units (10.063%) was significantly larger than that in the other units (5.078%). Comparatively, the most likely cluster of a higher rate of change of the density of licensed doctors was detected in nine units (Hubei, Henan, Hunan, Anhui, Jiangxi, Chongqing, Shaanxi, Jiangsu, and Zhejiang), with Hubei being the cluster center. An average annual increase of 4.908% in the licensed doctor density was observed within the most likely cluster, in comparison to the 3.086% outside of it. Regarding registered nurses, 10 provincial units (center: Sichuan) in central and western China showed a faster increase in the mean annual trend (10.262% annually) than outside the cluster (7.152% annually). The most likely clusters of pharmacists and interns were both detected in western China, with Yunnan and Qinghai being the cluster centers, respectively. In terms of technologists, 12 units in central and western China (center: Yunnan) experienced a faster growth than the other units (6.710% versus 3.733% annually).

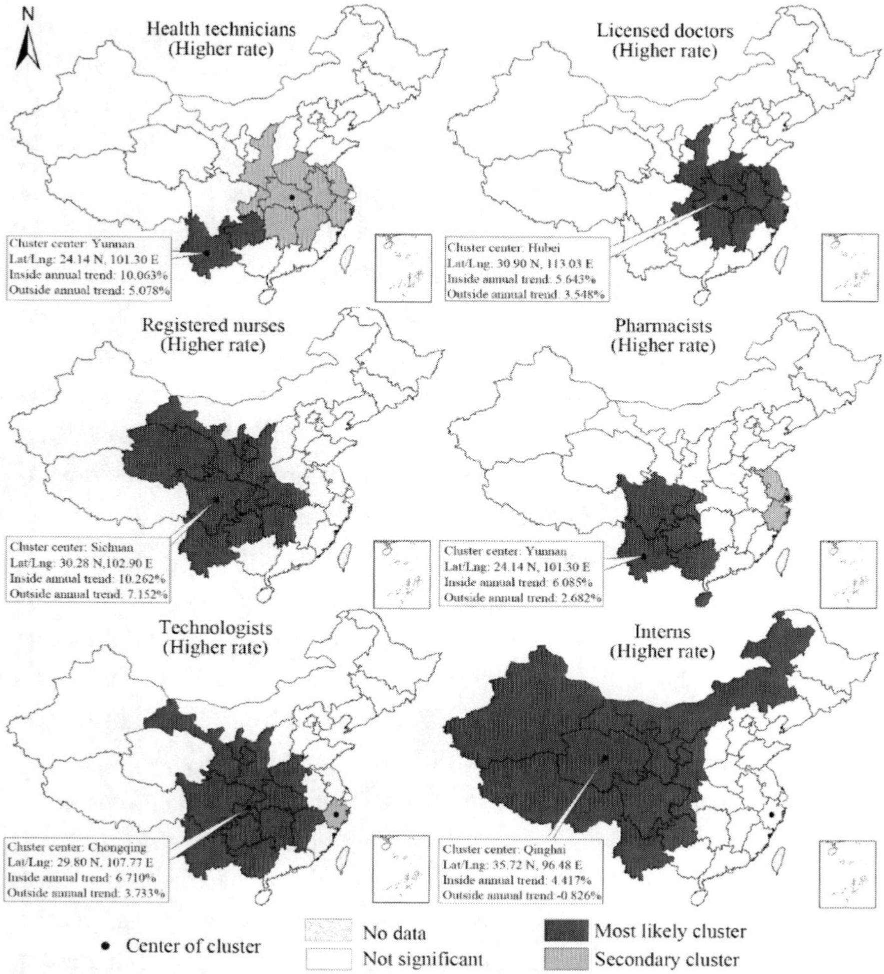

Note: Detailed information of the most likely clusters is noted on the maps.

Figure 4.8. Space-time clusters of higher rates of change of the densities of different subtypes of health technicians.

Figure 4.9 visualizes the space-time clusters of lower rates of change of densities of different subtypes of health technicians, which share numerous similarities. The most likely cluster centers of total health technicians, licensed doctors, registered nurses, pharmacists, and technologists were all located in the provincial unit of Heilongjiang, indicating that the units in northeast China experienced a slower increase in the densities of health technicians, licensed doctors, registered nurses, pharmacists, and technologists. Of these, the average rate of increase in the technologist density was very small, only 3.429%, while that in the other units could be as high as 6.007%. The most likely cluster of the lower change rate of interns was located in 10 provincial units in central and eastern China, with Hebei being the cluster center. The average density of interns among these units even decreased during 2012–2016. The mean annual percentage change in the rate was −3.590%, which was significantly lower than that outside the cluster (1.657% annually). In addition, one secondary cluster of lower rates of change was also detected for licensed doctors, registered nurses, pharmacists, and interns. More information about all the space-time clusters of higher and lower rates of change of health technician density can be found in Table 4.1, which presents the detailed parameters of all the space-time clusters.

Figure 4.10 visualizes the space-time clusters of higher rates of change of densities of different subtypes of licensed doctors. In short, the maps differ greatly in the units that included in the clusters. The most likely cluster of higher rates of change of clinicians was located in nine provincial units in central China, with Hubei being the cluster center. It was exactly the same as the most likely cluster of higher rates of change of total licensed doctors (Figure 4.6), which may be largely due to its larger proportion of licensed doctors. The mean annual rate of change for these nine provincial units reached 5.422%, which was almost twice that in other units (2.991% annually). An accelerated increase of TCM doctor density was observed in Jiangsu (center), Shandong, Henan, Shanghai, Anhui, and Zhejiang, with an average annual growth rate reaching 7.690%.

As for dentists, Heilongjiang was fund to be the center of the most likely cluster, which also included Jilin, Liaoning, and Beijing. A 9.386% average annual rate of increase was observed in these units. In addition, almost all the units in central and eastern China displayed a faster growth of dentist density than western China, which was evidenced by two secondary clusters that included 13 units. In terms of public health doctors, their density in 10 provincial units (center: Fujian) in southeast China increased 1.643% annually during 2012–2014, while a decreasing trend

(−1.506% annually) was observable outside the most likely cluster. Among general practitioners, a significantly higher increase in their density was observed in 10 provincial units in central and southern China (20.052% versus 13.000% annually).

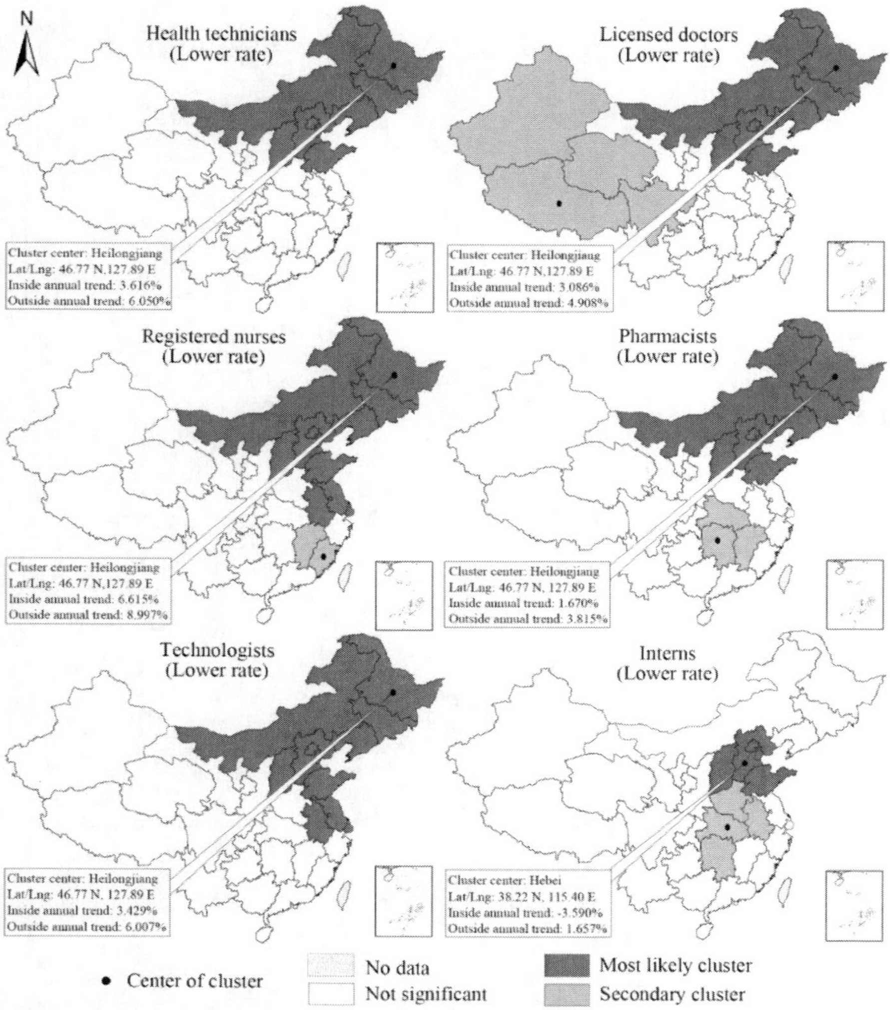

Note: Detailed information of the most likely clusters is noted on the maps.

Figure 4.9. Space-time clusters of lower rates of change of densities of different subtypes of health technicians.

Table 4.1. Space-time clusters of higher and lower rates of change of densities of different subtypes of health technicians during 2012–2016

Manpower	Cluster type	Units included	Coordinates of cluster center	Radius of cluster (Km)	Average density	Inside time trend (Annual)	Outside time trend (Annual)	LLR	p
Health technician*	Higher	Yunnan (center), Guizhou	24.14 N, 101.30 E	602.35	4.601	10.063%	5.078%	3834.69	0.001
Health technician	Higher	Hubei (center), Henan, Hunan, Anhui, Jiangxi, Chongqing, Shaanxi, Jiangsu, Zhejiang	30.90 N, 113.03 E	709.15	5.451	6.205%	4.780%	1625.56	0.001
Health technician*	Lower	Heilongjiang (center), Jilin, Liaoning, Beijing, Tianjin, Hebei, Shandong, Neimenggu, Shanxi	46.77 N, 127.89 E	1620.87	5.908	3.616%	6.050%	4246.94	0.001
Licensed doctor*	Higher	Hubei, Henan, Hunan, Anhui, Jiangxi, Chongqing, Shaanxi, Jiangsu, Zhejiang	30.90 N, 113.03 E	709.15	2.064	5.643%	3.548%	1363.95	0.001
Licensed doctor*	Lower	Heilongjiang, Jilin, Liaoning, Beijing, Tianjin, Hebei, Shandong, Neimenggu, Shanxi	46.77 N, 127.89 E	1620.87	2.387	3.086%	4.908%	954.72	0.001
Licensed doctor	Lower	Xizang, Qinghai, Xinjiang, Sichuan	31.10 N, 89.12 E	1319.29	2.202	2.646%	4.491%	363.03	0.001
Registered nurse*	Higher	Sichuan, Chongqing, Guizhou, Gansu, Shaanxi, Yunnan, Ningxia, Qinghai, Hunan, Hubei	30.28 N, 102.90 E	971.45	2.123	10.262%	7.152%	2453.76	0.001
Registered nurse*	Lower	Heilongjiang, Jilin, Liaoning, Beijing, Tianjin, Hebei, Shandong, Neimenggu, Shanxi, Jiangsu, Shanghai, Anhui	46.77 N, 127.89 E	1875.67	2.267	6.615%	8.997%	1763.84	0.001
Registered nurse	Lower	Fujian, Jiangxi	26.00 N, 118.02 E	305.25	2.016	6.599%	8.095%	153.69	0.001
Pharmacist*	Higher	Yunnan, Guizhou, Sichuan, Guangxi, Chongqing, Hainan	24.14 N, 101.30 E	1031.27	0.251	6.085%	2.682%	282.13	0.001
Pharmacist	Higher	Shanghai, Jiangsu, Zhejiang	31.21 N, 121.68 E	279.11	0.371	4.544%	2.978%	57.39	0.001

Manpower	Cluster type	Units included	Coordinates of cluster center	Radius of cluster (Km)	Average density	Inside time trend (Annual)	Outside time trend (Annual)	LLR	p
Pharmacist*	Lower	Heilongjiang, Jilin, Liaoning, Beijing, Tianjin, Hebei, Shandong, Neimenggu, Shanxi	46.77 N, 127.89 E	1620.87	0.309	1.670%	3.815%	182.27	0.001
Pharmacist	Lower	Hunan, Hubei, Jiangxi	28.02 N, 111.58 E	399.45	0.303	1.073%	3.506%	128.18	0.001
Technologist*	Higher	Chongqing, Guizhou, Hunan, Sichuan, Shaanxi, Hubei, Henan, Guangxi, Gansu, Jiangxi, Ningxia, Yunnan	29.80 N, 107.77 E	896.95	0.289	6.710%	3.733%	394.24	0.001
Technologist	Higher	Zhejiang	29.10 N, 120.10 E	0	0.351	6.171%	4.881%	13.74	0.001
Technologist*	Lower	Heilongjiang, Jilin, Liaoning, Beijing, Tianjin, Hebei, Shandong, Neimenggu, Shanxi, Jiangsu, Shanghai, Anhui	46.77 N, 127.89 E	1875.67	0.307	3.429%	6.007%	298.49	0.001
Interns*	Higher	Qinghai, Gansu, Sichuan, Xizang, Ningxia, Shaanxi, Xinjiang, Chongqing, Yunnan, Guizhou, Neimenggu	35.72 N, 96.48 E	1413.28	0.766	4.417%	−0.826%	2317.86	0.001
Interns*	Lower	Hebei, Tianjin, Beijing, Shanxi, Shandong	38.22 N, 115.40 E	351.28	0.638	−3.590%	1.657%	1788.72	0.001
Interns	Lower	Hubei, Henan, Hunan, Anhui	30.90 N, 113.03 E	413.08	0.515	−0.806%	0.978%	191.1	0.001

Note: Most likely cl.
usters are noted with *.

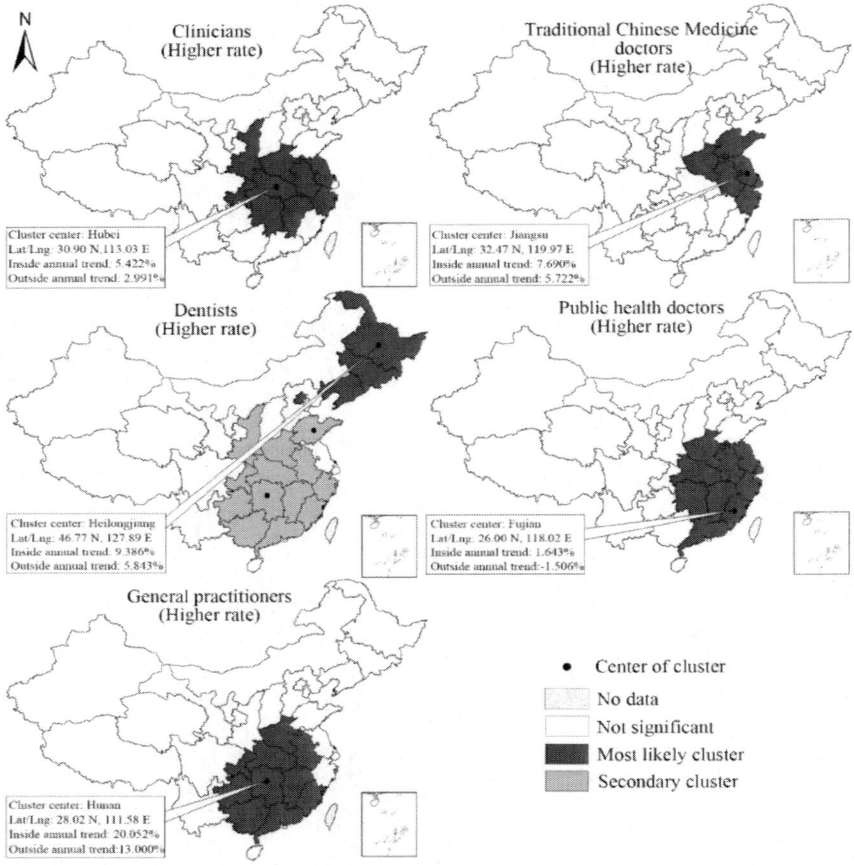

Note: Detailed information of the most likely clusters is noted on the maps.

Figure 4.10. Space-time clusters of higher rates of change of densities of different subtypes of licensed doctors.

Figure 4.11 visualizes the space-time clusters of lower rates of change of densities of different subtypes of licensed doctors. Two clusters displaying significantly lower increases were identified for clinician density. The most likely cluster comprised nine units in northwest China (center: Heilongjiang), while the secondary cluster was situated in four remote western units (Xinjiang, Xizang, Qinghai, and Sichuan), with Xizang being the cluster center. Similarly, a slower increase in dentist density was also detected in these four provincial units, the 6.248% annual increase rate among which being significantly slower than that observed in other units (8.937% annually).

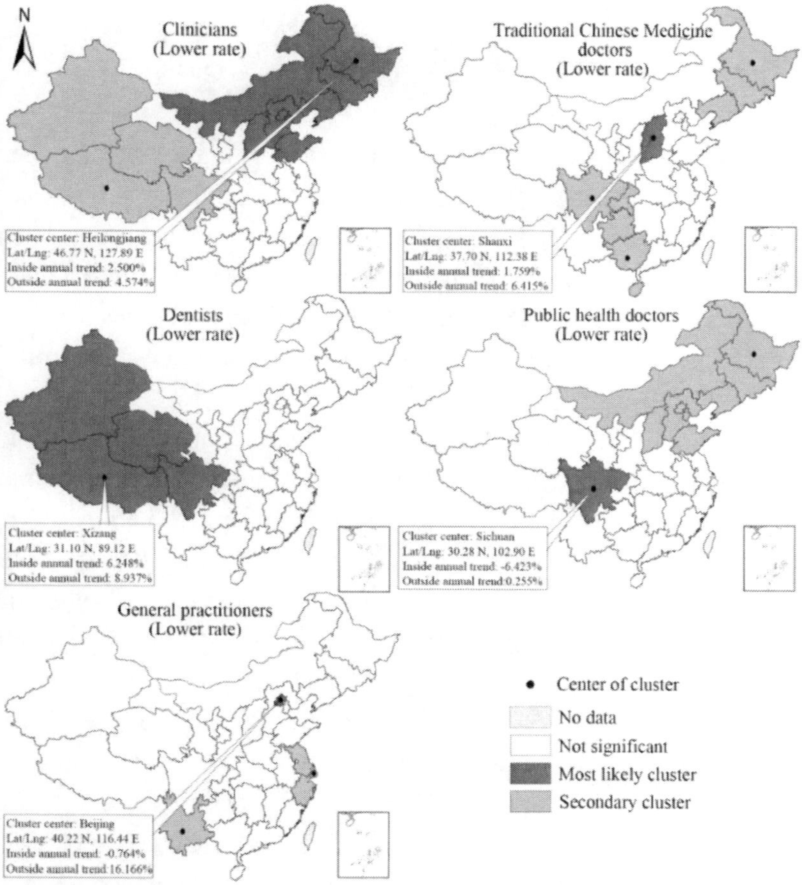

Note: Detailed information of the most likely clusters is noted on the maps.

Figure 4.11. Space-time clusters of lower rates of change of densities of different subtypes of licensed doctors.

As for TCM doctors, public health doctors, and general practitioners, the most likely clusters of lower rates of change were only detected in one provincial unit each, Shanxi, Sichuan, and Beijing, respectively. It was noteworthy that the public health doctor density in Sichuan even decreased 6.423% annually, which was in sharp contrast to the 0.255% annual increase among the other 30 provincial units. More information about all the space-time clusters of higher and lower rates of change of licensed doctor density can be found in Table 4.2.

4.3.2. Urban Health Manpower Distribution

Figure 4.12 visualizes the space-time clusters of higher rates of change of densities of different subtypes of urban health technicians. In general, the units that experienced a higher increase of urban health technician density were concentrated in southern China. Chongqing and Guizhou were included in the most likely clusters of all subtypes of health technicians, while secondary clusters were always detected in central and eastern China.

Regarding the total urban health technicians, the most likely cluster of higher rates of change of its density was detected in Chongqing and Guizhou, just as with urban registered nurses and interns. The mean annual rate of change in the total urban health technician density within Chongqing and Guizhou was as much as three times that of other units (13.892% versus 4.770% annually). The most likely cluster of higher increases in the density of urban licensed doctors was located in Chongqing, Guizhou, and Hunan, with a 10.627% average annual increase in urban licensed doctor density observed in these three units, significantly higher than the 3.988% among other units. In comparison, the urban registered nurse density in Chongqing and Guizhou increased 15.907% annually, in comparison to the 6.398% in other units. The average rate of increase of urban interns in Chongqing and Guizhou even reached 12.579%, while that in other units was only 0.978%. As for urban pharmacists, Chongqing, Guizhou, and Guangxi were included in the most likely cluster (center: Fujian), which experienced more rapid growth than the other units (9.853% versus 2.754% annually). In contrast, the most likely cluster of higher increases in technologist density was detected in Chongqing, Guizhou, Hunan, and Guangxi, in which the mean percentage rate reached 9.464%, which was significantly larger than that of other units (3.567% annually).

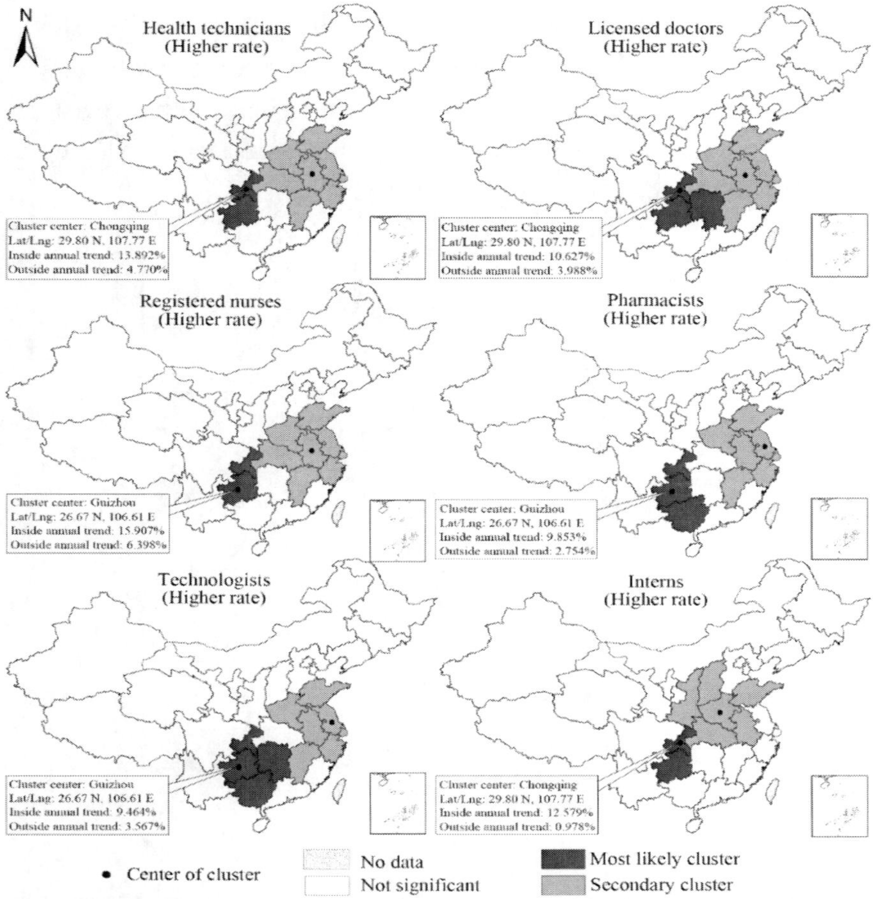

Note: Detailed information of the most likely clusters is noted on the maps.

Figure 4.12. Space-time clusters of higher rates of change of densities of different subtypes of urban health technicians.

Figure 4.13 visualizes the space-time clusters of lower rates of change of densities of different subtypes of urban health technicians. Beijing was detected as the most likely cluster center of lower rates of change of total rural health technician density, rural registered nurse density and rural intern density and secondary cluster center of lower rates of change of the pharmacist and technologist densities. The maps indicate that Beijing and provincial units nearby presented a slower increase in the densities of these subtypes of rural health manpower. More specifically, the average density of urban health technicians in Beijing, Tianjin, and Hebei displayed slower growth, with the annual growth rate being 1.564%, in contrast with 5.591% in other units. Meanwhile, a 2.582% annual increase in the urban registered nurse density was observed in Beijing, Tianjin, and Hebei, which was significantly lower than that in other units (4.950%).

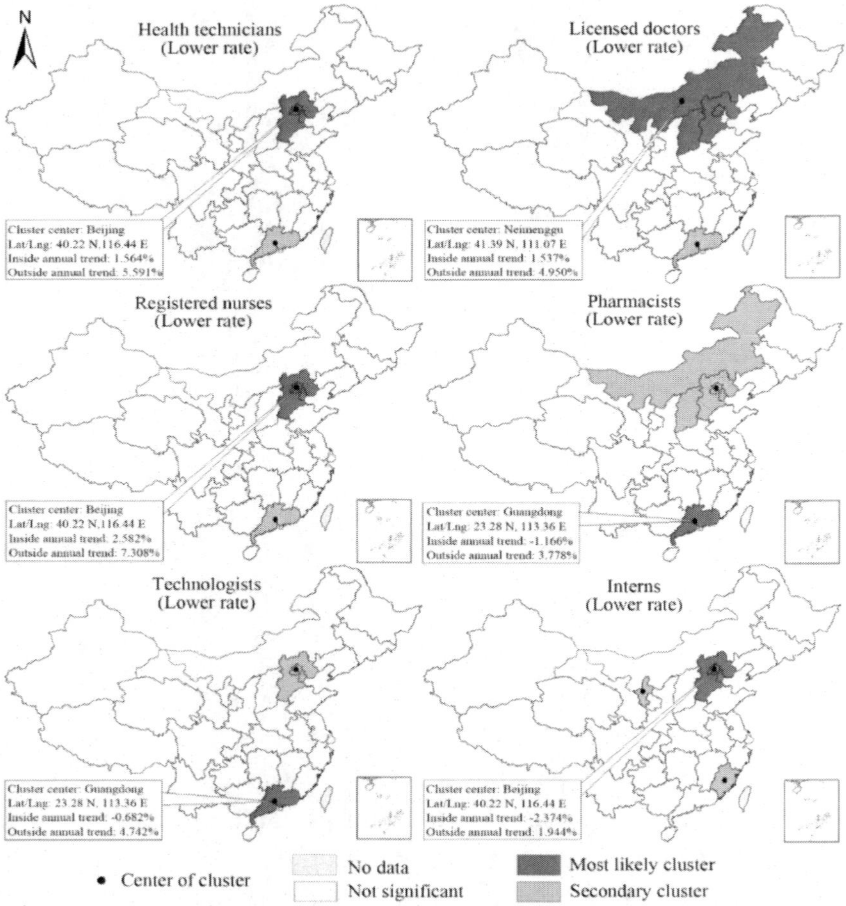

Note: Detailed information of the most likely clusters is noted on the maps.

Figure 4.13. Space-time clusters of lower rates of change of densities of different subtypes of urban health technicians.

The density of urban interns in these units decreased 2.374% annually, whereas that in other units maintained an upward trend. In contrast, a

1.537% average annual increase in the urban licensed doctor density was found in four units (Neimenggu, Shanxi, Hebei, and Beijing) in north China, which presented a sharp contrast with the value of 4.950% outside of the cluster. When it comes to pharmacists and technologists, the most likely clusters of lower rates of change of their densities were both located in Guangdong, which displayed a downtrend during 2012–2016. More information about all the space-time clusters of higher and lower rates of change of urban health technician density can be found in Table 4.2.

4.3.3. Rural Health Manpower Distribution

Figure 4.14 visualizes the space-time clusters of higher rates of change of densities of different subtypes of rural health technicians. Regarding the total rural health technicians, the most likely cluster of highest increase in its density was detected in nine provincial units (center: Guizhou), among which the average annual increase rate reached 6.171% (compared to the 3.206% outside of the cluster). It is worth noting that the units included in the most likely cluster of higher rates of change of registered nurse density were exactly same as those for total rural health technicians. A 10.475% annual increase in rural registered nurse density was observed among these nine provincial units, which was significantly higher than the 6.423% among other units. In contrast, the most likely cluster of higher rates of change of rural licensed doctor density was detected in Hunan and Hubei in central China. An average increase rate of 7.823% was observed within the cluster, while that of units outside of the cluster was only 2.613%. In addition, Jiangsu and its three neighbors (Shanghai, Anhui, and Zhejiang) were included in a secondary cluster, which also experienced a relatively more rapid growth of rural licensed doctor density than did the others. Comparatively, the most likely clusters of higher rates of change of rural pharmacist density, technologist density, and intern density were all detected among 11 western provincial units (center: Xizang).

Table 4.2. Space-time clusters of higher and lower rates of change of densities of different subtypes of licensed doctors during 2012–2016

Manpower	Cluster type	Units included	Coordinates of cluster center	Radius of cluster (Km)	Average density	Inside time trend (Annual)	Outside time trend (Annual)	LLR	p
Clinician*	Higher	Hubei (center), Henan, Hunan, Anhui, Jiangxi, Chongqing, Shaanxi, Jiangsu, Zhejiang	30.90 N, 113.03 E	709.15	1.625	5.422%	2.991%	1435.02	0.001
Clinicians*	Lower	Heilongjiang (center), Jilin, Liaoning, Beijing, Tianjin, Hebei, Shandong, Neimenggu, Shanxi	46.77 N, 127.89 E	1620.87	1.823	2.500%	4.574%	956.88	0.001
Clinicians	Lower	Xizang (center), Qinghai, Xinjiang, Sichuan	31.10 N, 89.12 E	1319.29	1.581	1.931%	4.099%	366.38	0.001
TCM doctor*	Higher	Jiangsu (center), Shanghai, Anhui, Zhejiang, Shandong, Henan	32.47 N, 119.97 E	611.70	0.279	7.690%	5.722%	142.04	0.001
TCM doctor*	Lower	Shanxi (center)	37.70 N, 112.38 E	0	0.383	1.759%	6.415%	135.03	0.001
TCM doctor	Lower	Heilongjiang (center), Jilin, Liaoning	46.77 N, 127.89 E	683.82	0.276	4.004%	6.426%	74.35	0.001
TCM doctor	Lower	Guangxi (center), Hainan, Guizhou	23.02 N, 108.41 E	444.67	0.233	8.957%	6.118%	70.25	0.001
TCM doctor	Lower	Sichuan (center), Chongqing	30.28 N, 102.90 E	471.25	0.485	5.560%	6.356%	13.27	0.001
Dentist*	Higher	Heilongjiang (center), Jilin, Liaoning, Beijing	46.77 N, 127.89 E	1172.90	0.180	9.386%	5.843%	105.95	0.001
Dentist	Higher	Hunan (center), Hubei, Jiangxi, Chongqing, Guizhou, Guangdong, Guangxi, Henan, Fujian, Anhui, Shaanxi, Zhejiang	28.02 N, 111.58 E	840.52	0.088	10.061%	7.806%	73.27	0.001
Dentist	Higher	Shandong (center)	36.18 N, 118.43 E	0	0.119	12.502%	8.412%	72.33	0.001
Dentist*	Lower	Xizang (center), Qinghai, Xinjiang, Sichuan	31.10 N, 89.12 E	1319.29	0.086	6.248%	8.937%	28.32	0.001
Public health doctor*	Higher	Fujian (center), Jiangxi, Zhejiang, Guangdong, Anhui, Hunan, Shanghai, Hubei, Jiangsu, Henan	26.00 N, 118.02 E	965.93	0.081	1.643%	−1.506%	137.03	0.001
Public health doctor*	Lower	Sichuan (center)	30.28 N, 102.90 E	0	0.063	−6.423%	0.255%	116.05	0.001
Public health doctor	Lower	Heilongjiang (center), Jilin, Liaoning, Beijing, Tianjin, Hebei, Shandong, Neimenggu, Shanxi	46.77 N, 127.89 E	1620.87	0.088	−2.146%	0.845%	105.81	0.001
Gereral practitioner*	Higher	Hunan (center), Hubei, Jiangxi, Chongqing, Guizhou, Guangdong, Guangxi, Henan, Fujian, Anhui	28.02 N, 111.58 E	698.79	0.094	20.052%	13.000%	649.50	0.001
Gereral practitioner*	Lower	Beijing (center)	40.22 N, 116.44 E	0	0.388	−0.764%	16.166%	968.41	0.001
Gereral practitioner	Lower	Shanghai (center), Jiangsu, Zhejiang	31.21 N, 121.68 E	279.11	0.283	12.777%	16.277%	149.60	0.001
Gereral practitioner	Lower	Yunnan (center)	24.14 N, 101.30 E	0	0.087	7.162%	15.478%	110.84	0.001

Note: Most likely clusters are noted with *.

Table 4.3. Space-time clusters of higher and lower rates of change of densities of different subtypes of urban health technicians during 2012–2016

Manpower	Cluster type	Units included	Coordinates of cluster center	Radius of cluster (Km)	Average density	Inside time trend (Annual)	Outside time trend (Annual)	LLR	p
Urban health technician*	Higher	Chongqing (center), Guizhou	29.80 N, 107.77 E	365.86	6.879	13.892%	4.770%	5266.90	0.001
Urban health technician	Higher	Anhui (center), Jiangsu, Henan, Hubei, Zhejiang, Shanghai, Shandong, Jiangxi	32.01 N, 117.19 E	498.51	9.289	6.013%	4.741%	669.49	0.001
Urban health technician*	Lower	Beijing (center), Tianjin, Hebei	40.22 N, 116.44 E	239.59	12.083	1.564%	5.591%	2995.16	0.001
Urban health technician	Lower	Guangdong (center)	23.28 N, 113.36 E	0	11.263	1.719%	5.559%	2575.97	0.001
Urban licensed doctor*	Higher	Chongqing (center), Guizhou, Hunan	29.80 N, 107.77 E	420.64	2.912	10.627%	3.988%	1884.68	0.001
Urban licensed doctor	Higher	Anhui (center), Jiangsu, Henan, Hubei, Zhejiang, Shanghai, Shandong, Jiangxi	32.01 N, 117.19 E	498.51	3.362	5.498%	3.972%	355.91	0.001
Urban licensed doctor*	Lower	Neimenggu (center), Shanxi, Beijing, Hebei	41.39 N, 111.07 E	510.10	4.852	1.537%	4.950%	1010.63	0.001
Urban licensed doctor	Lower	Guangdong (center)	23.28 N, 113.36 E	0	4.037	1.100%	4.871%	904.91	0.001
Urban registered nurse*	Higher	Guizhou (center), Chongqing	26.67 N, 106.61 E	365.86	3.100	15.907%	6.398%	2484.74	0.001
Urban registered nurse	Higher	Anhui (center), Jiangsu, Henan, Hubei, Zhejiang, Shanghai, Shandong, Jiangxi	32.01 N, 117.19 E	498.51	4.216	7.531%	6.452%	208.09	0.001
Urban registered nurse*	Lower	Beijing (center), Tianjin, Hebei	40.22 N, 116.44 E	239.59	5.034	2.582%	7.308%	1677.67	0.001
Urban registered nurse	Lower	Guangdong (center)	23.28 N, 113.36 E	0	4.830	3.428%	7.197%	1029.08	0.001
Urban pharmacist*	Higher	Guizhou (center), Chongqing, Guangxi	26.67 N, 106.61 E	444.67	0.362	9.853%	2.754%	283.72	0.001
Urban pharmacist	Higher	Jiangsu (center), Shanghai, Anhui, Zhejiang, Shandong, Henan, Jiangxi	32.47 N, 119.97 E	671.06	0.489	4.489%	2.717%	66.33	0.001
Urban pharmacist*	Lower	Guangdong (center)	23.28 N, 113.36 E	0	0.690	−1.166%	3.778%	270.86	0.001
Urban pharmacist	Lower	Beijing (center), Tianjin, Hebei, Shanxi, Neimenggu	40.22 N, 116.44 E	469.93	0.631	0.677%	3.716%	125.13	0.001
Urban technologis*	Higher	Guizhou (center), Chongqing, Guangxi, Hunan	26.67 N, 106.61 E	512.73	0.423	9.464%	3.567%	298.14	0.001
Urban technologist	Higher	Jiangsu (center), Shanghai, Anhui, Zhejiang, Shandong, Henan, Jiangxi	32.47 N, 119.97 E	671.06	0.511	5.264%	3.714%	51.95	0.001
Urban technologist*	Lower	Guangdong (center)	23.28 N, 113.36 E	0	0.604	−0.682%	4.742%	285.17	0.001
Urban technologist	Lower	Beijing (center), Tianjin, Hebei	40.22 N, 116.44 E	239.59	0.641	1.074%	4.535%	119.63	0.001
Urban intern*	Higher	Chongqing (center), Guizhou	29.80 N, 107.77 E	365.86	0.612	12.579%	0.978%	793.32	0.001
Urban intern	Higher	Henan (center), Hubei, Anhui, Shaanxi, Shanxi, Shandong	33.80 N, 113.59 E	514.06	0.727	2.830%	1.055%	93.73	0.001
Urban intern*	Lower	Beijing (center), Tianjin, Hebei	40.22 N, 116.44 E	239.59	1.081	−2.374%	1.944%	331.14	0.001
Urban intern	Lower	Fujian (center)	26.00 N, 118.02 E	0	0.727	−4.640%	1.674%	151.43	0.001
Urban intern	Lower	Ningxia (center)	37.37 N, 105.99 E	0	0.992	−6.811%	1.592%	105.36	0.001

Note: Most likely clusters are noted with *.

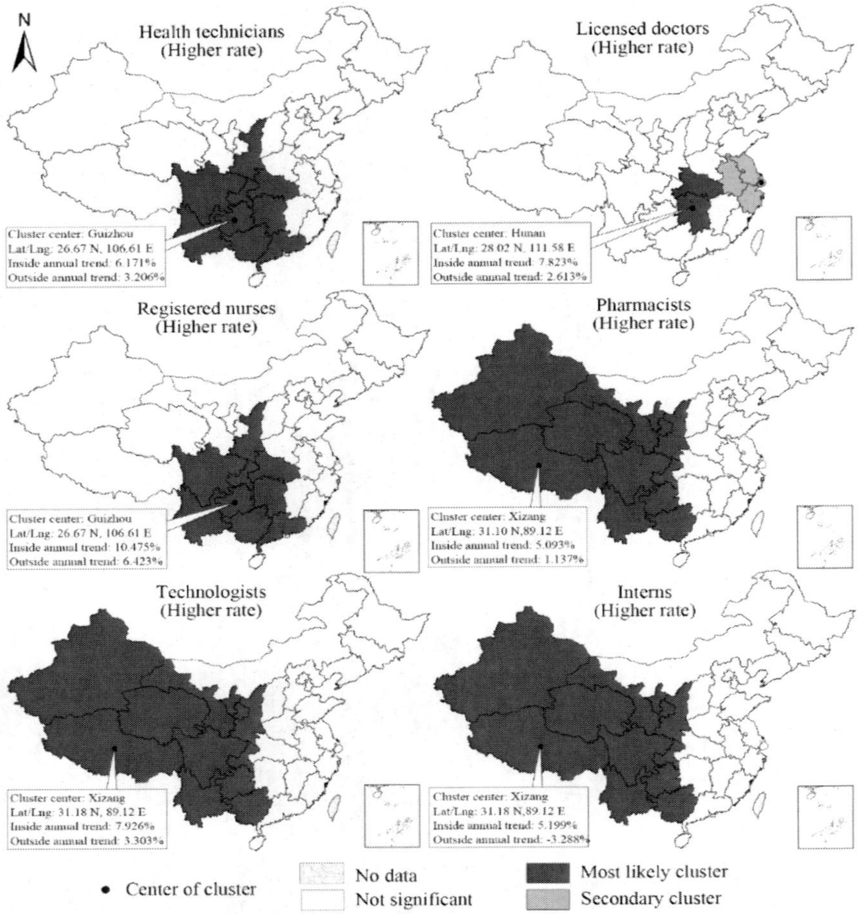

Note: Detailed information of the most likely clusters is noted on the maps.

Figure 4.14. Space-time clusters of higher rates of change of densities of different subtypes of urban health technicians.

Figure 4.15 visualizes the space-time clusters of lower rates of change of densities of different subtypes of rural health technicians. Heilongjiang was detected as the most likely cluster center for total rural health technicians and the four major subtypes besides interns. Among these, the units included in the most likely clusters for total rural health technicians, rural licensed doctors, rural registered nurses, and rural technologists were exactly the same, Heilongjiang, Jilin, Liaoning, Beijing, Tianjin, and Shandong, while that of technologists further included Neimenggu (Inner

Mongolia), Shanxi, Hebei, Jiangsu, Zhejiang, and Shanghai. The average annual rate of change within the clusters was roughly 3%–5% higher than outside of the cluster. As for interns, six provincial units (Tianjin, Beijing, Hebei, Shandong, Shanxi, Liaoning), with Tianjin being the cluster center, were included in the most likely cluster of lower increase of density. An 8.062% average annual decrease was observed among these units, compared to the 1.610% average annual increase among other units. More information about all the space-time clusters of higher and lower rates of change of rural health technician density can be found in table 4.7.

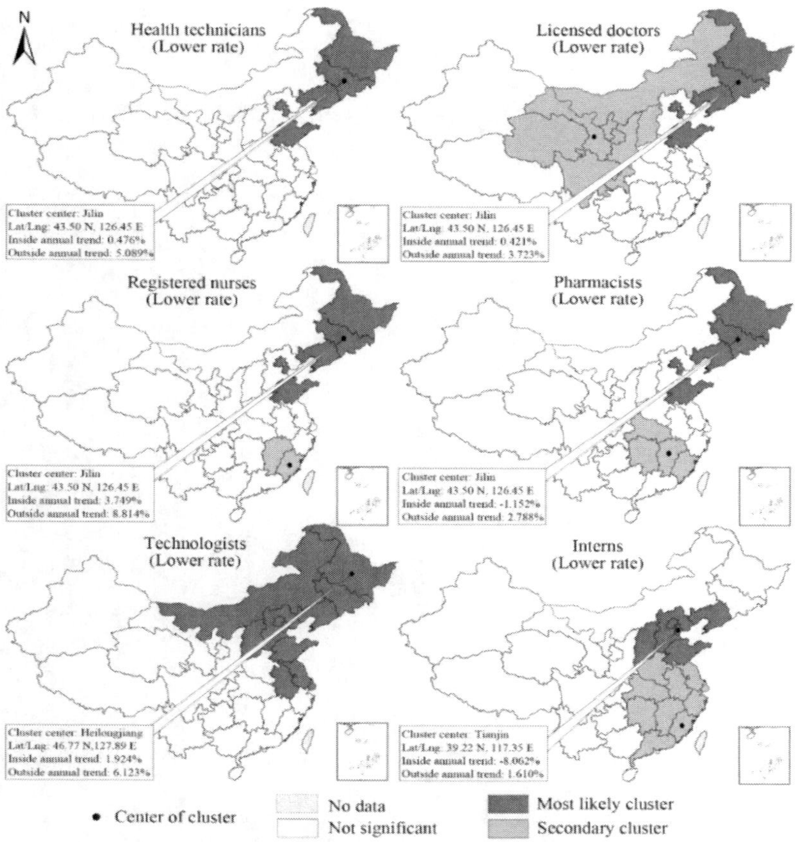

Note: Detailed information of the most likely clusters is noted on the maps.

Figure 4.15. Space-time clusters of lower rates of change of densities of different subtypes of urban health technicians.

Table 4.4. Space-time clusters of higher and lower rates of change of densities of different subtypes of rural health technicians during 2012–2016

Manpower	Cluster type	Units included	Coordinates of cluster center	Radius of cluster (Km)	Average density	Inside time trend (Annual)	Outside time trend (Annual)	LLR	p
Rural health technician*	Higher	Guizhou (center), Chongqing, Guangxi, Hunan, Sichuan, Yunnan, Guangdong, Hubei, Shaanxi	26.67 N, 106.61 E	852.87	3.604	6.171%	3.206%	3404.86	0.001
Rural health technician*	Lower	Jilin (center), Liaoning, Heilongjiang, Tianjin, Beijing, Shandong	43.50 N, 126.45 E	1062.23	4.375	0.476%	5.089%	4999.83	0.001
Rural licensed doctor*	Higher	Hunan (center), Hubei	28.02 N, 111.58 E	349.86	1.542	7.823%	2.613%	1710.52	0.001
Rural licensed doctor	Higher	Shanghai (center), Jiangsu, Zhejiang, Anhui	31.21 N, 121.68 E	434.36	1.727	4.508%	2.917%	225.29	0.001
Rural licensed doctor*	Lower	Jilin (center), Liaoning, Heilongjiang, Tianjin, Beijing, Shandong	43.50 N, 126.45 E	1062.23	1.768	0.421%	3.723%	1048.75	0.001
Rural licensed doctor	Lower	Gansu (center), Ningxia, Shaanxi, Sichuan, Qinghai, Chongqing, Shanxi, Neimenggu	35.95 N, 103.80 E	873.17	1.546	1.740%	3.502%	330.11	0.001
Rural registered nurse*	Higher	Guizhou (center), Chongqing, Guangxi, Hunan, Sichuan, Yunnan, Guangdong, Hubei, Shaanxi	26.67 N, 106.61 E	852.87	1.279	10.475%	6.423%	2058.32	0.001
Rural registered nurse*	Lower	Jilin (center), Liaoning, Heilongjiang, Tianjin, Beijing, Shandong	43.50 N, 126.45 E	1062.23	1.501	3.749%	8.814%	1931.54	0.001
Rural registered nurse	Lower	Fujian (center), Jiangxi	26.00 N, 118.02 E	305.25	1.274	6.084%	8.102%	138.59	0.001
Rural pharmacist*	Higher	Xizang (center), Qinghai, Xinjiang, Sichuan, Yunnan, Gansu, Ningxia, Guizhou, Chongqing, Shaanxi, Guangxi	31.10 N, 89.12 E	2106.09	0.186	5.093%	1.137%	281.69	0.001
Rural pharmacist*	Lower	Jilin (center), Liaoning, Heilongjiang, Tianjin, Beijing, Shandong	43.50 N, 126.45 E	1062.23	0.249	−1.152%	2.788%	215.10	0.001
Rural pharmacist	Lower	Jiangxi (center), Fujian, Hunan, Hubei	27.73 N, 115.63 E	432.79	0.236	0.321%	2.541%	76.46	0.001
Rural technologist*	Higher	Xizang (center), Qinghai, Xinjiang, Sichuan, Yunnan, Gansu, Ningxia, Guizhou, Chongqing, Shaanxi, Guangxi	31.10 N, 89.12 E	2106.09	0.201	7.926%	3.303%	377.17	0.001
Rural technologist*	Lower	Heilongjiang (center), Jilin, Liaoning, Beijing, Tianjin, Hebei, Shandong, Neimenggu, Shanxi, Jiangsu, Shanghai, Anhui	46.77 N, 127.89 E	1875.67	0.205	1.924%	6.123%	362.67	0.001
Rural intern*	Higher	Xizang (center), Qinghai, Xinjiang, Sichuan, Yunnan, Gansu, Ningxia, Guizhou, Chongqing, Shaanxi, Guangxi	31.10 N, 89.12 E	2106.09	0.566	5.199%	−3.288%	3536.54	0.001
Rural intern*	Lower	Tianjin (center), Beijing, Hebei, Shandong, Shanxi, Liaoning	39.22 N, 117.35 E	579.04	0.467	−8.062%	1.610%	3369.81	0.001
Rural intern	Lower	Fujian (center), Jiangxi, Zhejiang, Guangdong, Anhui, Hunan, Shanghai, Hubei, Jiangsu, Henan	26.00 N, 118.02 E	965.93	0.365	1.474%	0.409%	182.56	0.001

Note: Most likely clusters are noted with *.

4.4. Spatial Changing Patterns

4.4.1. Total Health Manpower Distribution

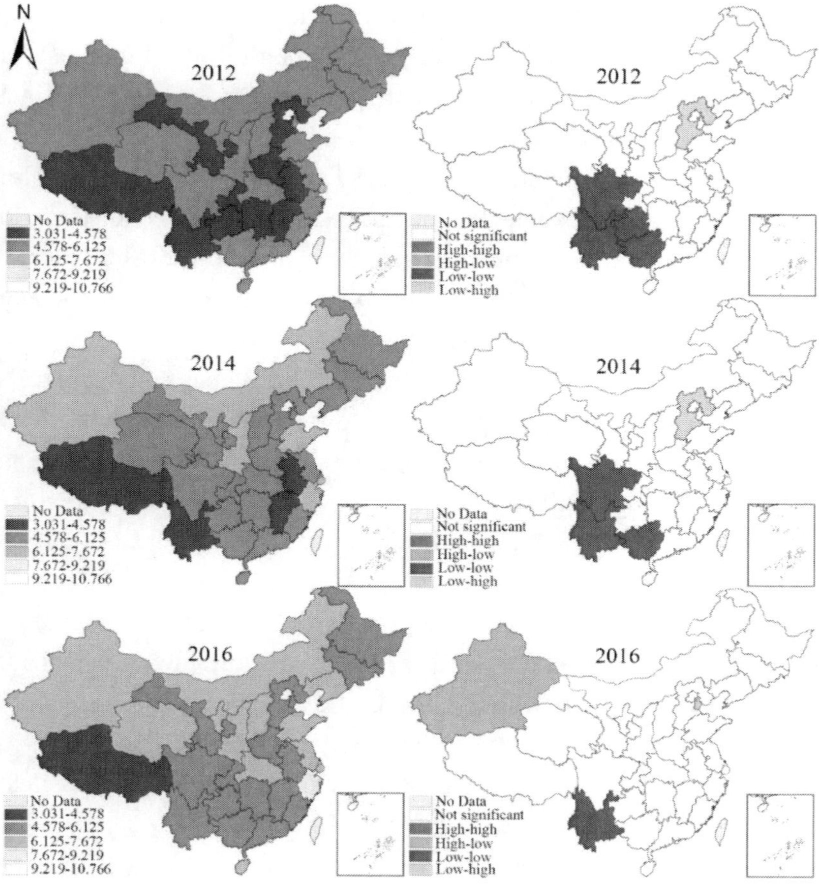

Figure 4.16. Hierarchical maps and univariate LISA cluster maps of the densities of health technicians.

Figure 4.16 displays the hierarchical maps and univariate LISA cluster maps for total health technicians in 2012, 2014, and 2016. The hierarchical maps in Figure 4.16 show the increasing health technician density in almost all the provincial units during 2012–2016. As the changes in color in the hierarchical maps show the change in health manpower density quite clearly and vividly, this section will only focus on the interpretations of univariate LISA cluster maps. In 2012, four low-low cluster units (Sichuan, Yunnan, Guangxi, Guizhou) in southwest China were identified across the country, and Hebei was categorized as a low-high cluster unit. During the first subperiod (2012–2014), Guizhou Province moved out of the low-low cluster area, and Sichuan and Guangxi followed in the second subperiod (2014–2016). In the year 2016, Yunnan was the only provincial unit displaying a low-low cluster feature, indicating the relative lack of health technicians in Yunnan and its adjacent units. Moreover, the low-high cluster feature of Hebei lost significance during the second subperiod. It is important to note that Xinjiang displayed a high-low cluster feature in 2016, indicating that Xinjiang was in a better situation than its adjacent units (Xizang, Qinghai, and Gansu) on average.

Figures 4.17 and 4.18 display the hierarchical maps and univariate LISA cluster maps, respectively, for different subtypes of health technicians. In the case of licensed doctors, six provincial units (Yunnan, Guangxi, Guangdong, Guizhou, Hubei, and Hunan) were associated with the low-low type, whereas Sichuan displayed a high-low cluster feature at the very beginning. The high-low and high-high types were only found in Hebei and Tianjin, respectively. The clustering pattern remained almost unchanged during the first subperiod, with only the low-low cluster feature of Sichuan changing to high-low. During 2014–2016, Hunan turned from low-low cluster type into high-low cluster type, Guangxi moved out the low-low cluster area, while Sichuan was included in the low-low cluster area again.

The univariate LISA cluster map view indicates that the clustering pattern of registered nurses remained relatively stable. The high-low cluster feature of Xinjiang Province remained significant across the whole research period, while the low-low cluster area gradually moved towards the west during the second period, with Qinghai replacing Guizhou to display low-low cluster feature during the second period.

Turning to pharmacists, Xinjiang was the only provincial unit to display a high-low cluster feature during the whole research period, whereas Shandong began to display a high-low cluster feature during the first subperiod. The low-high cluster type was only found in Hebei, where it was significant at the first time point. In particular, the low-low cluster area changed slightly during the research period. Qinghai moved out of the low-low cluster area during the first period but displayed the low-low cluster feature again in 2016, while the low-low cluster feature of Guizhou became no longer significant during 2012–2014.

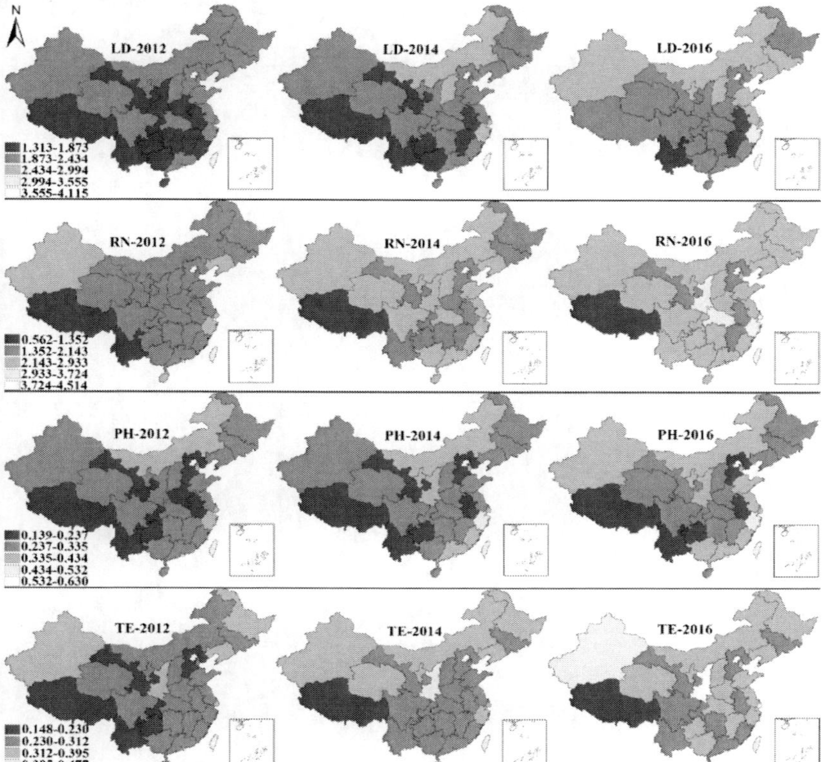

Note: LD = licensed doctors, RN = registered nurses, PH = Pharmacists, TE = technologists, IN=interns, the same below.

Figure 4.17. Hierarchical maps of the densities of different subtypes of health technicians.

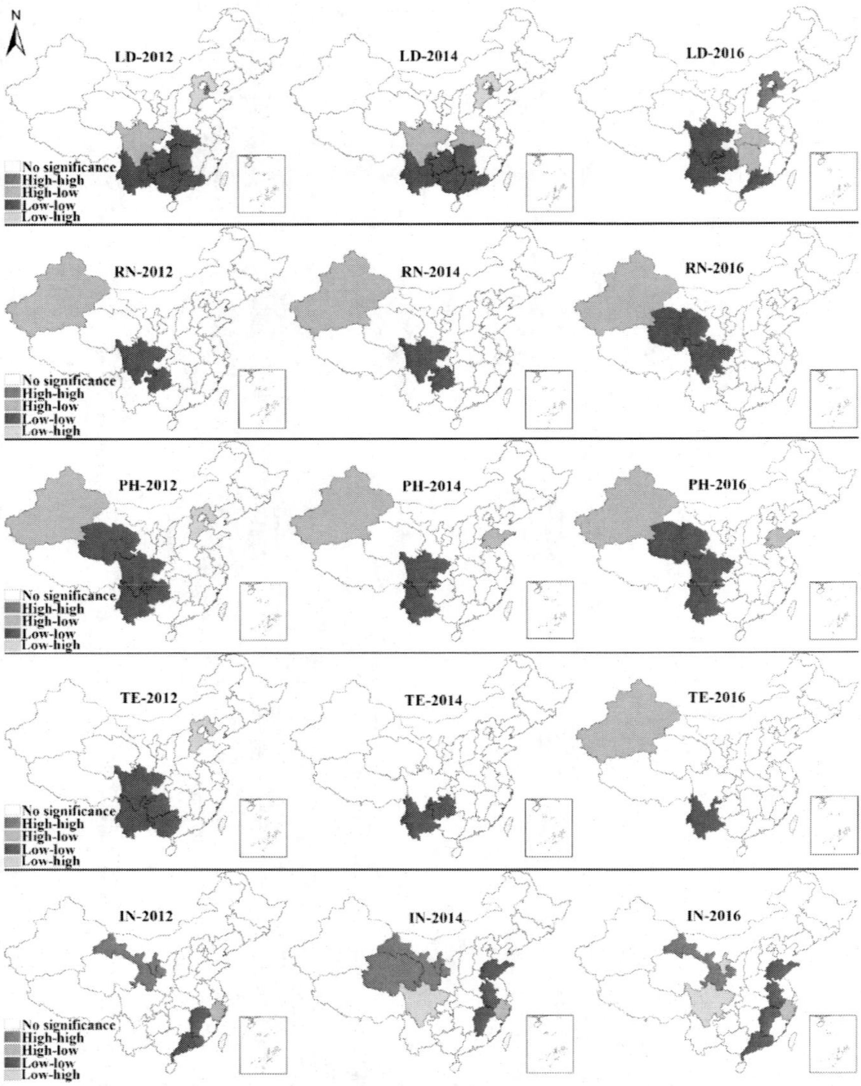

Note: LD = licensed doctors, RN = registered nurses, PH = Pharmacists, TE = technologists, IN = interns, the same below.

Figure 4.18. Univariate LISA cluster maps of the densities of different subtypes of health technicians.

Regarding the technologists, four southwest provinces (Guangxi, Yunnan, Guizhou, and Sichuan) were identified with a low-low cluster feature in 2012, whereas the low-high type was found in Hebei. Guangxi and Sichuan moved out of the low-low cluster area in the first subperiod, and Guizhou followed in the second subperiod. In 2016, only Yunnan remained in the low-low cluster area. In contrast, the low-high cluster feature was only significant in Hebei in 2012, and the high-low type was only associated with Xinjiang in 2016.

By contrast, the spatial cluster features of interns were much more complex, as all types of spatial clusters could be found on the univariate LISA cluster maps. Ningxia and Gansu showed a high-high cluster feature in 2012, and two southern units (Jiangxi, Guangdong) were identified with a low-low cluster feature in the same year. During 2012–2016, the spatial cluster areas changed greatly over time. In the end, all four provincial units (Shandong, Anhui, Jiangxi, Guangdong) included in the low-low cluster area were located in central and eastern China. The high-high type was only found in Gansu, which was adjacent to two low-high cluster units (Ningxia, Sichuan). In addition, Zhejiang displayed a high-low cluster feature throughout the period.

Figures 4.19 and 4.20 display the hierarchical maps and univariate LISA cluster maps, respectively, for different subtypes of licensed doctors. The clustering pattern of clinicians displayed strong consistency during 2012–2016. Sichuan exhibited a low-low cluster feature during 2012–2016. Similarly, the high-low cluster feature in Hubei achieved statistical significance across the whole period. However, Guizhou only exhibited a high-low cluster feature in 2012.

The clustering pattern of TCM doctors was much simpler; only the high-low cluster type was detected. Sichuan displayed a high-low cluster feature during the whole research period, while the high-low cluster feature in Guizhou was only significant in 2014.

The clustering pattern of dentists remained unchanged during the research period. Sichuan showed a low-low cluster feature at all three time points, while the high-low cluster type was always found in three provincial units (Ningxia, Hubei, Guizhou).

As for public health doctors, Sichuan was the only provincial unit included in the high-low cluster area and significant all the time. Henan and Hubei each displayed a high-low cluster feature only in 2014 and

2016, respectively. In addition, the low-low type was only detected in Henan in 2016, and the low-high cluster feature was only significant in Fujian at the first two time points.

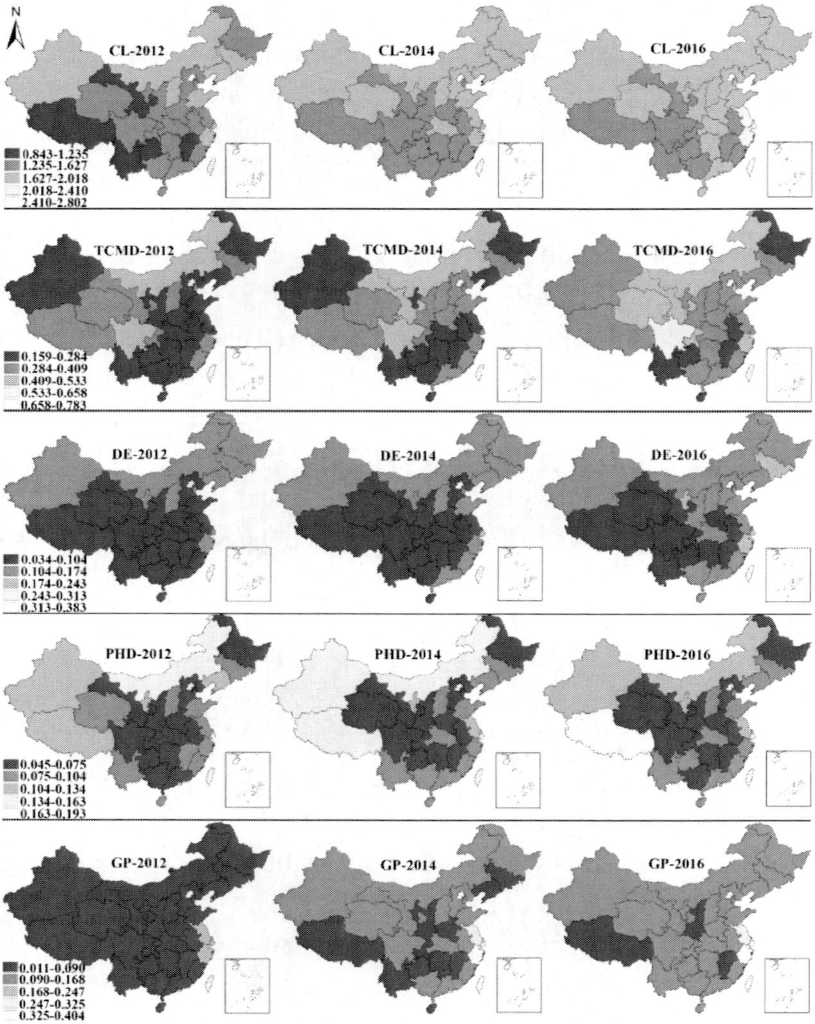

Note: CL = clinicians, TCMD = TCM doctors, DE = dentists, PHD = public health doctors, GP = general practitioners.

Figure 4.19. Hierarchical maps of the densities of different subtypes of licensed doctors.

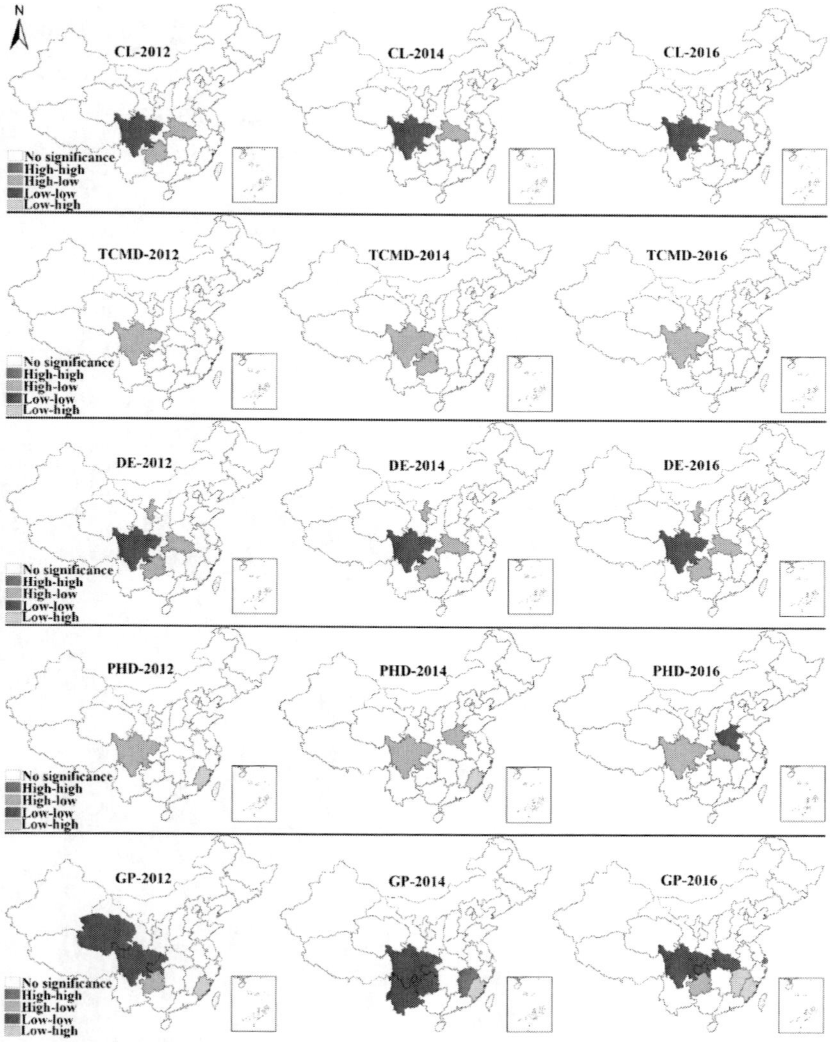

Note: CL = clinicians, TCMD = TCM doctors, DE = dentists, PHD = public health doctors, GP = general practitioners.

Figure 4.20. Univariate LISA cluster maps of the densities of different subtypes of licensed doctors.

Last but not least, the density of general practitioners in Sichuan and Chongqing displayed a low-low cluster feature from 2012 on, while those in Qinghai, Yunnan, Guizhou, and Hubei were only significant at certain time points. The only significant high-low cluster area could be found in

Jiangxi in 2014. Fujian was identified with a low-low cluster feature at three time points, while Jiangxi turned from a high-low cluster feature to low-high during 2014–2016. In 2016, the high-high and high-low types were found in Shanghai and Guizhou, respectively.

4.4.2. Urban Health Manpower Distribution

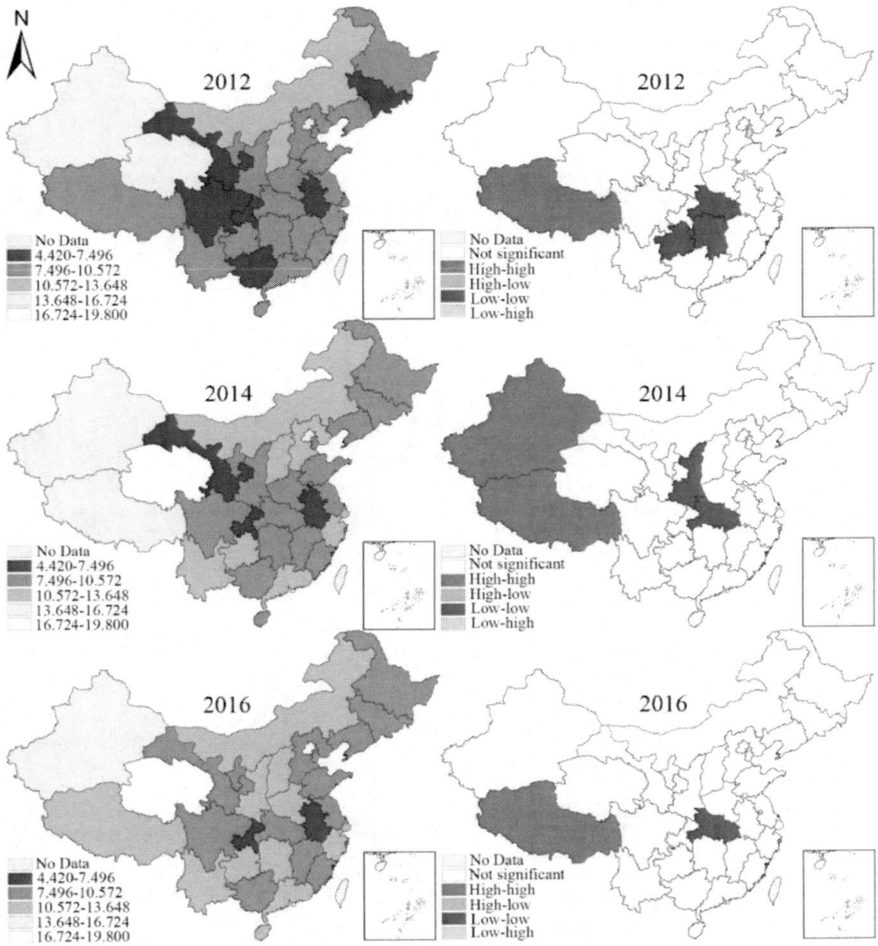

Figure 4.21. Hierarchical maps and univariate LISA cluster maps of the densities of urban health technicians.

Figure 4.21 displays the hierarchical maps and univariate LISA cluster maps for urban health technicians in 2012, 2014, and 2016. Only high-high and low-low cluster types could be found on the univariate LISA cluster maps. In 2012, almost all the low-low cluster units were located in south China, namely, Guizhou, Hubei, and Hunan. Xizang displayed a high-high cluster feature that continued until 2016. During the first subperiod, the low-low cluster feature of Hunan and Guizhou became no longer significant, while Shaanxi began to exhibit a low-high cluster feature. In the second subperiod, Shaanxi moved out of the low-low cluster area, leaving only Hubei displaying a low-low cluster feature in 2016. It is noteworthy that the high-high cluster feature was significant in Xinjiang in 2014 but lost statistical significance after that.

Figures 4.22 and 4.23 display the hierarchical maps and univariate LISA cluster maps, respectively, for different subtypes of urban health technicians. As with urban licensed doctors, Xinjiang was identified with a high-high cluster feature, while four provincial units (Hubei, Hunan, Chongqing, and Guizhou) were associated with a low-low cluster type at the very beginning. The high-high cluster area expanded during 2012–2014, with Xinjiang being identified as high-high cluster unit as well. As the high-high cluster area gradually shrank thereafter, Xinjiang was removed from the high-high cluster area during 2014–2016. In contrast, the low-low cluster area gradually shrank and moved from south China to north China. By 2016, only Hubei and Shaanxi remained in the low-low cluster area.

In comparison, the complexity of the urban registered nurses' clustering pattern reduced over time. In 2012, Xizang and Tianjin were included in the low-high cluster area, whereas Guizhou was the only unit identified with a low-low cluster feature. During the first subperiod, Shaanxi replaced Guizhou to be included in the low-low cluster area, while it lost statistical significance in the second subperiod. In addition, Tianjin and Xizang were both removed from the low-high cluster area during 2012–2014, and a high-high cluster feature was detected in Xizang in 2014. Interestingly, Xizang returned to displaying a low-high cluster feature in 2016.

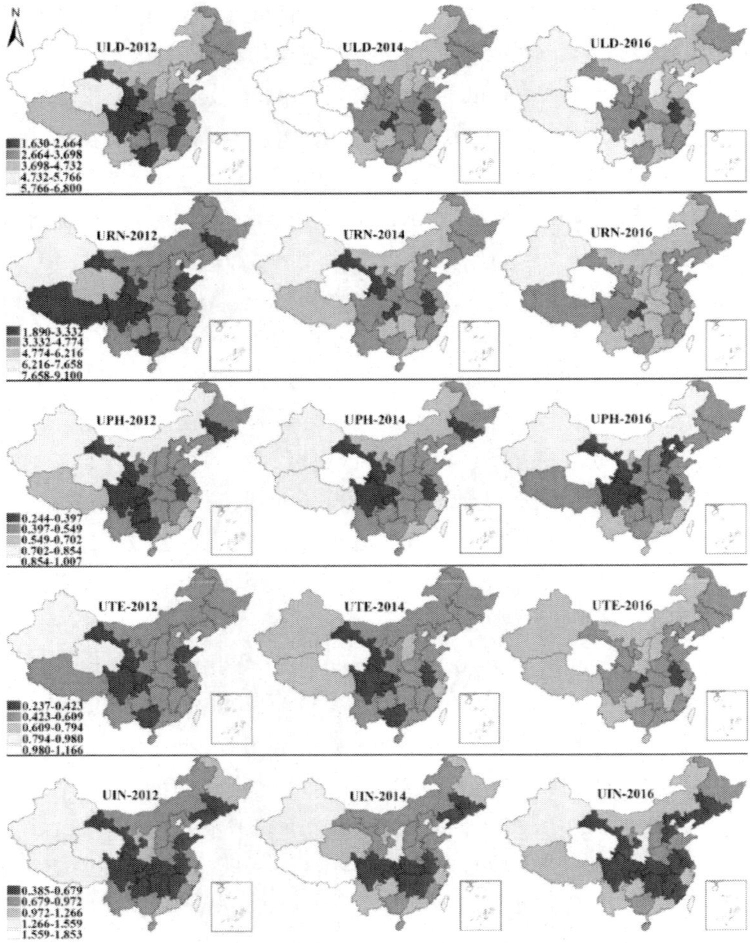

Note: ULD = urban licensed doctors, URN = urban registered nurses, UPH = urban pharmacists, UTE = urban technologists, UIN = urban interns, the same below.

Figure 4.22. Hierarchical maps of the densities of different subtypes of urban health technicians.

By contrast, only two cluster types (high-low and low-low) could be found on the univariate LISA cluster maps of urban pharmacists, with the changing pattern of the latter being more complex. As for the high-low type, only Neimenggu displayed a high-low cluster feature in 2014 and 2016, while the units in the low-low cluster area had been changing over time. A total of nine province-times of low-low clusters were detected among five provincial units (Guizhou, Chongqing, Hubei, Henan, and Shandong) at three time points. Chongqing only exhibited a low-low cluster feature in 2012 and Guizhou was identified with a low-low cluster feature in 2012 and 2014, while the low-low cluster feature in Henan reached statistical significance in 2014 and 2016. In contrast, the low-low cluster feature in Hubei was invariably significant. In 2016, Shandong also exhibited a low-low cluster feature.

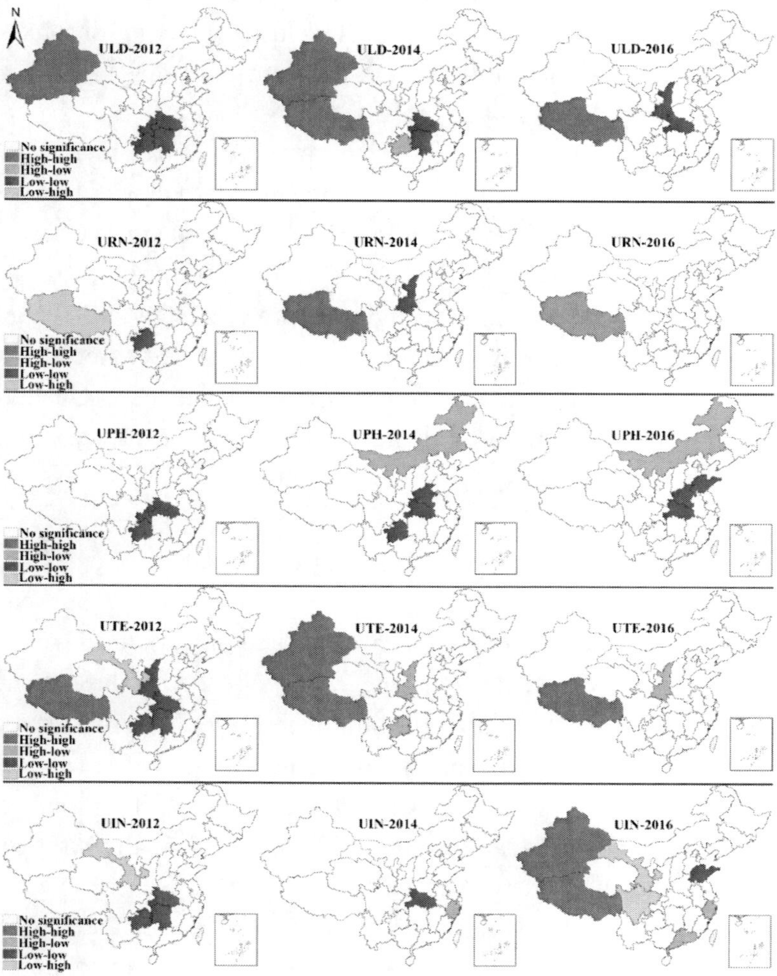

Figure 4.23. Univariate LISA cluster maps of the densities of different subtypes of urban health technicians.

Regarding urban technologists, four provincial units displayed a low-low cluster feature, while Xinjiang displayed a high-high cluster feature in 2012. In addition, Gansu was characterized by a low-high cluster feature. The changing pattern of the high-high cluster area was exactly the same as that of total urban health technicians. The high-high cluster feature of Xinjiang was no longer significant in 2016, while Xizang stopped displaying the high-high cluster feature in 2016. In contrast, the low-low and low-high cluster area disappeared from the univariate LISA cluster map during 2012–2014. Furthermore, the cluster type in Shaanxi and Guizhou changed from low-low to high-low, but only that in the former was maintained until 2016.

Similar to total interns, the clustering pattern of urban interns varied greatly over time. At the first two time points, only two cluster types were identified, while all four types of clusters passed the significance test in 2016. At the end of the study period, the high-high cluster type was found in Xinjiang and Xizang and the low-high type was detected in Sichuan and Gansu. By contrast, Shandong was the only provincial unit associated with the low-low type in 2016, while two eastern provincial units (Guangdong and Zhejiang) showed a high-low cluster feature in the meantime.

4.4.3. Rural Health Manpower Distribution

Figure 4.24 displays the hierarchical maps and univariate LISA cluster maps for rural health technicians in 2012, 2014, and 2016. Throughout the ensuing five years, the rural health technician density increased dramatically in almost all provincial units. The most noticeable characteristic was that the low-low cluster area gradually shrank from Sichuan, Yunnan, Guangxi, and Hunan from 2012 and finally disappeared in 2016. In parallel fashion, the other three types of clusters were not significant throughout the whole research period either. At the end of the research period, only Xinjiang displayed a high-low cluster feature and Jiangsu a high-high cluster feature, indicating a relatively balanced distribution regarding the total quantity of rural health technicians.

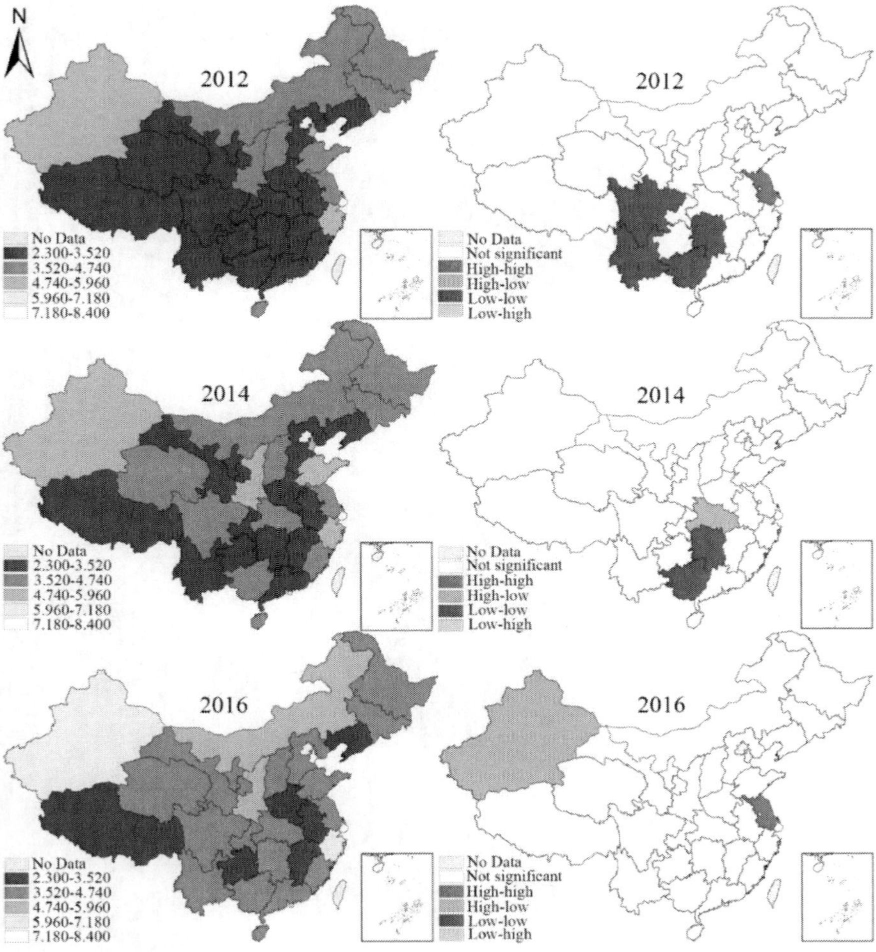

Figure 4.24. Hierarchical maps and univariate LISA cluster maps of the densities of rural health technicians in 2012, 2014, and 2016.

Figures 4.25 and 4.26 display the hierarchical maps and univariate LISA cluster maps, respectively, for different subtypes of rural health technicians. In general, the number of provincial units included in the low-low cluster area of rural licensed doctors dropped significantly during the observation period. In the beginning, most of the low-low cluster units were concentrated in south China, namely, Yunnan, Guangxi, Guangdong, Hunan, Hubei, and Sichuan. Meanwhile, Jiangsu exhibited a high-high cluster feature. As time passed, the cluster features in Guangxi and

Guangdong lost significance, and Hubei moved from the low-low cluster area to the high-low cluster area after 2014.

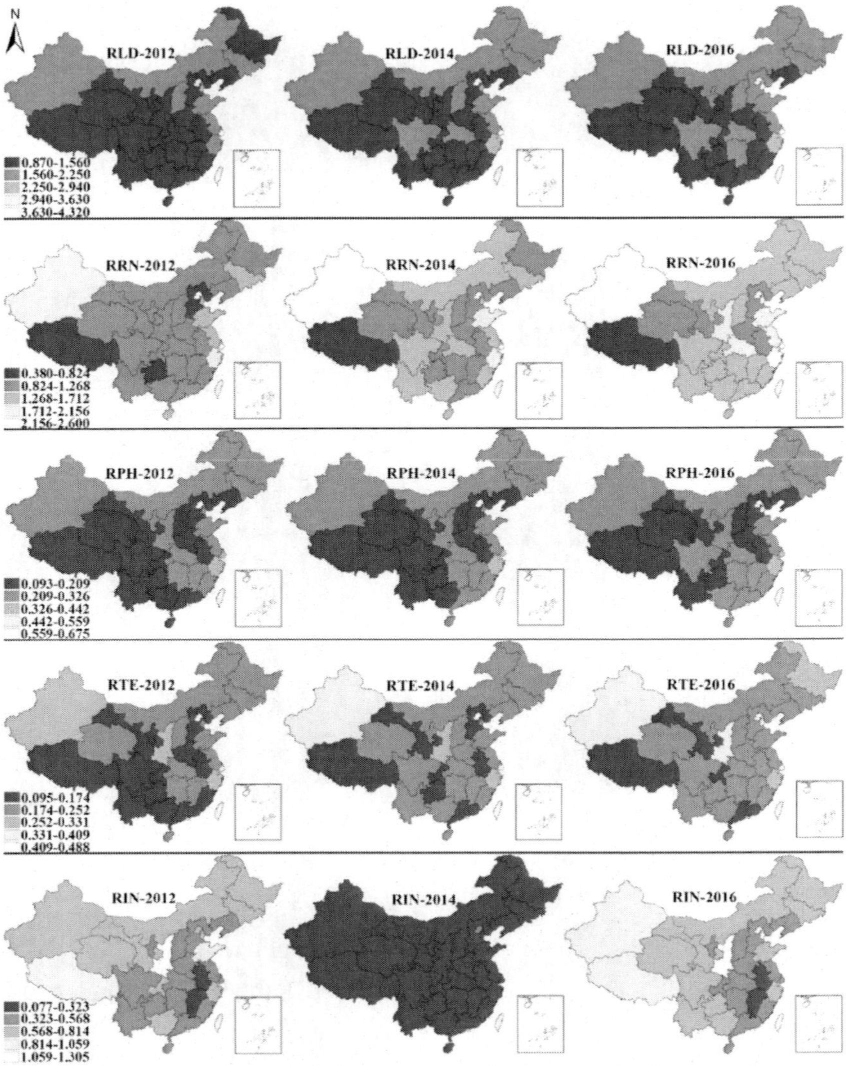

Note: RLD = rural licensed doctors, RRN = rural registered nurses, RPH = rural pharmacists, RTE = rural technologists, RIN = rural interns.

Figure 4.25. Hierarchical maps of the densities of different subtypes of health technicians.

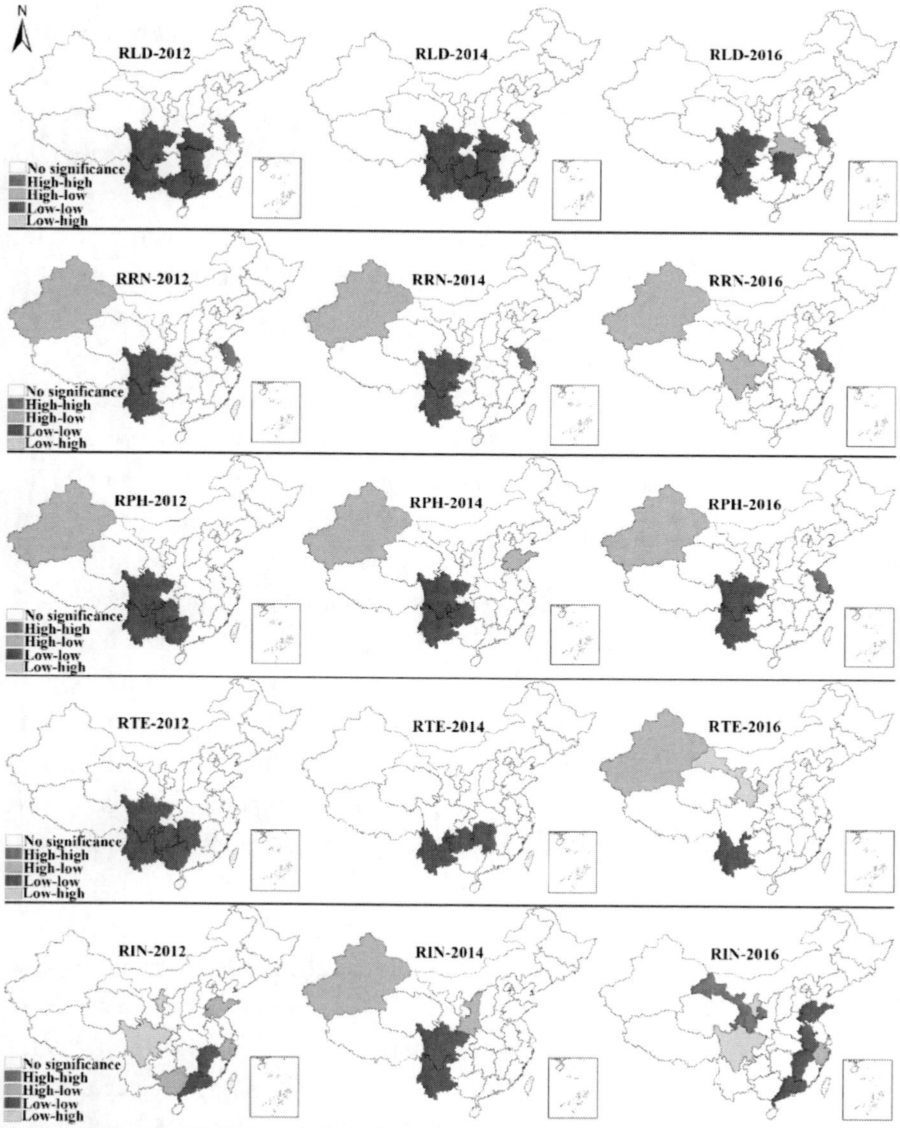

Note: RLD = rural licensed doctors, RRN = rural registered nurses, RPH = rural pharmacists, RTE = rural technologists, RIN = rural interns.

Figure 4.26. Univariate LISA cluster maps of the densities of different subtypes of health technicians.

The clustering pattern of rural registered nurses was much simpler than that of rural licensed doctors. Since 2012, Xinjiang displayed a high-low cluster feature, and Sichuan joined it during 2014–2016, while the low-low cluster area gradually shrank and completely disappeared during 2014–2016. By comparison, Jiangsu displayed a high-high cluster feature throughout the research period, and the same cluster type appeared in Shanghai in 2016.

As for rural pharmacists, four provincial units (Sichuan, Yunnan, Guangxi, and Guizhou) were included in the low-low cluster area in 2012. After that, Sichuan and Yunnan stood out as low-low cluster units throughout the whole research period. The LISA maps also highlight Xinjiang, which displayed high-low cluster feature during 2012–2016. By contrast, the low-high type could only be found in univariate LISA cluster maps. Even though Shandong displayed a high-low cluster feature in 2014, its cluster feature did not persist with time. In 2016, except for Sichuan (low-low), Yunnan (low-low), and Xinjiang (high-low), only the high-high cluster feature in Jiangsu and Shanghai passed the significance test.

Regarding rural technologists, five provincial units (Sichuan, Yunnan, Guizhou, Guangxi, and Hunan) in southwest China were identified with a low-low cluster feature in 2012. Sichuan and Guangxi first moved out the cluster area during 2012–2014, while Guizhou and Hunan followed during 2014–2016. By the end, only Yunnan was still situated in the low-low cluster area. In the meantime, two adjacent units, namely Xinjiang and Gansu, showed high-low and low-high cluster features in 2016, respectively.

In comparison, the clustering pattern of rural interns changed greatly during 2012–2016. It is important to note that the clustering pattern in 2014 was quite different due to the sharp decrease in the rural intern density in all the provincial units. In the end, the high-high cluster feature was only detected in Gansu, with its two adjacent units (Sichuan and Ningxia) displaying a low-high cluster feature. By contrast, the low-low cluster area included four provincial units (Shandong, Anhui, Jiangxi, and Guangdong) in central and eastern China, and Zhejiang displayed a high-low cluster feature.

4.5. Chapter Summary

On the basis of a 5-year (2012–2016) panel dataset, this chapter visualized and compared the temporal trends, spatial variation in temporal trends, and changing spatial patterns of different subtypes of health manpower in China. Overall, China's health system quite simply experienced an extraordinary period, which is evidenced by the steady and rapid increase of health manpower quantity and its density among the people. As reported in the boxplots, almost all subtypes of health manpower, especially in the urban sectors, maintained a rapid increase during the research period. However, health manpower misdistribution reduced the equity of the health systems in China throughout this period.

At the very beginning of the research period (2012–2016), different subtypes of health manpower appeared in the spatial distribution patterns, in which the western and southern provincial units were usually the hardest hit by health manpower shortage and were thus associated with a low-low cluster type. Fortunately, the low-low cluster area gradually shrank for most subtypes of health manpower, indicating a more balanced distribution of health manpower in later years. Unfortunately, some provincial units (Yunnan, Sichuan, etc.) were left behind in the distribution of almost all subtypes of health manpower. Besides this, great urban-rural disparities were detected in the distribution of health manpower in China. The density of each subtype of health manpower in urban areas can be 2–4 times greater in rural areas, and the gap was even larger in western China.

Chapter 5

DETERMINANTS OF THE HEALTH MANPOWER DISTRIBUTION IN CHINA

Based on China's 5-year (2012–2016) panel dataset, this chapter investigates and compares the determinants of the health manpower distribution in China. The first section of this chapter displays the descriptive statistics of the dependent and independent variables. By taking total health technicians as an example, the second section presents the preliminary estimation results of spatial panel econometric models and interprets the model slection procedures. The third section decomposes the relationship between independent and dependent variables into direct, spillover, and total effects and further compares the results for different subtypes of health manpower.

5.1. DESCRIPTIVE STATISTICS

Table 5.1 reports the descriptive statistics of the main variables employed in the study of determinants. In total, there are 11 dependent variables and 5 independent variables. Their relationships will be tested with different spatial panel econometric models.

Table 5.1. Descriptive statistics of the variables

Variable	Obs	Mean	Std err	Min.	Max.	Unit
HTD	155	5.658	1.156	3.031	10.766	Persons/1000 population
LDD	155	2.163	0.431	1.313	4.115	Persons/1000 population
RND	155	2.219	0.572	0.562	4.514	Persons/1000 population
PHD	155	0.306	0.082	0.139	0.630	Persons/1000 population
TED	155	0.307	0.066	0.148	0.559	Persons/1000 population
OHTD	155	0.663	0.197	0.345	1.384	Persons/1000 population
CDD	155	1.640	0.299	0.843	2.802	Persons/1000 population
TCMDD	155	0.324	0.109	0.159	0.783	Persons/1000 population
DDD	155	0.111	0.058	0.034	0.383	Persons/1000 population
PHDD	155	0.089	0.028	0.045	0.193	Persons/1000 population
GPD	155	0.120	0.084	0.011	0.404	Persons/1000 population
OVPA	155	5.317	1.794	3.007	10.716	Times/person
IVPA	155	0.143	0.031	0.047	0.223	Times/person
GHEPA	155	918.4	363.2	498.2	2584.3	Yuan/person
SHEPA	155	1142.9	839.7	281.2	5739.7	Yuan/person
MGD	155	2.644	1.024	0.491	5.430	Person/10000 population

5.2. Empirical Results of the Spatial Panel Econometric Models

Following the procedures specified in the methodology section (Figure 3.4), this study first estimated four SDPM models: The SDPM with spatial fixed effects (Column 2 in each table), with time fixed effects (Column 3 in each table), with spatial and time fixed effects (Column 4 in each table), and with random effects (Column 5 in each table).

The model selection principles were then followed to choose the best model. In the context of this study, the SDPM with spatial fixed effects was preferred to the time fixed and both fixed models, as the dataset belonged to the short panel ($n > T$). Therefore, the Hausman test was conducted to make a choice between the SDPM with fixed effects and the random effect model. After the Hausman test, the LR and Wald tests were conducted successively to determine whether the SDPM model could be simplified. After this step, the best model was obtained.

Table 5.2. Estimation results of spatial panel econometric models for health technician density

Variable	SDPM with spatial fixed effects (Best)	SDPM with time fixed effects	SDPM with spatial and time fixed effects	SDPM with random effects	SEPM with spatial fixed effects	SLPM with spatial fixed effects
ln(OV)	0.583***	0.037	0.534***	0.426***	0.549***	0.347***
	(0.076)	(0.039)	(0.078)	(0.076)	(0.075)	(0.077)
ln(IV)	0.101***	0.207***	0.151***	0.143***	0.121***	0.144***
	(0.036)	(0.041)	(0.039)	(0.036)	(0.035)	(0.041)
ln(GHE)	0.087**	0.156***	0.115***	0.090**	0.117***	0.032
	(0.039)	(0.035)	(0.040)	(0.040)	(0.032)	(0.038)
ln(SHE)	0.035	0.237***	0.057**	0.075***	0.065***	0.061**
	(0.024)	(0.025)	(0.025)	(0.029)	(0.023)	(0.024)
ln(MGD)	0.015	0.007	0.014	0.024	0.013	0.026
	(0.015)	(0.022)	(0.015)	(0.017)	(0.016)	(0.017)
W*	−0.674***	−0.094	−0.693***	−0.438***		
ln(OV)	(0.127)	(0.064)	(0.174)	(0.122)		
W*	−0.055	−0.555***	0.127	−0.109		
ln(IV)	(0.072)	(0.076)	(0.096)	(0.069)		
W*	−0.111*	−0.232***	−0.003	−0.052		
ln(GHE)	(0.062)	(0.071)	(0.083)	(0.065)		
W*	0.059	−0.130***	0.148***	0.004		
ln(SHE)	(0.047)	(0.067)	(0.057)	(0.052)		
W*	0.065**	0.073*	0.093**	0.050		
ln(MGD)	(0.029)	(0.041)	(0.036)	(0.031)		
ρ	0.655***	0.049	0.560***	0.548***		0.369***
	(0.074)	(0.112)	(0.087)	(0.087)		(0.072)
λ					0.681***	
					(0.078)	
LL	394.7047	180.0270	400.0931	292.6357	386.4250	374.8943
R_w^2	0.9118	0.0818	0.9011	0.9168	0.9116	0.9102
R_b^2	0.4522	0.8415	0.4083	0.5367	0.3880	0.3265
R^2	0.5222	0.6255	0.4491	0.6027	0.4461	0.4130
Obs	155	155	155	155	155	155
Test	Hausman test				LR test	Wald test
	H_0: difference in coefficients not systematic					
	$\chi^2(11) = 20.9$ $p = 0.034$				$\chi^2 = 43.9$	$\chi^2 = 16.7$
					$p = 0.000$	$p = 0.005$

Note: Standard error in parentheses, ***p < 0.01,**p < 0.05,*p < 0.1

This section takes the health technician density as an example to demonstrate the model selection procedures for spatial panel econometric models. Table 5.2 reports the estimation results of spatial panel econometric models for total health technicians. The Hausman test (its outcomes are given at the bottom of Columns 2 to 5) showed that the

SDPM with spatial fixed effects was significantly superior to the SDPM with random effects. To further determine whether the SDPM model with spatial fixed effects was the best model, this study estimated the SEPM and SLPM with spatial fixed effects to see whether the SDPM could be simplified into SEPM and SLPM. According to the results of LR and Wald test (the outcomes are listed at the bottom of Columns 6 and 7), both null hypotheses were rejected at the 0.05 significance level, indicating that the SDPM with spatial fixed effects was the best spatial panel econometric model for health technician density.

The estimation results of spatial panel econometric models for different subtypes of health manpower are listed in Appendix C. In this study, the SDPM was the best model in most cases, namely, those of health technicians, licensed doctors, clinicians, public health doctors, registered nurses, dentists, and technologists. For pharmacists, the SEPM with spatial fixed effects proved to be the best, as the null hypothesis of the LR test cannot be rejected. As for TCM doctors, the SLPM with random effects was selected as the results could not pass the Hausman and Wald tests. When making estimates for interns, the SDPM with random effects was better than the SDPM with fixed effects, and it could not be further simplified. It is noteworthy that, based on the results of the Hausman, Wald, and LR tests, the density of general practitioners should not be estimated via spatial panel econometric models, and that the non-spatial panel model was shown to be a better one. Therefore this study estimated the non-spatial model for general practitioners and conducted the Hausman test to make a choice between models with fixed effects and random effects.

After all the best models were identified, the relationship between dependent variables and independent variables (positive or negative, significant or not) were clear at a glance. However, the coefficients of variables in SDPM could not be explained directly as the effects of percentage variation in independent variables on dependent variables thanks to the unique characteristics of spatial panel econometric models, which have been mentioned in the methodology section. Thus I decomposed the effects of the independent variables on the dependent variables into direct, spillover, and total effects based on the selected best models.

5.3. Decomposition of the Direct, Spillover and Total Effects

Table 5.3 displays the direct effects of the independent variables on the densities of different subtypes of health technicians (licensed doctors, registered nurses, pharmacists, technologists, interns, and their sum) and their associated *t*-statistics, which were calculated based on the selected best models. When all the independent variables were incorporated into the model, outpatient visits per capita played a leading role in determining the densities of all subtypes of health technicians and their sum, with all the estimates being significant at the 0.01 significance level.

Table 5.3. Direct effects of independent variables on the densities of different subtypes of health technicians and their sum

Variable	Health technicians	Licensed doctors	Registered nurses	Pharmacist	Technologist	Interns
OV	0.509***	0.544***	0.374***	0.536***	0.393***	0.427***
	(0.081)	(0.078)	(0.118)	(0.113)	(0.110)	(0.149)
IV	0.105**	0.178***	0.315***	0.105*	0.024	−0.080
	(0.045)	(0.040)	(0.064)	(0.054)	(0.062)	(0.093)
GHE	0.074*	0.088**	0.152**	0.015	−0.092*	0.223**
	(0.041)	(0.039)	(0.060)	(0.047)	(0.056)	(0.099)
SHE	0.055*	0.067**	0.075*	0.054	0.074*	−0.009
	(0.028)	(0.026)	(0.041)	(0.033)	(0.038)	(0.074)
MGD	0.034**	0.023	0.026	0.033	0.066**	0.025
	(0.017)	(0.016)	(0.024)	(0.024)	(0.023)	(0.046)

Note: t-statistics in parentheses, ***p < 0.01, **p < 0.05, *p < 0.1

Overall, a 1% increase in outpatient visits per capita in the local unit contributed to an average increment of 0.509% of health technician density in the same unit. In the case of licensed doctors and pharmacists, the coefficients were even larger, so that a 1% increase in outpatient visits per capita in one provincial unit was likely to result in a 0.544% and 0.536%

increase of licensed doctor density and pharmacist density in the same provincial unit, respectively. Comparatively, a 1% increase in the number of outpatient visits per capita was associated with a 0.374% increase in registered nurse density and 0.393% in technologist density, slightly less than the figure of 0.427% for interns. The results upheld Hypothesis 1, indicating that the demand in health services can generally help increase the health manpower stock in a provincial unit.

Also, the analytical results supported the significant direct effects of inpatient visits per capita on health technician density, especially the densities of licensed doctors and registered nurses. The results showed that a larger value of inpatient visits per capita would contribute to a relatively higher density of registered nurses. A roughly 1% increase in inpatient visits per capita led to a 0.178% increase in the density of licensed doctor density, which was almost half the effect on registered nurse density (0.315%). Moreover, a 1% increase in inpatient visits per capita was associated with a 0.105% increase in pharmacist density, but this was significant only at the 0.1 level.

The influence of the government health expenditure per capita on the density of health manpower was mixed. The results showed that higher per capita government health expenditure would contribute to a higher density of total health technician density; a 1% increase led to a 0.074% increase in the density of health technicians in the same unit. The coefficients increased to 0.088% and 0.152% for licensed doctors and registered nurses, respectively. More importantly, a 1% increase of government health investment per capita in one unit yielded a 0.223% increase in intern density in the same unit. However, this study failed to obtain a significant positive relationship between government health expenditure per capita and the density of pharmacists and technologists, which contradicted Hypothesis 2.

The direct effects of social health expenditure per capita on the health manpower density were akin to those of government health expenditure. A significant positive relationship was detected between the social health expenditure per capita and the densities of health technicians, licensed doctors, registered nurses, and technologists, though only the estimate of the relationship between licensed doctor density and social health expenditure per capita was significant at the 0.05 level; to-wit, a 1% increase in the social health expenditure per capita in one provincial unit led to a 0.067% increase in the density of licensed doctors in that unit.

The results further show that the medical graduate density had a significantly positive effect on the density of health technicians, as expected under Hypothesis 4. However, among the subtypes of health technicians, only the density of technologists was significantly related to the medical graduate density, whereby a 1% increase in the medical graduate density in one unit was associated with a 0.066% increase in the density of technologists in the same unit, significant at the 0.05 level.

Table 5.4. Spillover effects of independent variables on the densities of different subtypes of health technicians and their sum

Variable	Health technicians	Licensed doctors	Registered nurses	Pharmacist	Technologist	Interns
OV	−0.801**	−0.396**	−0.746*	—	−0.476	−0.302
	(0.352)	(0.182)	(0.413)		(0.415)	(0.309)
IV	0.033	−0.241**	0.063	—	−0.275	0.447*
	(0.197)	(0.104)	(0.234)		(0.266)	(0.249)
GHE	−0.160	0.003	−0.233	—	−0.214	0.261
	(0.177)	(0.086)	(0.213)		(0.214)	(0.225)
SHE	0.231	0.081	0.295*	—	0.456**	−0.418**
	(0.144)	(0.071)	(0.172)		(0.183)	(0.178)
MGD	0.204**	0.098**	0.214**	—	0.168*	−0.078
	(0.083)	(0.042)	(0.098)		(0.100)	(0.121)

Note: t-statistics in parentheses, ***p < 0.01, **p < 0.05, *p < 0.1. "—"means not applicable.

Table 5.4 reports the spillover effects of the independent variables on the average density of different subtypes of health technicians in adjacent units. In the first place, the findings support the negative effect of outpatient visits per capita on the density of health technicians in adjacent units. Overall, a 1% increase in outpatient visits per capita in the local provincial unit would on average lead to a 0.801% decrease in health technician density in all the neighboring units. More specifically, a 1% increase in the number of outpatient visits per capita in one unit was associated with a 0.396% decrease in the licensed doctor density and

0.746% in the registered nurse density in adjacent units, though the latter was significant only at the 0.1 level. Results also showed that a 1% increase in the inpatient visits per capita in one unit was associated with a 0.241% decrease in the licensed doctor density of adjacent units. Nevertheless, a 1% increase of inpatient visits per capita in the local unit could result in an increase as high as 0.447% in the intern density in neighboring units, which was significant at the 0.1 level.

For health expenditure, the spillover effects of government health expenditure were not significant, while the spillover effects of social health expenditure were mixed. Results showed that a higher investment in social health expenditure would contribute to a higher density of registered nurses and technologists in adjacent units; a 1% increase led to a 0.295% increase in registered nurse density (significant at the 0.1 level) and 0.456% in technologist density (significant at the 0.05 level), while a 1% increase in social health expenditure per capita in the local provincial unit would on average lead to a 0.418% decrease in the intern density of all the neighboring units.

Regarding the medical graduate density, it exerted positive spillover effects on the density of health technicians and almost all its subtypes except pharmacists and interns. More exactly, a 1% increase in the medical graduate density in one unit yielded a 0.204% increase in the health technician density of adjacent units (0.098% for licensed doctors and 0.214% for registered nurse). Both these estimates were significant at the 0.05 significance level. In addition, a 1% increase in the medical graduate density in one unit was also associated with 0.168% increase in technologist density in neighboring units, which only reached the 0.1 significance level.

Table 5.5 reports the total effects of independent variables on the density of different subtypes of health technicians for reference. The total effects were significant when one independent variable exerted simultaneously strong and consistent direct and spillover effects. Obviously, only the social health expenditure per capital and medical graduate density displayed significant total effects. For example, if the social health expenditure per capita increased 1% in all the provincial units, the technologist density in each unit would tend to increase by 0.530%, which was in sharp contrast to the 0.427% decrease in the intern density. At the same time, it is important to note that the total effects of medical graduate density were significant under most circumstances. A 1% increase in medical graduate density in all the provincial units contributed to a 0.238% increase in health technician density, 0.121% increase in licensed doctor density, 0.240% increase in registered nurse density, and 0.235% increase in technologist density. The findings upheld Hypothesis 2, indicating the significant effect of medical education on the health manpower distribution.

Table 5.5. Total effects of independent variables on the densities of different subtypes of health technicians and their sum

Variable	Health technicians	Licensed doctors	Registered nurses	Pharmacist	Technologist	Interns
OV	−0.293	0.148	−0.372	—	−0.084	0.125
	(0.391)	(0.197)	(0.461)		(0.466)	(0.314)
IV	0.137	−0.063	0.377	—	−0.251	0.367
	(0.228)	(0.121)	(0.274)		(0.308)	(0.275)
GHE	−0.086	0.091	−0.080	—	−0.306	0.485*
	(0.199)	(0.095)	(0.240)		(0.242)	(0.258)
SHE	0.285*	0.148*	0.369*	—	0.530***	−0.427**
	(0.159)	(0.077)	(0.190)		(0.202)	(0.200)
MGD	0.238**	0.121***	0.240**	—	0.235**	−0.053
	(0.092)	(0.045)	(0.109)		(0.111)	(0.133)

Note: t-statistics in parentheses, ***$p < 0.01$, **$p < 0.05$, *$p < 0.1$. "—"means not applicable.

Table 5.6 reports the direct effects of independent variables on the density of different subtypes of licensed doctors. The outpatient visits per capita played a huge role in driving the densities of almost all subtypes of licensed doctors except dentists. A 1% increase of outpatient visits per capita corresponded to a 0.628% increase in clinician density, with figures as high as 0.959% and 0.756% for public health doctors and general practitioners, respectively. However, a 1% increase in the number of outpatient visits per capita was only associated with a 0.10% increase in the density of TCM doctors. All these estimates reached significance at the 5% level.

Table 5.6. Direct effects of independent variables on the densities of different subtypes of licensed doctors

Variable	Clinicians	TCM doctors	Dentists	Public health doctors	General Practitioners
OV	0.628***	0.194**	0.223	0.959***	0.756***
	(0.090)	(0.096)	(0.141)	(0.178)	(0.211)
IV	0.256***	−0.094	−0.014	0.344***	0.703***
	(0.047)	(0.058)	(0.067)	(0.090)	(0.161)
GHE	0.085*	0.139***	0.035	0.260***	0.302**
	(0.045)	(0.052)	(0.070)	(0.088)	(0.144)
SHE	0.041	0.158***	0.210***	−0.041	0.445***
	(0.031)	(0.037)	(0.047)	(0.060)	(0.117)
MGD	0.035*	−0.005	0.028	0.018	0.013
	(0.019)	(0.026)	(0.028)	(0.036)	(0.086)

Note: t-statistics in parentheses, ***$p < 0.01$, **$p < 0.05$, *$p < 0.1$.

Regarding the inpatient visits per capita, the estimated results showed a significant relationship between the inpatient visits per capita and the densities of clinicians, public health doctors, and general practitioners, which were significant at the 0.01 significance level. A 1% increase in inpatient visits per capita led to a 0.256% increase in the density of clinicians, 0.344% in public health doctor density, and 0.703% in general practitioner density in the same unit.

Government and social health expenditures per capita showed both similarities and differences in driving the densities of subtypes of licensed doctors. They were both significantly related to the TCM doctor density and general practitioner density. A 1% increase in government health expenditure in the local unit could lead to a 0.139% (0.158% by social health expenditure) increase in TCM doctor density in the same unit. In contrast, a 1% increase of government and social health expenditure per capita in the local unit could respectively result in a 0.302% and 0.425% increase in general practitioner density in the same unit. Government health expenditure also affected the clinician density (a 1% increase in expenditure corresponds to a 0.085% increase in clinician density) and public health doctor density (a 1% increase in expenditure corresponds to a 0.260% increase in public health doctor density). By comparison, a 1% increase in social expenditure per capita was also related to a 0.210%

increase in dentist density in one unit. As for the medical graduate density, only the density of clinicians was significantly correlated with the medical graduate density at the 0.1 significance level.

Table 5.7. Spillover effects of independent variables on the densities of different subtypes of licensed doctors

Variable	Clinicians	TCM doctors	Dentists	Public health doctors	General Practitioners
OV	−0.461**	0.066	−0.155	−0.330	—
	(0.217)	(0.051)	(0.206)	(0.352)	
IV	−0.306**	−0.032	0.050	−0.489**	—
	(0.125)	(0.028)	(0.101)	(0.191)	
GHE	0.030	0.043*	0.019	−0.162	—
	(0.103)	(0.024)	(0.099)	(0.165)	
SHE	0.063	0.050**	0.144*	−0.102	—
	(0.085)	(0.022)	(0.077)	(0.133)	
MGD	0.090*	−0.003	0.200***	0.103	—
	(0.050)	(0.010)	(0.045)	(0.078)	

Note: t-statistics in parentheses, ***$p < 0.01$, **$p < 0.05$, *$p < 0.1$. "—"means not applicable.

Table 5.7 reports the spillover effects of the independent variables on the densities of different subtypes of licensed doctors in adjacent units. As for the clinicians, the findings showed that the spillover effects of outpatient and inpatient visits per capita and medical graduate density were both significant for clinicians. It was estimated that a 1% increase in outpatient and inpatient visits per capita in one provincial unit would lead to a 0.461% and 0.306% decrease in clinician density in adjacent units, respectively, while a 1% increase in medical graduate density accompanied a 0.090% increase in clinician density in adjacent units. Concerning TCM doctors, the spillover effects of government and social health expenditure were positive and significant. A 1% increase in government health expenditure per capita in the local provincial unit would on average lead to a 0.043% (0.050% by social health expenditure per capita) increase in TCM doctor density in all the neighboring units. In the case of dentists, a 1% increase in social health expenditure per capita in the local unit could lead to a 0.144% increase in dentist density in the neighboring units, which only reached the 0.1 significance level. In contrast, a 1% increase in medical graduate density in the local unit could result in a 0.200% increase in dentist density in the neighboring units, which was significant at the 0.01 significance level. Surprisingly, a 1% increase in inpatient visits per capita could result in a 0.489% decrease in public health doctor density in adjacent units.

Table 5.8. Total effects of independent variables on the density of different types of licensed doctors

Variable	Clinicians	TCM doctors	Dentists	Public health doctors	General Practitioners
OV	0.167	0.261*	0.068	0.629*	—
	(0.236)	(0.138)	(0.171)	(0.361)	
IV	−0.051	−0.126	0.036	−0.145	—
	(0.146)	(0.082)	(0.102)	(0.220)	
GHE	0.115	0.182***	0.054	0.097	—
	(0.114)	(0.065)	(0.084)	(0.175)	
SHE	0.104	0.208***	0.355***	−0.143	—
	(0.092)	(0.046)	(0.066)	(0.138)	
MGD	0.125**	−0.009	0.228***	0.121	—
	(0.054)	(0.035)	(0.039)	(0.081)	

Note: t-statistics in parentheses, ***$p < 0.01$, **$p < 0.05$, *$p < 0.1$. "—"means not applicable.

Table 5.8 reports the total effects of the independent variables on the density of different subtypes of health technicians for reference. Regarding health service demand, only the outpatient visits exerted significant total effects on TCM doctor density and public health doctor density, whereby a 1% increase in outpatient visits per capita in all the units accompanied a 0.261% increase in TCM doctor density and 0.629% increase in public health doctor density in each unit, but these two estimates were only significant at the 0.1 level. In relation to the health expenditure, the total effects of government and social health expenditure per capita were both significant in driving the TCM doctor density. A 1% increase in the government and social health expenditure per capita in all the units could respectively result in 0.182% and 0.208% increases in the TCM doctor density in each unit. In addition, a 1% increase in government and social health expenditure per capita in all the units could also lead to 0.355% increase in the dentist density in each unit. Regarding the medical graduate density, a 1% increase in the medical graduate density in all the units was correlated with a 0.125% increase in the clinician density and a 0.228% increase in the dentist density in each unit.

5.4. Comparison and Visualization of the Direct and Spillover Effects

Figures 5.1 and 5.2 summarize the direct (left side) and spillover effects (right side) of outpatient and inpatient visits per capita, respectively, on the densities of different subtypes of health manpower. The findings confirmed the significant direct effects of both outpatient and inpatient health services per capita on the density of health technicians as a whole, indicating that the health services demand was pivotal in driving the health manpower density.

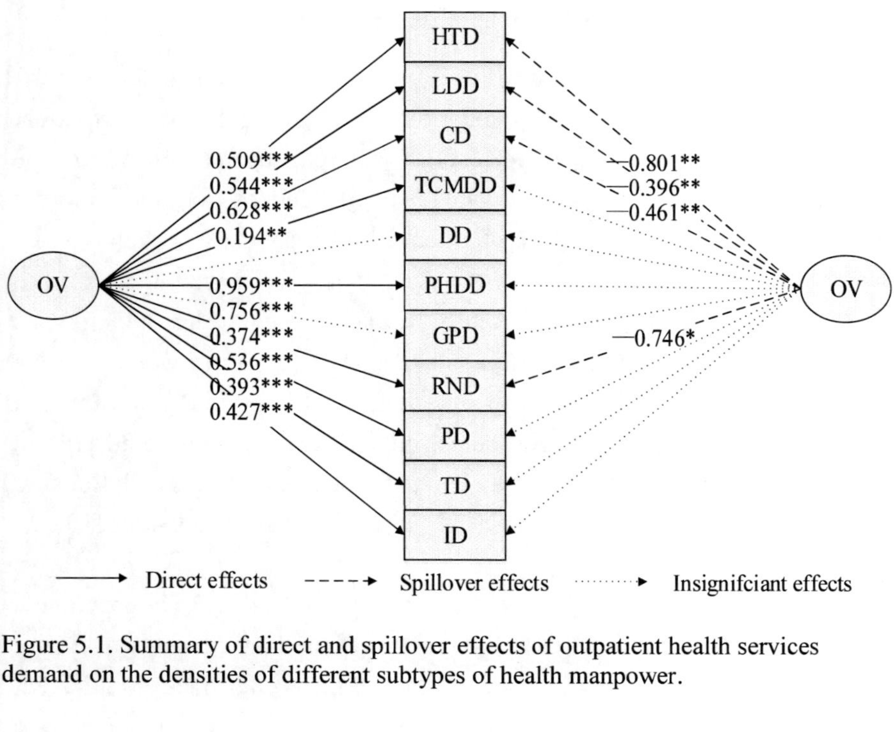

Figure 5.1. Summary of direct and spillover effects of outpatient health services demand on the densities of different subtypes of health manpower.

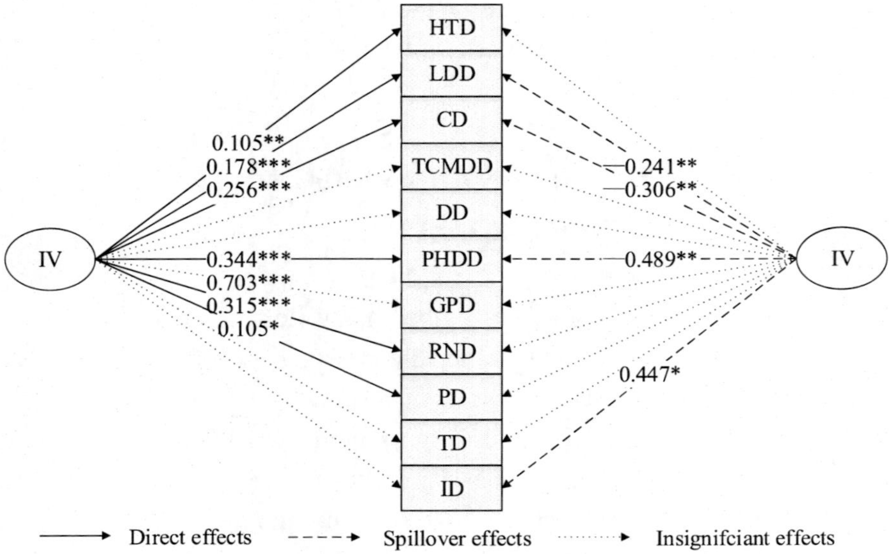

Figure 5.2. Summary of direct and spillover effects of inpatient health services demand on the densities of different subtypes of health manpower.

As for the five main categories of health technicians (licensed doctors, registered nurses, pharmacists, technologists, and interns), outpatient health service demand (direct effects) was significantly related to the densities of all of them, with the coefficient of licensed doctors being the largest. In contrast, the growth in inpatient health services per capita in one unit only significantly increased the densities of licensed doctors and registered nurses in the unit, especially the latter. Regarding the subtypes of licensed doctors, the regression results suggested a significantly positive correlation between outpatient and inpatient health services per capita in one unit and the densities of clinicians, public health doctors, and GPs in the same unit, while this study failed to find a significant relationship between inpatient health services per capita and the density of TCM doctors.

As shown on the right side of Figures 5.1 and 5.2, a province's increased health service demand adversely affected the densities of core types of health manpower (licensed doctors, registered nurses) in adjacent units, which implied that the increase in the health service demand in one province had a negative impact on its neighboring provinces. More specifically, if there were high medical needs in one unit, this not only accompanied higher health manpower density in the respective unit, but that unit was also more likely to attract the clinicians and registered nurses from adjacent units. Unexpectedly, the increase of inpatient health service demand could also help attract public health doctors from adjacent units.

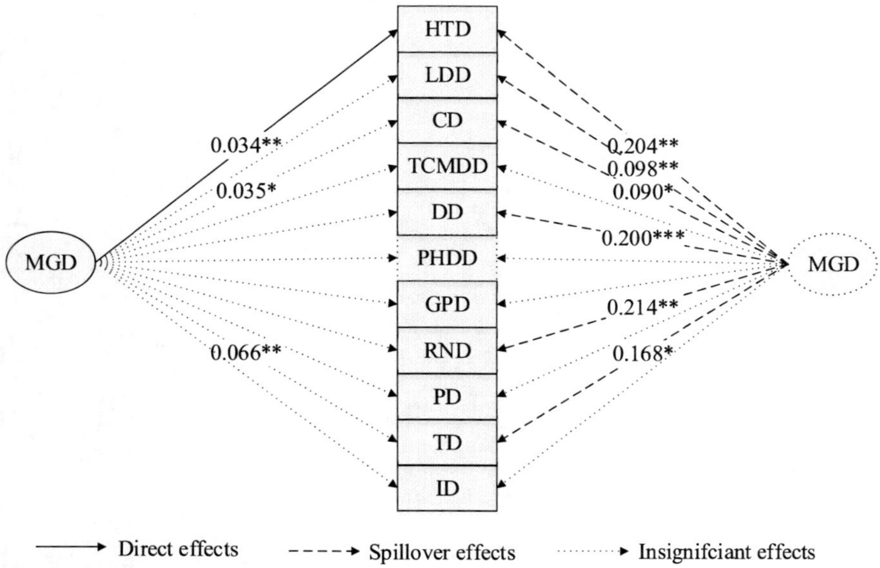

Figure 5.3. Summary of direct and spillover effects of medical graduate density on the densities of different subtypes of health manpower.

Figure 5.3 summarizes the direct (left side) and spillover effects (right side) of medical graduate density on the densities of different subtypes of health manpower. Although the effect of medical education capacity was not explored by existing studies, this study considered the medical graduate density an important independent variable and then observed a significant relationship between it and the density of total health technicians in the same unit. This was consistent with Hypothesis 3 that the supply of health manpower was built upon the education strength in a region. With regard to the subtypes of health technicians, however, matters varied greatly. Only the density of limited subtypes of health manpower (technologists at the 0.05 level and clinicians at the 0.1 level) were significantly related to the density of medical students in local units. Intriguingly, the medical education capacity had relatively strong spillover effects on adjacent units compared to its direct effects. The results confirmed the positive and significant spillover effects of medical education capacity on some major subtypes of health manpower, like clinicians and registered nurses.

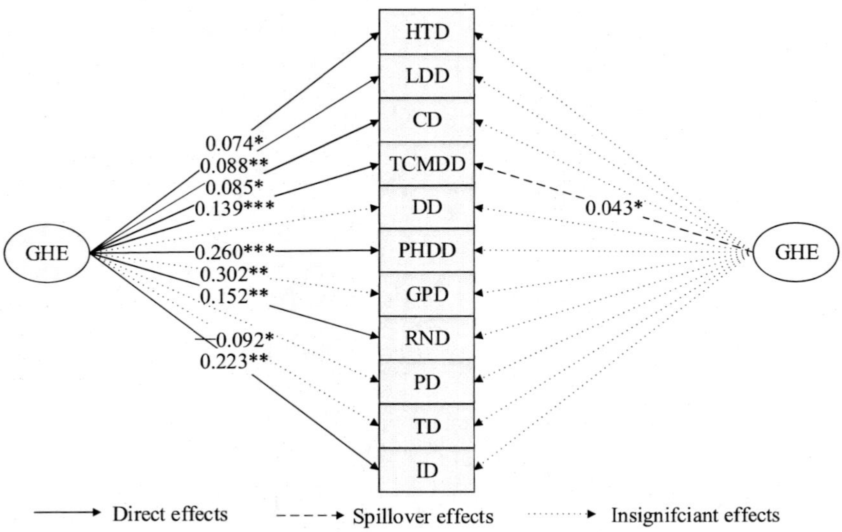

Figure 5.4. Summary of direct and spillover effects of government health expenditure on the densities of different subtypes of health manpower.

Figures 5.4 and 5.5 summarize the direct and spillover effects of government and social health expenditure per capita, respectively, on the densities of different subtypes of health manpower. The regression results suggested a significantly positive correlation between the density of health technicians and both government and social health expenditure per capita. As for the direct effects, different subtypes of health technicians showed different sensitivities to government and social health expenditure. First, government and social health expenditure per capita in one unit were both potent predictors of the density of health technician density, licensed doctor density, registered nurse density, TCM doctor density, and GP density. These practitioners provide health services directly and thus by their nature are a major concern of the government and target of social health expenditure. Second, some subtypes of health technicians were sensitive to the investment of only one type of health expenditure. That is, the densities of clinicians, public health doctors, and interns were only sensitive to government health expenditure, while the densities of technologists and dentists were only significantly related to the social health expenditure per capita. Regarding the spillover effects, the social health expenditure in one unit exerted much more pronounced spillover effects on adjacent units than the government health expenditure. An increase of government health expenditure per capita in one unit only served to increase the density of TCM doctors in the adjacent units, but the increase of social health expenditure per capita in one unit was associated with increases in the densities of TCM doctors, registered nurses, technologists, and dentists in the adjacent units. This indicates that the social health expenditure investment in one unit could also benefit its neighbors more through spillover effects.

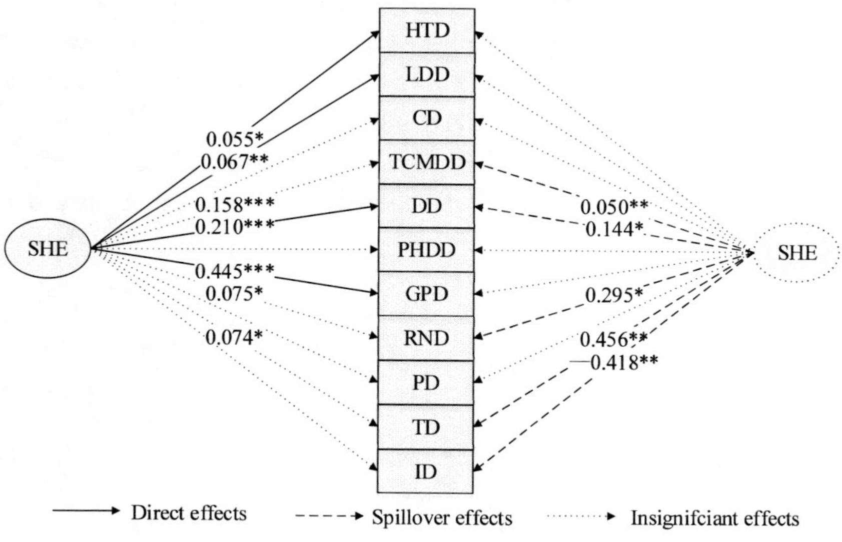

Figure 5.5. Summary of direct and spillover effects of social health expenditure on the densities of different subtypes of health manpower.

5.5. Chapter Summary

On the basis of a 5-year (2012–2016) panel dataset, this chapter empirically measured the determinants of densities of different subtypes of health manpower in China. In general, the direct and spillover effects of all the independent variables achieved statistical significance for at least one subtype of health manpower, which confirms the rationality and validity of the theoretical model, while the coefficients for the effects of the independent variables on the densities of different subtypes of health manpower varied greatly.

On the demand side, inpatient and outpatient health service demand forcefully drove the densities of almost all subtypes of health manpower. Due to the larger scale of their demand, outpatients exerted a broader and more intense influence on health manpower density than did inpatients, affecting more subtypes of health manpower and driving more of the health manpower densities (in terms of the coefficients between variables). On the supply side, medical graduate density was significantly related to the densities of several subtypes of health manpower, while its power was relatively limited in increasing the health manpower density in local units when compared to its spillover effects on neighboring units. Government and social health expenditure played different roles in the health labor market, government health expenditure exerting stronger direct effects while the spillover effects of social health expenditure were much broader.

Chapter 6

DISCUSSION

Chapters 4 and 5 report the characteristics and determinants of the health manpower distribution in China. The results show that spatial variations exist in the upward trend of health manpower density in China, and its spatial clustering patterns vary with time and across subtypes of health manpower. Behind the scenes, various factors from the supply side and demand side and spillover effects from adjacent units drive the variation in health manpower density in each unit. In the following sections, the main findings and their implications will be thoroughly discussed.

6.1. CHARACTERISTICS

Reviewing the past decade, the problem of health manpower misdistribution in China was characterized as a "crisis" due to the shortage of qualified health technicians (Mandeville et al. 2016). However, China has experienced a transition from a shortage to a rapid growth in the numbers of healthcare workers. According to the *Long-Term Medical Personnel Development Plan of China (2011–2020)*, the health manpower stock in China (10,694 thousand in 2015) has overfulfilled the goal for

2015 (9,530 thousand) and is closing in on the final 2020 target (12,550 thousand) inch by inch. Thus, scarcity is no longer a problem; uneven distribution is now at the center of discussions.

The present study has shown that the regional differences in the densities of each subtype of health manpower remain relatively high, indicating some provincial units are lagging behind. Compared to other regions, the eastern provincial units with their great economic strength are unlikely to suffer health manpower shortage and are better positioned to cope with shortages of health manpower (Zhu, Hsieh, Zhang 2018). Due to their backward economies and disadvantaged locations in Western China, the low-low and low-high cluster features gradually disappeared from east to west during the research period for most subtypes of health manpower. Sichuan and Yunnan, which are located in the southeast border area, were low-low cluster overlap area for various subtypes of health manpower, indicating a relative lack of health manpower in them and adjacent units. In addition, the Beijing-Tianjin-Hebei region is once again in the spotlight as in many regional studies (P. S. Zhao et al. 2013; H. Zhao et al. 2016). In the earlier research period, the significant high-high and low-high cluster features in this region showed that health manpower in Hebei had a tendency to move to Beijing and Tianjin. Hebei is connected to Beijing and Tianjin not only geographically but also socially and economically. Beijing, the capital of China, and Tianjin, one municipality directly under the Central Government, possess remarkable economic advantages and may thus attract health manpower from Hebei Province. Later, the low-high cluster feature in Hebei either became insignificant or turned into a high-high cluster type, meaning that Hebei Province had progressively eliminated its health manpower shortage in spite of the brain drain to Beijing and Tianjin.

More specifically, this study revealed the urban-rural imbalances of health manpower distribution in China, indicating that China faces a tougher challenge in equally distributing rural health manpower than urban health manpower. Overall, the density of each subtype of health manpower in urban areas can be 2–4 times greater than in rural areas. Surprisingly, the urban health manpower density in some sparsely populated western areas, like Xinjiang, Xizang, and Qinghai, displayed high-high cluster features across the research period, indicating a sufficient urban health manpower stock in these units. With respect to rural health manpower, a totally different picture of health manpower clustering was revealed, as the low-low cluster feature was always detected in western provincial units. For instance, Sichuan and Yunnan exhibited a low-low cluster feature for rural licensed doctor density and rural pharmacist density at almost all the time points. In addition, Xinjiang displayed a high-low cluster feature, indicating the relative lack of health manpower in its neighbors (Xizang, Gansu, Qinghai).

The huge gaps in urban and rural health manpower densities in western China compel us to rethink the efficacy and rationality of the past health manpower allocation policies. For a long time, the western provincial units have been supposed to be disadvantaged in various aspects, such as the education, attraction, and retention of health manpower. Accordingly, the Central Government has always given a certain preference to these units when planning health manpower allocation (B. Zhu, Fu, Liu, He, et al. 2018). Nevertheless, as it turns out, health manpower in these units tends to concentrate in urban areas, evidenced by the extremely high health manpower density and high-high cluster feature only for the urban health manpower in these units. In contrast, health institutions in the rural area only retain a small number of health workers. That is to say, the policy inclinations of the Central Government did translate into effective health coverage of health manpower in rural west China, but only attracted more health workers to work in the urban areas. In addition, the vast area in these units further reduces the health manpower accessibility in sparsely populated rural areas, such as Tibet, Xinjiang, and Qinghai. As a result, the contemporary policy instruments are far from sufficient to channel health manpower into the rural and remote areas of west China, let alone ensure an influx of all subtypes of personnel with a balanced skill mix. Another case that should draw our attention is three provincial units in rural northeast China (Heilongjiang, Jilin, and Liaoning). As reported for the results of spatial variations in temporal trends, these units displayed lower increases than the average of all other units, which may be related to the sluggish economy of northeast China. The unfavorable outcome of urban and rural comparison is mainly attributed to the lower increase of its rural composition. On current trends, rural health manpower in northeast China may soon face a shortage.

We can draw some take-away lessons from the above-mentioned spatio-temporal dynamics and spatial clusters of the health manpower distribution in China.

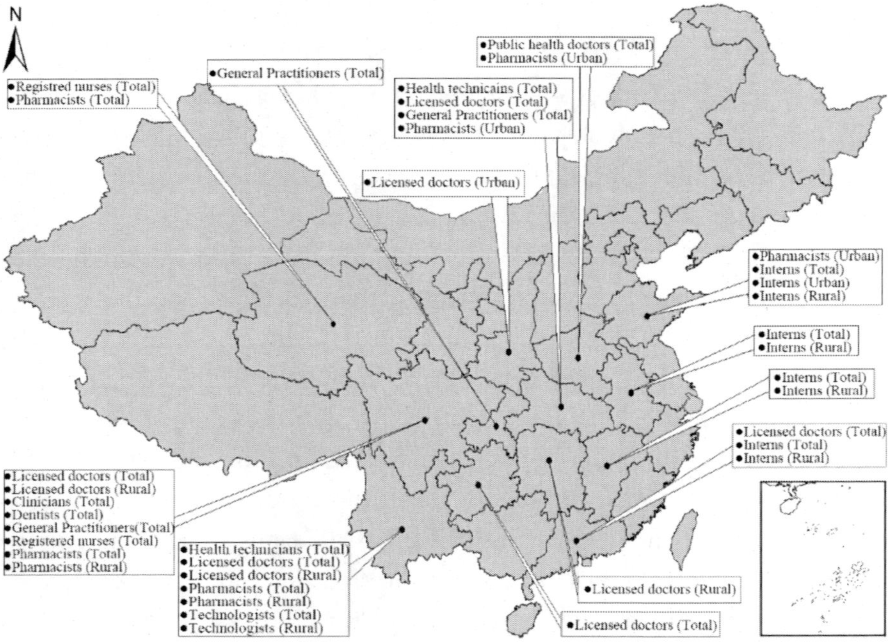

Figure 6.1. Summary of locations and manpower types that display low-low cluster feature in 2016.

First, the low-low and low-high cluster areas should be given priority in corresponding policy formulation. Compared with the spread of infectious diseases and air pollutants (B. Zhu et al. 2017; Hao and Liu 2016), health manpower distribution, affected by multiple geographical, economic, and social factors, shows distinctive spatial clustering features in different areas rather than a single pattern across the whole country. As reported previously, various types of spatial clustering can be observed in the univariate LISA cluster maps, indicating the complex distribution patterns of health manpower in China. As far as policy planning is concerned, the government should pay extra attention to the low-low and low-high cluster types. The low-low cluster type indicates that the health manpower shortage has gone beyond the provincial level and exhibits a trend of regionalization, while the low-high cluste type means that the central unit is at a disadvantage when compared to its neighbors. For the units (Figures 6.1 and 6.2) included in low-low, low-high cluster areas and their neighbors, cooperation, not confrontation, should be strengthened, such as collaborative policy design for the education of medical students and measures to attract health manpower.

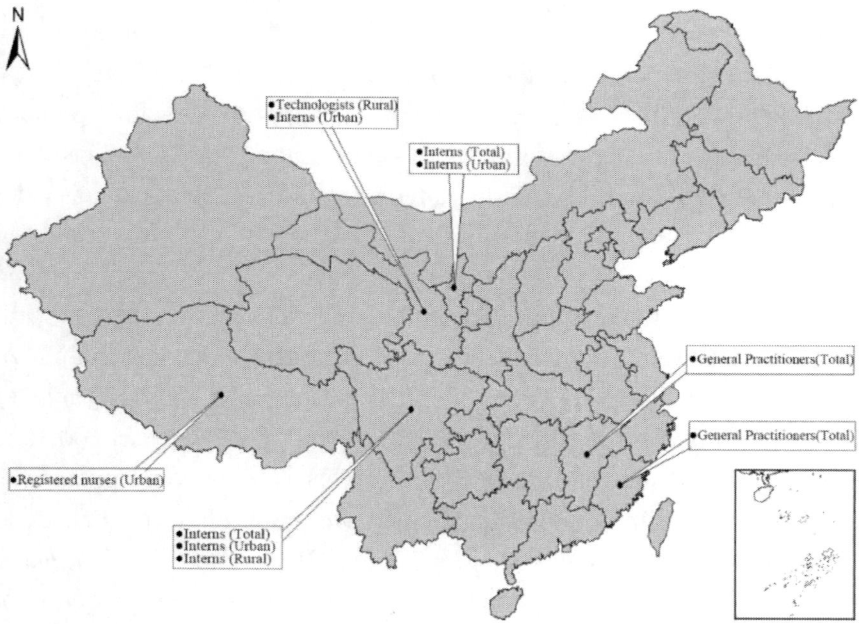

Figure 6.2. Summary of locations and manpower types that display low-high cluster feature in 2016.

Second, the huge urban-rural imbalances are making inroads on the basic health care needs of the rural population. The lack of health manpower in rural and remote areas is a worldwide problem. However, there are many successful examples, such as Australia, from which China can learn in order to better promote health manpower flow to rural and remote areas. The Australian geographical classifications of the Remoteness Area (ASGC-RA) system divided the whole country into five scales bye remoteness (McGrail and Humphreys 2009) and health professionals in remote and rural areas are provided with supplementary salary and benefits. Such geographical classification systems with discrimination in the salary packages of different regions have been introduced in many developed countries to support the rural and remote areas.

Third, the pursuit of total quantity balance may obscure the imbalances of certain subtypes of health manpower. Different subtypes of health manpower displayed relatively different spatio-temporal dynamics and spatial clustering patterns, which may be attributed to the relatively different cultivation channels and job requirements of different subtypes of health manpower. It also suggests that health manpower allocation policies should probably vary across subtypes of health manpower. As indicated by the differentiated spatial clustering patterns of different subtypes of health manpower, the balanced distribution of total health manpower tends to obscure the imbalances of its subtypes. For instance, both the low-low and low-high clusters are not significant in the univariate cluster maps of rural health technicians in 2016, indicating the relatively even distribution of rural health manpower. However, low-low cluster units can be found for three major subtypes of rural health manpower (rural licensed doctors, rural pharmacists, and rural technologists). That is, if we only pursue the balance of total health manpower quantity, we may ignore imbalances in its subtypes. However, the current *Long-Term Medical Personnel Development Plan of China (2011–2020)* only sets quantitative goals for total health technicians, total licensed doctors, and total registered nurses. This practice may cover over imbalances in certain subtypes of health manpower, like the subtypes of licensed doctors, pharmacists, and technologists.

Fourth, the characteristic differences across subtypes of health manpower reveal another health manpower dimension that is often ignored—skill mix imbalances. Effective and efficient health service delivery requires not only a sufficient quantity of health manpower but also proper teamwork in which each member contributes different skills and performs different functions. The key issue sometimes may not be the quantity but the variety and composition of mixed skilled personnel. In effect, the differences among the spatial clustering patterns of different subtypes of health manpower result from the different proportions and variegated composition of health manpower in each provincial unit. In both high- and low-income countries and in different medical institutions, there are numerous examples of the mismatch between the capability of the workforce and their current positions (WHO 2006b). For instance, skilled nurses are doing technologists' tasks because of a lack of technologists. Practicing medical personnel are burdened with management duties regardless of having no expertise in these areas. This may all lead to low efficiency and excessive workload for certain kinds of health manpower (Fulton et al. 2011). Nevertheless, the proper skill mix is contextual, correlated with geography, demography, and the level of medical services in each specific region. There is therefore no one-size-fits-all approach to determining the skill mix for all the provincial units (WHO 2013). However, there is no doubt that an appropriate and sustainable skill mix should go beyond the cadres of doctors and nurses and cover all types of health manpower due to the complex health manpower classification and medical service requirements in China.

6.2. Determinants

On the demand side, health service demand forcefully drove the health manpower density at the provincial level, while outpatient and inpatient health service demand exerted relatively different influences, which also differed across subtypes of health manpower.

Based on the empirical results of spatial panel econometric models, the densities of almost all the subtypes of health manpower were significantly related to the outpatient health service demand in the same units, while the results for licensed doctors and registered nurses are more significant than for pharmacists (significant at 0.1 level) and technologists (not significant). Undoubtedly the pharmacists and technologists are also indispensable in inpatient health services delivery, as inpatients usually need to take medical examinations and medicine, tasks that involve pharmacists and technologists. The outpatient service demand tends to have a greater influence on the densities of pharmacists and technologists, as a population's outpatient service demand can far the inpatient service demand. More specifically, the effect of average outpatient services per capita (5.317) during 2012–2016 across the nation was as much as 37 times greater than that of inpatient services (0.143)[3]. Therefore, the workload of pharmacists and technologists may mainly come from outpatient health services, which also provide interns more internship opportunities. It is not surprising that this study failed to find a significant relationship between inpatient health services per capita and the density of TCM doctors, which can be attributed to the relatively weak role of TCM doctors in inpatient services. That is, TCM doctors usually adopt non-surgical treatment methods, like herbal medicine, acupuncture, massage, and dietary therapy, for which patients do not need to stay in health institutions overnight. In addition, neither outpatient nor inpatient health service demand is significantly correlated with dentist density. This may result from the undifferentiated measurement of the health services demand. Due to data availability, this study only adopted total health service visits per capita rather than oral care service visits to predict the dentist density. However, dentists only provide a small proportion of health services and serve a smaller number of patients (X. Sun et al. 2017).

With regard to spillover effects, the uneven health service demand indicated in the results is likely to induce a brain drain of health manpower by siphoning off the health talents of surrounding regions. However, only the density of licensed doctors and its largest component (clinicians) were significantly related to the outpatient and inpatient health service demand in adjacent units. This may also be attributed to the direct role of clinicians in outpatient and inpatient service delivery even though outpatient and

[3] See the summary statistics in Table 5.1.

inpatient health services correspond to different aspects of the population's medical needs and thus call for a different skill mix of health manpower. But what outpatient and inpatient services have in common is that they directly connect patients and health manpower. The more important a subtype of health manpower is in health service delivery, the more likely this subtype of health manpower is to be attracted to a high-demand area. Accordingly, only the attraction and enrollment of clinicians can help meet the health service demands in local units more efficiently.

These findings suggest that the government should take health service demand into consideration in health manpower planning. At present, China only uses the health manpower density to determine manpower requirements and fails to take into consideration the wide local variations in health service demand. More specifically, extreme health service demand differences could be observed at the provincial level ([3.007, 10.716] for the OVPA range and [0.047, 0.223] for the IVPA range[4]), indicating that the workload of health workers differs across regions. Following WHO suggestions, the Workload Indicators of Staffing Need (WISN) is a complementary, systematic way to manage health manpower well (WHO 2010c). It calculates health worker requirements based on health workers' workload, with activity (time) standards applied for each workload component. I believe that it holds promise for resolving the problems of allocating health manpower in China due to the significant role of health service delivery in driving health manpower distribution. The finding indicates that a balanced health manpower distribution cannot be achieved only with efforts from the supply side. At first sight, the government is powerless on the demand side, as the population's health services demand looks like the people's own business. In fact, the population's health services demand can also be stimulated by means of related health policies, like health insurance and medical assistance, as these medical needs have never been fully met. Based on these findings, if the medical needs repressed by economic conditions can be better satisfied, health manpower densities will increase. Although the three basic health

[4] See the summary statistics in Table 5.1.

insurance schemes (*Urban Employee Basic Medical Insurance, Urban Residents Basic Medical Insurance and New Rural Cooperative Medical Care*) have gradually covered 1214 million residents[5] (*nearly 90%*) since the public-welfare-oriented medical system reform launched in 2007 (K. Zhou et al. 2015), there are also some problems that result in weak risk protection of health insurance schemes. More efforts are required to target health insurance and medical needs towards the most-in-need population.

On the supply side, medical education benefits not only the local health system but also the surrounding regions. The spillover effects of education have been shown and explored by many existing studies (Yajuan 2010). This study for the first time proved the spillover effects of medical education on the recruitment of health manpower in adjacent units. Furthermore, the spillover effects of medical education on neighboring units are stronger among the core types of health manpower (i.e., clinicians, registered nurses etc.). This may indicate the strong mobility of medical graduates. That is, it is common for medical students to prefer a workplace in an adjacent provincial unit after graduation for personal reasons, like socioeconomic factors, family, or good career prospects (Hou et al. 2016). However, investment in the health system requires time to achieve substantial progress (G Dussault and Vujicic 2008). On the one hand, it takes years to nurture medical students. In 2013, China launched a nationwide reform of medical education, called 5+3 (5-year undergraduate and 3-year standardized residency training), to ensure education quality, but which also takes more time for medical students to formally enter the health labor market (J. Zhu, Li, and Chen 2016). Second, medical graduates should master the matching skills appropriate to the positions. These both require the education sector to plan ahead.

When it comes to health expenditure, this study showed a significant relationship between either government or social health expenditure and total health technician density in a given unit. This finding echoes studies using GNI per capita and government health expenditure to predict the

---

[5] See the Statistical Bulletin on National Economic and Social Development of the PRC in 2018. http://www.stats.gov.cn/tjsj/zxfb/201902/t20190228_1651265.html.

density of health manpower (Freed, Nahra, and Wheeler 2004; Kanchanachitra et al. 2011; Zaman, Gemmell, and Lievens 2014) and fortifies the notion that the investment of financial resources can improve the accessibility of healthcare services (WHO 2010b).

However, different subtypes of health manpower showed different sensitivities to government and social investment health. This seemingly surprising result, I suspect, may be attributed to the differing focus of government and social capital and competition between public and proprietary hospitals in recruiting health workers. Solicitude for the common good is an essential character of the government health expenditure, causing it to be focused on the health manpower subtypes that are committed to the public welfare. For instance, public health doctors rely heavily on subsidies from the government as they provide non-profit public health services like establishing health records; screening for major diseases in elderly people; and providing health education and managing chronic non-communicable diseases (Ding et al. 2013; T. Li et al. 2016). In contrast, social health expenditure tends to invest in dentists and technologists, who are essential in high-profit health examination and oral care services. Besides, due to the narrower supply channel of doctors mentioned above, competition is particularly keen in the recruitment of doctors. Therefore, proprietary hospitals may be disadvantaged in the attraction and retention of some subtypes of health manpower, such as clinicians. Tang et al. (2014) found that many doctors in proprietary hospitals used to work in public hospitals, which reveals that proprietary hospitals may develop at the expense of public hospitals, especially when competing for the services of clinicians. Therefore, the total number of clinicians in a region may not increase with the growth of social health expenditure there, as it may only change clinicians' place of practice. Last but not least, the density of pharmacists is correlated with neither government nor social health expenditure per capita. This may be attributed to the limited demand for pharmacists due to the fact that only a set number of pharmacists are required and enrolled in each institution.

We can draw some take-away lessons from the above-mentioned determinants of the distribution of different subtypes of health manpower in China.

First, different subtypes of health manpower responded differently to the determinants of the health labor market. The supply-side factors, demand-side factor jointly drive how health manpower is distributed, while the determinants of the health manpower distribution differ across subtypes of health manpower, which may be attributed to their different roles in healthcare delivery and different supply channels. For instance, the closer is one subtype of health manpower related to the outpatient health services; the more likely is its density being driven by the outpatient visits. The findings echo the study of characteristics and point to subtype-specific health manpower allocation policies in China.

Second, spillover effects matter in driving the distribution of all subtypes of health manpower. With the help of spatial panel econometric models, this study measured the spillover effects in the distribution of different subtypes of health manpower and found that strong spillover effects exist between regions, which were even stronger than the direct effects. For some units with lower health service demand, the health worker are likely to be attracted to adjacent units, while units bordering with provincial units rich in medical graduates can also benefit from the spillover effects. Now that the geographical units can not get rid of the influence of spillover effects from other units, the health sectors should take them into consideration when educating, attracting and retaining health workers.

Third, precisely because government and social health investment differ in their fundamental nature (the common good versus profitability), they play different but complementary roles in health manpower allocation (Tang et al. 2014; C. Wang and Chen 2017). With different preferences, government and social health expenditures keep a watchful eye on different subtypes of health manpower and have their own different strengths. For instance, government health expenditure is stronger in allocating clinicians, while social health expenditure exerts more spillover effects. Therefore, the path to higher coverage of health manpower requires the collaboration of government and social health investment (B. Zhu, Fu, Liu, and Mao 2018). If only the government is involved, it is very likely that the health labor market will face a shortage of funds, while in the case of the exclusive involvement of social health expenditure, markets may fail due to the constrained reactions of the health manpower supply and demand to price signals in the health labor market (McPake et al. 2014).

Chapter 7

CONCLUSION

As the world's most populous nation, 0.

China has the world's largest troop of health manpower as well as a diverse health manpower composition across provincial units (J. Zhu, Li, and Chen 2016). Understanding the status of this large share of global human resources for health is of vital importance. However, existing studies have paid little attention to the spatial-temporal dynamics of the health manpower distribution and its causes at the regional level. The findings of this study will therefore supplement previous studies and serve the interest of policy makers, as the need to address health manpower misdistribution has become increasingly urgent. The major findings, policy and theoretical implications, limitations, and suggested directions for future research are elaborated in this chapter.

7.1. MAJOR FINDINGS

This study aims to reveal the spatial distribution of health manpower in China and answer the following two research questions:

1. *How is health manpower distributed in China?*

2. *What factors may contribute to regional differences in the health manpower distribution in China?*

Overall, this study provides cogent evidence for the spatial clustering of different subtypes of health manpower in China as well as revealing their determinants at the provincial level. To answer the first research question, this study explored the spatial distribution characteristics of health manpower in China and found that it exhibited three major characteristics.

First, spatial disparities and spatial clusters exist in the distribution of health manpower in China. Regional differences and various types of spatial clustering can be observed in the hierarchical maps and univariate LISA cluster maps above, indicating that some provincial units are extremely disadvantaged in providing effective coverage of health manpower. The health manpower shortage in southwest China has even transcended the provincial level to exhibit a trend of regionalization.

Second, huge urban-rural imbalances are seen in the distribution of health manpower in China, reflected not only in the huge urban-rural gaps in health manpower densities, but also between the spatial clustering patterns of urban and rural health manpower. As it is precisely western China, disadvantaged in various aspects (position, economy, education system, etc.), that has a poorer stock of rural health manpower, the imbalanced distribution of rural health manpower poses greater challenges to the Chinese government.

Third, spatial distribution characteristics vary across different subtypes of health manpower. That is the case for both the urban and rural health manpower distributions, whose differences may be attributable to the different supply channel and training requirements of different subtypes of health manpower. At present, the pursuit of total quantity balance tends to obscure the imbalances of certain subtypes of health manpower, which is also hindering the attainment of the right mix of health manpower in China. As previously mentioned, the provincial units displaying low-low cluster features have gradually been reduced and either became insignificant or turned into other types. However, the elimination of licensed doctors was relatively slow. More administrative units are identified as low-low cluster units in the distribution of licensed doctors than registered nurses and fewer units moved out of the low-low cluster units, which may be attributed to the narrow supply channel and long training cycle of licensed doctors (J. Zhu, Li, and Chen 2016).

To answer the second research question, this study constructed the theoretical "supply-demand-spillover" research model (Figure 2.2) to map out the determinants of the health manpower distribution. With the help of spatial panel econometric models, this study empirically measured the direct effects of within-province factors but also the spillover effects of factors in adjacent provincial units. The findings serve as the basis for understanding the spatio-temporal dynamics and spatial clustering patterns of the health manpower distribution in China and provide new information for evidence-based health manpower allocation policy making in China. Both the direct effects and spillover effects of all the variables reached statistical significance for several subtypes of health manpower, which verifies the rationality and validity of the proposed research model. The determinants of the health workforce distribution may be summarized as follows.

First, the health services demand forcefully drives the health manpower distribution across the nation due to the inherent and direct driving role of the demand-side factors, as expected. For precisely this reason, the health service demand increase in a province could significantly help one unit attract licensed doctors and registered nurses, who are direct providers of health services, from adjacent units. Among these, the inpatient and outpatient service demand differently affects the densities of different subtypes of health manpower, which may be attributed to their distinct roles in health services delivery. Moreover, due to the larger scale of outpatient demand, outpatients exert a broader and more intense influence on health manpower density than do inpatients, affecting more subtypes of health manpower and driving health manpower densities more strongly (in terms of the coefficients between variables).

Second, medical education is making significant contributions to the health care industry by educating medical graduates. Unexpectedly but intriguingly, the power of medical education is relatively limited in increasing the health manpower density in local units compared to its spillover effects on neighboring units. It would thus be an effective strategy to increase the supply of health manpower through coordinated efforts across the provincial boundaries.

Third, government and social health expenditures play different roles in the health labor market. They collectively drive the health manpower density but differ in two ways: 1) Government and social health expenditure have different strengths in attracting different subtypes of health manpower: Government health investment plays a unique role in increasing the stock of clinicians and public health doctors at home, while social health investment does better in dentists and general practitioners. 2) Social health investment exerts stronger positive spillover effects on adjacent units.

To summarize, China is still faced with the challenge of health manpower misdistribution, which demands more attention from policy makers. As Mandeville and colleagues (Mandeville et al. 2016) urged the developing world to search for sustainable solutions for healthcare disparities, it is of paramount importance to effectively tackle the issue of misdistribution in the foreseeable future.

7.2. Policy Implications

Maintaining the well-being of all citizens regardless of where they live requires the equitable distribution of properly trained healthcare workers. Just as stated in *Healthy China 2030*, China would have no national health without a rational distribution of health manpower (W. Wang and Zakus 2016). Has China reached this goal yet? This research shows remarkable achievements as well as areas needing improvement.

Based on the characteristics and determinants of health manpower distribution in China, the misdistribution of health manpower is not merely a local problem; it is, in fact, a national problem. To address the problem of health manpower misdistribution, collaboration across provincial boundaries should be initiated through effective institutional arrangements, such as deliberative policy design and effective human resource management initiatives to educate, recruit, and retain healthcare workers and prevent a brain drain of health manpower from disadvantaged units.

In the short term, subtype-specific and region-oriented health manpower planning and allocation policies are suggested, aimed at urban and rural health manpower, respectively, by prioritizing the identified up-to-date low-low and low-high cluster areas (Figures 6.1 and 6.2). This includes but is not limited to preferential policies to channel the most-needed manpower subtypes to the most-in-need provincial units. More specifically, the identified low-low and low-high clusters should be precisely the priority areas for existing area-targeted health manpower programs in China. For example, the ongoing "Rural-Oriented Medical Education Scheme" (RMES) has been educating health manpower for disadvantaged rural and remote areas. RMES provides scholarships and tuition waivers for medical students with a rural background, who will in return work in primary-level medical and health care institutions in their hometowns for a couple of years after graduation. This has proven to be an effective strategy to promote the balanced distribution of health manpower, as it is much more difficult to urge the health manpower in other provincial units to migrate to the remote provinces or attract urban health manpower to the countryside (Somers, Strasser, and Jolly 2007; King et al. 2016). The identified cluster areas will sharpen the focus of RMES by channeling the most-needed manpower subtype to the most-in-need provincial units.

Another example is the "Medical Pairing-Assistance Scheme." It has been a tradition in China to pair some eastern provincial units or units with sufficient skilled health manpower stock with disadvantaged western units. The detection of low-low and low-high cluster areas will make such pairings more accurate by pairing up the provincial units that are most in need and those units which have a comparatively abundant stock of certain subtypes of health manpower. For the remote regions whose problems cannot be solved by the previous long-term policies, some expediency can be afforded with the assistance of emerging technologies. For example, telemedicine is one possible solution to support the remote or border provinces that have a high demand for some kinds of health manpower. Although less effective for serious diseases, telemedicine will save time and energy for both patients and physicians in subsequent visits and during the recovery period (Cai et al. 2016).

In the long run, the results demonstrate the significance and necessity of generating more collaborative efforts involving multiple government sectors (e.g., the health, economic, and human resources sectors) to mobilize domestic resources to combat the uneven distribution of health manpower (Zhu, Hsieh, Zhang 2018). In the first place, the *Long-Term Medical Personnel Development Plan of China (2011–2020)* is currently the only working health manpower plan. Planning the health manpower development every decade has failed to capture the quick changes of health manpower distribution in China and renders the goals of the plan inoperative in the later stages of the planning period. Moreover, it only sets quantitative goals for total health technicians, total licensed doctors, and total registered nurses, which may obscure imbalances in certain subtypes of health manpower, such as the subtypes of licensed doctors, pharmacists, and technologists. Therefore, a more detailed medical personnel development plan for China that includes each subtype of urban and rural health manpower should be made based on the current status of the health manpower distribution in China. It should set a clear goal for health manpower allocation; be renewable over time; and specify the duties of all the respective government sectors.

Second, this study also highlights that the health sector should proactively allocate health manpower via health service demand. The low health manpower density in some units may also result from the population's inability to meet their medical needs. In those disadvantaged units, the government is supposed to take a stronger role to meet more of the population's needs and strengthen the financial protection they have to avoid people falling into poverty because of illnesses. The more people's needs are satisfied, the more power health institutions can obtain to attract and recruit health workers.

Third, due to the significant supporting role of medical education in neighboring regions, coordinated actions across borders are suggested for remote units to improve their medical education capacity together. The education sector is suggested to increase quotas for medical universities located in disadvantaged low-low and low-high units. It is also the duty of the education sector to plan ahead to match medical student skills with the subtypes of health manpower in most need.

Four, there is no doubt that the financial sector should keep prompting the influx of government and private capital into the health manpower market. The inflow of non-government capital to support proprietary hospitals also requires partnership between the public and private sectors. That is, the government can give social entrepreneurs tax exemptions or take other measures to encourage building proprietary hospitals while enlarging the recruitment pool of healthcare workers. More importantly, the different focuses of government and social capital make it possible to adjust the densities of certain subtypes of health manpower.

7.3. Theoretical Implications

In most instances, health geography has focused on the geographies of infectious diseases and cancers, involving spatial epidemiology to quantifying disease incidence and distributions, and on the analysis of the causes of the factors that may contribute to an individual or population's diseases. This study provides an example of the application of spatial analysis methods to health economic research and provides methodological reference for future studies of health equity. With the introduction of two complementary spatial statistics (space-time scan statistics and Moran's I statistics), this study thoroughly explored the spatial variations in the temporal trends and the spatial clustering patterns of the health manpower distribution, which can easily be understood and compared when displayed on maps.

This study has further theoretical implications by building a framework to understand the underlying factors of the health manpower distribution. Supply and demand theory has been widely used for understanding the dynamics of the labor market, but has rarely been applied to the health field. Besides, little studies tried to empirically validate the use of supply and demand theory. Based on the Chinese context, this study refined the supply-side and demand-side factors and measured their indicators in five consecutive years (2012–2016). As validated by the results, supply and demand theory works well in exploring the behaviors of health manpower at the macro level. This study therefore provides a theoretical framework to understand the health manpower distribution in China and also has merits in explaining the health manpower distribution in other contexts similar to that of China.

Last but not least, spillover effects, which have been widely discussed in the new economic geography, are reexamined and incorporated into the research model to understand their contribution to the health manpower distribution for the first time. On account of the stronger connections between provincial units, this study reasonably suspected that spillover effects may exist between adjacent units. As shown by the results, the health service demand, medical education, and social health investment in one unit could significantly influence the health manpower stock in adjacent units. This study provides a theoretical reference for understanding the flow and brain drain of health manpower between different regions and highlights an important research direction for further in-depth studies. In addition, the consideration of spillover effects also advances the application of the supply and demand theory. The neglected spillover effects in existing studies are missing pieces in our understanding of the distribution of health manpower. This study therefore made up the shortcomings of previous studies by optimizing the use of the supply and demand theory in the Chinese context.

7.4. Limitations and Future Research Directions

As an exploratory study attempting to investigate the issue of health manpower misdistribution in China, the present study surely has limitations that should be acknowledged. Due to issues of data availability, this study only investigated the characteristics and determinants of health manpower distribution at the provincial level. It therefore cannot avoid the problem of scale, which is a classical issue in geography, namely, the modifiable areal unit problem (MAUP) (Pietrzak 2014). In any analysis of geography, the research scales matter greatly. Just as we cannot find two identical leaves in the world, every geographical unit is different from all the others. As shown in Figure 7.1, a provincial research scale means that the provincial average is adopted to represent the whole unit, which may thus obscure the diversity of its components. A new and nuanced picture might be drawn when zooming into smaller research scales. Moreover, this study of health manpower focuses on its quantity without a due consideration of its quality. As quantity does not equate to quality, disadvantaged areas may have not only a lower density of health manpower but also less well-educated workforces (Anand et al. 2008).

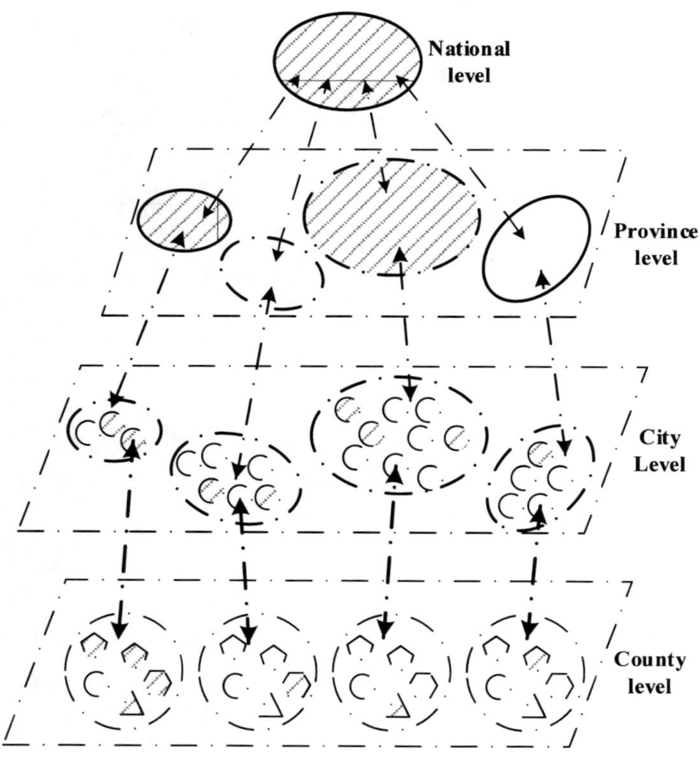

Figure 7.1. Research scales in geography.

Regarding the determinants of the health manpower distribution, this study chose only five independent variables to predict the density of health manpower at the provincial level due to data availability. I certainly believe that more socioeconomic factors should be considered, but they were not included in this study. The existing variables can also be measured more precisely by classifying different levels of medical graduates, outpatient visits, inpatient visits and health expenditures. Moreover, this study only considered the spillover effects of adjacent units. In fact, the spillovers can exert effects at greater distances due to political and economic factors. For instance, health workers are more likely to be attracted to the capital or larger cities no matter where in China they are.

More research is encouraged to delve into this important area and contribute to the better living of mankind, in China as well as in other nations. Future studies are suggested to zoom in to smaller geographical scales, like the city or county level, and take the quality of health manpower into consideration. It is also important to note that the spatial analysis is not restricted to application to the national sample; it can be conducted for each geographical unit at each time point on condition that the data at smaller scales are available. But there is no doubt that a larger geographic context and a smaller research scale contribute exponentially to the applicability and significance of the analysis.

REFERENCES

Abbas, Tariq, Muhammad Younus, and Sayyad Aun Muhammad. 2015. "Spatial Cluster Analysis of Human Cases of Crimean Congo Hemorrhagic Fever Reported in Pakistan." *Infectious Diseases of Poverty* 4 (1): 9. https://doi.org/10.1186/2049-9957-4-9.

Abdullayev, Rakif, Ian Kracalik, Rita Ismayilova, Narmin Ustun, Ayden Talibzade, and Jason K Blackburn. 2012. "Analyzing the Spatial and Temporal Distribution of Human Brucellosis in Azerbaijan (1995 - 2009) Using Spatial and Spatio-Temporal Statistics." *BMC Infectious Diseases* 12: 185. https://doi.org/10.1186/1471-2334-12-185.

Ahmed, Syed Masud, Md Awlad Hossain, Ahmed Mushtaque RajaChowdhury, and Abbas Uddin Bhuiya. 2011. "The Health Workforce Crisis in Bangladesh: Shortage, Inappropriate Skill-Mix and Inequitable Distribution." *Human Resources for Health* 9: 1–7. https://doi.org/10.1186/1478-4491-9-3.

Altman, Isidore. 1961. "Changes in Physician-Population Ratios Among the States." *Public Health Reports* 76 (12): 1051–55.

Amin, Ariane. 2016. "Exploring the Role of Economic Incentives and Spillover Effects in Biodiversity Conservation Policies in Sub-Saharan Africa." *Ecological Economics* 127: 185–91. https://doi.org/10.1016/j.ecolecon.2016.03.018.

Anand, Sudhir, and Till Bärnighausen. 2004. "Human Resources and Health Outcomes: Cross-Country Econometric Study." *The Lancet* 364 (9445): 1603–9. https://doi.org/10.1016/S0140-6736(04)17313-3.

Anand, Sudhir, Victoria Y. Fan, Junhua Zhang, Lingling Zhang, Yang Ke, Zhe Dong, and Lincoln C. Chen. 2008. "China's Human Resources for Health: Quantity, Quality, and Distribution." *The Lancet*.

Anselin, L. 1988. *Spatial Econometrics: Methods and Models*. Dordrecht: Kluwer Academic Plublishers. http://www.citeulike.org/group/206/article/201692.

Anselin, L. 1995. "Local Indicators of Spatial Association—Lisa." *Geographical Analysis* 27 (2): 93–115.

Anselin, Luc. 2002. "Under the Hood:Issues in the Specification and Interpretation of Spatial Regression Models." *Agricultural Economics* 27: 247–67. https://doi.org/10.1111/j.1574-0862.2002.tb00120.x.

Anselin, Luc, and K. Bera Bera. 1998. "Spatial Dependence in Linear Regression Models with an Introduction to Spatial Econometrics." *Statistics Textbooks and Monographs* 155: 237–90.

Anselin, Luc, Ibnu Syabri, and Youngihn Kho. 2006. "Geoda: An Introduction to Spatial Data Analysis." *Geographical Analysis* 38: 5–22. https://doi.org/10.1111/j.0016-7363.2005.00671.x.

Asante, Augustine Danso, Anthony Barry Zwi, and Maria Theresa Ho. 2006. "Equity in Resource Allocation for Health: A Comparative Study of the Ashanti and Northern Regions of Ghana." *Health Policy* 78 (2–3): 135–48. https://doi.org/10.1016/j.healthpol.2006.03.013.

Belotti, Federico, and Gordon Hughes. 2017. "XSMLE: Stata Module for Spatial Panel Data Models Estimation." *The Stata Journal* 17 (1): 139–80.

Belt, Economic. 2017. *"Available Online at Www.Sciencedirect.Com Spatial Spillover Effects of Transport Infrastructure in Chinese New Silk Road"* 6: 1–8.

Bigbee, Jeri L, and Jody DeMeyer. 2007. "The Relationship Between Nurse To Population Ratio and Population Density: A Pilot Study in Rural/Frontier State." *Online Journal of Rural Nursing and Health Care* 7 (2): 36–43.

Bonenberger, Marc, Moses Aikins, Patricia Akweongo, and Kaspar Wyss. 2014. "The Effects of Health Worker Motivation and Job Satisfaction on Turnover Intention in Ghana : A Cross-Sectional Study." *Human Resources for Health* 12 (1): 1–12. https://doi.org/10.1186/1478-4491-12-43.

Braveman, Paula. 2006. "Health Disparities and Health Equity: Concepts and Measurement." *Annual Review of Public Health* 27: 167–94. https://doi.org/10.1146/annurev.publhealth.27.021405.102103.

Cai, Hui, Hongjing Wang, Tiankang Guo, and Guoxian Bao. 2016. "Application of Telemedicine in Gansu Province of China." *PLoS ONE* 11 (6): 1–11. https://doi.org/10.1371/journal.pone.0158026.

Campbell, James, James Buchan, Giorgio Cometto, Benedict David, Gilles Dussault, Helga Fogstad, Inês Fronteira, et al. 2013. "Human Resources for Health and Universal Health Coverage: Fostering Equity and Effective Coverage." *Bulletin of the World Health Organization* 91 (11): 853–63. https://doi.org/10.2471/BLT.13.118729.

Catalano, Michael, Tanya Leise, and Thomas Pfaff. 2009. "Measuring Resource Inequality: The Gini Coefficient." *Numeracy* 2 (2). https://doi.org/10.5038/1936-4660.2.2.4.

Chen, Lincoln. 2010. "Striking the Right Balance: Health Workforce Retention in Remote and Rural Areas." *Bulletin of the World Health Organization* 88 (5): 323. https://doi.org/10.2471/BLT.10.078477.

Chen, Lincoln, Timothy Evans, Sudhir Anand, Jo Ivey Boufford, Hilary Brown, Mushtaque Chowdhury, Marcos Cueto, et al. 2004. "Human Resources for Health: Overcoming the Crisis." *Lancet*. https://doi.org/10.1016/S0140-6736(04)17482-5.

Chen, Rui, Yali Zhao, Juan Du, Tao Wu, Yafang Huang, and Aimin Guo. 2014. "Health Workforce Equity in Urban Community Health Service of China." *PLoS ONE* 9 (12): 1–15. https://doi.org/10.1371/journal.pone.0115988.

Cheng, Yeqing, Zheye Wang, Xinyue Ye, and Yehua Wei. 2014. "Spatiotemporal Dynamics of Carbon Intensity from Energy Consumption in China." *Journal of Geographical Sciences* 24 (4): 631–50. https://doi.org/10.1007/s11442-014-1110-6.

Chuai, Xiaowei, Xianjin Huang, Wanjing Wang, Jiqun Wen, Qiang Chen, and Jiawen Peng. 2012. "Spatial Econometric Analysis of Carbon Emissions from Energy Consumption in China." *Journal of Geographical Sciences* 22 (4): 630–42. https://doi.org/10.1007/s11442-012-0952-z.

Culyer, A. J., and Adam Wagstaff. 1993. "Equity and Equality in Health and Health Care." *Journal of Health Economics* 12 (4): 431–57. https://doi.org/10.1016/0167-6296(93)90004-X.

Ding, Yan, Helen J. Smith, Yang Fei, Biao Xu, Shaofa Nie, Weirong Yan, Vinod K. Diwan, Rainer Sauerborn, and Hengjin Dong. 2013. "Factors Influencing the Provision of Public Health Services by Village Doctors in Hubei and Jiangxi Provinces, China." *Bulletin of the World Health Organization* 91 (1): 64–69. https://doi.org/10.2471/BLT.12.109447.

Doull, Linda, and Fiona Campbell. 2008. "Human Resources for Health in Fragile States." *The Lancet* 371 (9613): 626–27. https://doi.org/10.1016/S0140-6736(08)60278-0.

Dussault, G, and M Vujicic. 2008. "Demand and Supply of Human Resources for Health." *International Encyclopedia of Public Health* 2: 77–84.

Dussault, Gilles, and Maria Cristina Franceschini. 2006. "Not Enough There, Too Many Here: Understanding Geographical Imbalances in the Distribution of the Health Workforce." *Human Resources for Health* 4 (1): 12. https://doi.org/10.1186/1478-4491-4-12.

Elhorst, J. Paul. 2010. "Applied Spatial Econometrics: Raising the Bar." *Spatial Economic Analysis* 5 (1): 9–28. https://doi.org/10.1080/17421770903541772.

Elhorst, Paul, Gianfranco Piras, and Giuseppe Arbia. 2010. "Growth and Convergence in a Multiregional Model with Space—Time Dynamics." *Geographical Analysis* 42 (3): 338–55. http://dx.doi.org/10.1111/j.1538-4632.2010.00796.x.

Fischer, Manfred M., and Daniel A. Griffith. 2008. "Modeling Spatial Autocorrelation in Spatial Interaction Data: An Application to Patent Citation Data in the European Union." *Journal of Regional Science* 48 (5): 969–89. https://doi.org/10.1111/j.1467-9787.2008.00572.x.

Fischer, Manfred M, and Arthur Getis. 2010. *Handbook of Applied Spatial Analysis Software Tools, Methods and Applications*. Berlin, Heidelberg: Springer. https://doi.org/10.1007/978-3-642-03647-7_1.

Freed, Gary L., Tammie A. Nahra, and John R C Wheeler. 2004. "Relation of per Capita Income and Gross Domestic Product to the Supply and Distribution of Pediatricians in the United States." *Journal of Pediatrics* 144 (6): 723–28. https://doi.org/10.1016/j.jpeds.2004.02.043.

Fu, Y, and S Gabriel. 2009. "Human Capital Spillovers, Labor Migration and Regional Development in China." *IRES Working Paper Series*. http://papers.ssrn.com/sol3/papers.cfm?abstract_id=1417281.

Fulton, Brent D, Richard M Scheffler, Susan P Sparkes, Erica Yoonkyung Auh, Marko Vujicic, and Agnes Soucat. 2011. "Health Workforce Skill Mix and Task Shifting in Low Income Countries: A Review of Recent Evidence." *Human Resources for Health* 9: 1. https://doi.org/10.1186/1478-4491-9-1.

Greene, William H. 2012. *Econometric Analysis*. 7th ed. Upper Saddle River: Prentice Hall.

Gupta, N., P. Zurn, K. Diallo, and M.R. Dal Poz. 2003. "Uses of Population Census Data for Monitoring Geographical Imbalance in the Health Workforce: Snapshots from Three Developing Countries." *International Journal for Equity in Health* 2: 11.

Haddad, Mônica A., and Zorica Nedović-Budić. 2007. "Using Spatial Statistics to Analyze Intra - Urban Inequalities and Public Intervention in São Paulo, Brazil." *Journal of Human Development ISSN:* 7 (1): 85–109. https://doi.org/10.1080/14649880500502102.

Hajizadeh, Mohammad, M. Karen Campbell, and Sisira Sarma. 2016. "A Spatial Econometric Analysis of Adult Obesity: Evidence from Canada." *Applied Spatial Analysis and Policy* 9 (3): 329–63. https://doi.org/10.1007/s12061-015-9151-5.

Hao, Yu, and Yi Ming Liu. 2016. "The Influential Factors of Urban PM2.5 Concentrations in China: A Spatial Econometric Analysis." *Journal of Cleaner Production* 112: 1443–53. https://doi.org/10.1016/j.jclepro.2015.05.005.

Hausman, JA. 1976. "Specification Tests in Econemetrics." *Working Papers* 46 (6): 1251–71.

Hawkins, Linette, Martin Ryan, Helen Murray, Marty Grace, Glad Hawkins, Phillip Mendes, and Bernie Chatley. 2000. "Supply and Demand: A Study of Labour Market Trends and the Employment of New Social Work Graduates in Victoria." *Australian Social Work* 53 (1): 35–42. https://doi.org/10.1080/03124070008415555.

Hazarika, Indrajit. 2013. "Health Workforce in India: Assessment of Availability, Production and Distribution." *WHO South-East Asia Journal of Public Health* 2 (2): 106. https://doi.org/10.4103/2224-3151.122944.

Honarmand, Rasoul, Mostafa Mozhdehifard, and Zahra Kavosi. 2017. "Geographic Distribution Indices of General Practitioners, Midwives, Pediatricians, and Gynecologists in the Public Sector of Iran." *Electronic Physician* 9 (6): 4584–89. https://doi.org/10.14661/2015.1069-1072.

Hou, Jianlin, Maoyi Xu, Joseph C. Kolars, Zhe Dong, Weimin Wang, Amy Huang, and Yang Ke. 2016. "Career Preferences of Graduating Medical Students in China: A Nationwide Cross-Sectional Study." *BMC Medical Education* 16 (1): 1–7. https://doi.org/10.1016/j.cct.2004.12.010.

Huang, Jianhuan, and Jiejin Xia. 2016. "Regional Competition, Heterogeneous Factors and Pollution Intensity in China: A Spatial Econometric Analysis." *Sustainability.* 8 (2). https://doi.org/10.3390/su8020171.

Huang, Li, Xin-Xu Li, Eniola Michael Abe, Lin Xu, Yao Ruan, Chun-Li Cao, and Shi-Zhu Li. 2017. "Spatial-Temporal Analysis of Pulmonary Tuberculosis in the Northeast of the Yunnan Province, People's Republic of China." *Infectious Diseases of Poverty* 6 (1): 53. https://doi.org/10.1186/s40249-017-0268-4.

Jiang, Lei, and Minhe Ji. 2016. "China's Energy Intensity, Determinants and Spatial Effects." *Sustainability.* 8 (6): 544. https://doi.org/10.3390/su8060544.

Jiang, Xiushan, Lei Zhang, Chenfeng Xiong, and Ruijun Wang. 2016. "Transportation and Regional Economic Development: Analysis of Spatial Spillovers in China Provincial Regions." *Networks and Spatial Economics* 16 (3): 769–90. https://doi.org/10.1007/s11067-015-9298-2.

Jin, Jian, Jianxiang Wang, Xiaoyi Ma, Yuding Wang, and Renyong Li. 2015. "Equality of Medical Health Resource Allocation in China Based on the Gini Coefficient Method." *Iranian Journal of Public Health* 44 (4): 445–57.

Kanchanachitra, Churnrurtai, Magnus Lindelow, Timothy Johnston, Piya Hanvoravongchai, Fely Marilyn Lorenzo, Nguyen Lan Huong, Siswanto Agus Wilopo, and Jennifer Frances Dela Rosa. 2011. "Human Resources for Health in Southeast Asia: Shortages, Distributional Challenges, and International Trade in Health Services." *The Lancet* 377 (9767): 769–81. https://doi.org/10.1016/S0140-6736(10)62035-1.

Kang, Yan Qing, Tao Zhao, and Peng Wu. 2016. "Impacts of Energy-Related CO2 Emissions in China: A Spatial Panel Data Technique." *Natural Hazards.* 81 (1): 405–21. https://doi.org/10.1007/s11069-015-2087-x.

King, K. R., R. A. Purcell, Stephen J. Quinn, A. M. Schoo, and L. K. Walters. 2016. "Supports for Medical Students during Rural Clinical Placements: Factors Associated with Intention to Practise in Rural Locations." *Rural and Remote Health* 16 (2): 1–9.

Kreng, Victor B, and Chi-Tien Yang. 2011. "The Equality of Resource Allocation in Health Care under the National Health Insurance System in Taiwan." *Health Policy* 100: 203–10. https://doi.org/10.1016/j.healthpol.2010.08.003.

Laurence, Caroline O, and Jonathan Karnon. 2016. "Improving the Planning of the GP Workforce in Australia: A Simulation Model Incorporating Work Transitions, Health Need and Service Usage." *Human Resources for Health* 14: 13. https://doi.org/10.1186/s12960-016-0110-2.

Lee, Donghoon, and Kenneth I. Wolpin. 2010. "Accounting for Wage and Employment Changes in the US from 1968-2000: A Dynamic Model of Labor Market Equilibrium." *Journal of Econometrics* 156 (1): 68–85. https://doi.org/10.1016/j.jeconom.2009.09.008.

Lesage, James, and R. Kelly Pace. 2009. *Introduction to Spatial Econometrics*. Boca Raton: CRC Press.

Li, Dan, Zhongliang Zhou, Yafei Si, Yongjian Xu, Chi Shen, Yiyang Wang, and Xiao Wang. 2018. "Unequal Distribution of Health Human Resource in Mainland China: What Are the Determinants from a Comprehensive Perspective?" *International Journal for Equity in Health* 17 (1): 1–12. https://doi.org/10.1186/s12939-018-0742-z.

Li, Qian, Jinping Song, Enru Wang, Hao Hu, Jianhui Zhang, and Yeyao Wang. 2014. "Economic Growth and Pollutant Emissions in China: A Spatial Econometric Analysis." *Stochastic Environmental Research and Risk Assessment* 28 (2): 429–42. https://doi.org/10.1007/s00477-013-0762-6.

Li, Tongtong, Trudy Lei, Zheng Xie, and Tuohong Zhang. 2016. "Determinants of Basic Public Health Services Provision by Village Doctors in China: Using Non-Communicable Diseases Management as an Example Health Policy, Reform, Governance and Law." *BMC Health Services Research* 16 (1): 1–10. https://doi.org/10.1186/s12913-016-1276-y.

Liu, Jinlin, Bin Zhu, and Ying Mao. 2018. "Association between Rural Clinical Clerkship and Medical Students' Intentions to Choose Rural Medical Work after Graduation: A Cross-Sectional Study in Western China." *PloS ONE* 13 (4): e0195266. https://doi.org/10.1371/journal.pone.0195266.

Liu, Wen, Ying Liu, Peter Twum, and Shixue Li. 2016. "National Equity of Health Resource Allocation in China: Data from 2009 to 2013." *International Journal for Equity in Health* 15 (1): 68. https://doi.org/10.1186/s12939-016-0357-1.

Liu, Yu, Hongwei Xiao, Precious Zikhali, and Yingkang Lv. 2014. "Carbon Emissions in China: A Spatial Econometric Analysis at the Regional Level." *Sustainability* 6 (9): 6005–23. https://doi.org/10.3390/su6096005.

Long, Ruyin, Tianxiang Shao, and Hong Chen. 2016. "Spatial Econometric Analysis of China's Province-Level Industrial Carbon Productivity and Its Influencing Factors." *Applied Energy* 166: 210–19. https://doi.org/10.1016/j.apenergy.2015.09.100.

Lv, Yipeng, Chen Xue, Yang Ge, Feng Ye, Xu Liu, Yuan Liu, and Lulu Zhang. 2016. "Analysis of Factors Influencing Inpatient and Outpatient Satisfaction with the Chinese Military Health Service." *PLoS ONE* 11 (3): 1–13. https://doi.org/10.1371/journal.pone.0151234.

Mandeville, Kate L., Mylène Lagarde, Kara Hanson, and Anne Mills. 2016. "Human Resources for Health: Time to Move out of Crisis Mode." *The Lancet* 388 (10041): 220–22. https://doi.org/10.1016/S0140-6736(16)30952-7.

McGrail, Matthew R, and John S Humphreys. 2009. "Geographical Classifications to Guide Rural Health Policy in Australia." *Australia and New Zealand Health Policy* 6 (1): 28. https://doi.org/10.1186/1743-8462-6-28.

McPake, Barbara, Anthony Scott, Ijeoma Edoka, Barbara McPake, and Anthony Scott. 2014. *Analyzing Markets for Health Workers: Insights from Labor and Health Economics*. Washington, D.C.: World Bank. https://doi.org/10.1596/978-1-4648-0224-9.

McRae, Ian, and James R G Butler. 2014. "Supply and Demand in Physician Markets: A Panel Data Analysis of GP Services in Australia." *International Journal of Health Care Finance and Economics* 14 (3): 269–87. https://doi.org/10.1007/s10754-014-9148-7.

Murphy, Tomblin Gail, Adrian MacKenzie, Joan Guy-Walker, and Claudette Walker. 2014. "Needs-Based Human Resources for Health Planning in Jamaica: Using Simulation Modelling to Inform Policy Options for Pharmacists in the Public Sector." *Human Resources for Health.* 12 (1): 67. https://doi.org/10.1186/1478-4491-12-67.

National Health and Family Planning Commission of the PRC. 2011. "*Long-Term Medical Personnel Development Plan (2011-2020)*." Beijing.

National Health and Family Planning Commission of the PRC. 2018. *China Health and Family Planning Statistical Yearbook 2018*. Beijing: Chinese Peking Union Medical College Press.

National Ministry of Health of the PRC. 2007. *China Health Statistical Yearbook 2007*. Beijing: Chinese Peking Union Medical College Press.

O'Brien-Pallas, Linda, Andrea Baumann, Gail Donner, Gail Tomblin Murphy, Jacquelyn Lochhaas-Gerlach, and Marcia Luba. 2001. "Forecasting Models for Human Resources in Health Care." *Journal of Advanced Nursing* 33 (1): 120–29. https://doi.org/10.1046/j.1365-2648.2001.01645.x.

Parsons, Donna. 2010. "Medical-Workforce Planning:An Art or Science?" *Human Resource Management International Digest* 18 (5): 36. https://doi.org/10.1108/09670731011060289.

Pietrzak, Michał Bernard. 2014. "The Modifiable Areal Unit Problem—Analysis of Correlation and Regression." *Quarterly Journal of Economics and Economic Policy* 9 (4): 87–100.

Qi, Jiangyi. 2016. "Government Education Expenditure, Third-Party Spillover Effect and Economic Growth in China." *Journal of Sustainable Development* 9 (2): 145. https://doi.org/10.5539/jsd.v9n2p145.

Ranson, Michael Kent, Mickey Chopra, Salla Atkins, Mario Roberto Dal Poz, and Sara Bennett. 2010. "Priorities for Research into Human Resources for Health in Low- and Middle-Income Countries." *Bulletin of the World Health Organization* 88 (6): 435–43. https://doi.org/10.2471/BLT.09.066290.

Scholz, Stefan, Johann-Matthias Schulenburg, and Wolfgang Greiner. 2015. "Regional Differences of Outpatient Physician Supply as a Theoretical Economic and Empirical Generalized Linear Model." *Human Resources for Health* 13 (1): 85. https://doi.org/10.1186/s12960-015-0088-1.

Serneels, Pieter, Magnus Lindelow, Jose Garcia-Montalvo, and Abigail Barr. 2007. "For Public Service or Money: Understanding Geographical Imbalances in the Health Workforce." *Health Policy and Planning* 22 (3): 128. http://www.gprg.org/.

Shadmi, Efrat, William C W Wong, Karen Kinder, Iona Heath, and Michael Kidd. 2014. "Primary Care Priorities in Addressing Health Equity: Summary of the WONCA 2013 Health Equity Workshop." *International Journal for Equity in Health* 13: 104. https://doi.org/10.1186/s12939-014-0104-4.

Shamian, Judith, Gail Tomblin Murphy, Annette Elliott Rose, and Lianne Jeffs. 2015. "Human Resources for Health: A New Narrative." *The Lancet* 386 (9988): 25–26. https://doi.org/10.1016/S0140-6736(15)61195-3.

Sheldon, Trevor A., and Peter C. Smith. 2000. "Equity in the Allocation of Health Care Resources." *Health Economics* 9 (7): 571–74. https://doi.org/10.1002/1099-1050(200010)9:7<571::AID-HEC555>3.0.CO;2-8.

Shetty, Anil, and Shraddha Shetty. 2014. "The Correlation of Physician to Population Ratio and Life Expectancy in Asian Countries." *Journal of Medical Science and Clinical Research* 2 (4): 699–706.

Somers, George T., Roger Strasser, and Brian Jolly. 2007. "What Does It Take? The Influence of Rural Upbringing and Sense of Rural Background on Medical Students' Intention to Work in a Rural Environment." *Rural and Remote Health* 7 (2): 706. https://doi.org/706 [pii].

Song, Peige, Zhenghong Ren, Xinlei Chang, Xuebei Liu, and Lin An. 2016. "Inequality of Paediatric Workforce Distribution in China." *International Journal of Environmental Research and Public Health* 13 (7). https://doi.org/10.3390/ijerph13070703.

Sun, Jian, and Hongye Luo. 2017. "Evaluation on Equality and Efficiency of Health Resources Allocation and Health Services Utilization in China." *International Journal for Equity in Health* 16 (1): 127. https://doi.org/10.1186/s12939-017-0614-y.

Sun, Xiangyu, Eduardo Bernabé, Xuenan Liu, Shuguo Zheng, and Jennifer E. Gallagher. 2017. "Meeting the Oral Health Needs of 12-Year-Olds in China: Human Resources for Oral Health." *BMC Public Health* 17 (1): 1–12. https://doi.org/10.1186/s12889-017-4384-7.

Tang, Chengxiang, Yucheng Zhang, Lieping Chen, and Yongqiang Lin. 2014. "The Growth of Private Hospitals and Their Health Workforce in China: A Comparison with Public Hospitals." *Health Policy and Planning* 29 (1): 30–41. https://doi.org/10.1093/heapol/czs130.

Tao, Y, K Henry, Q Zou, and X Zhong. 2014. "Methods for Measuring Horizontal Equity in Health Resource Allocation: A Comparative Study." *Health Econ Rev* 4 (1): 10. http://www.ncbi.nlm.nih.gov/pubmed/26054400.

Theodorakis, Pavlos N., Georgios D. Mantzavinis, Llukan Rrumbullaku, Christos Lionis, and Erik Trell. 2006. "Measuring Health Inequalities in Albania: A Focus on the Distribution of General Practitioners." *Human Resources for Health* 4: 1–9. https://doi.org/10.1186/1478-4491-4-5.

Thongdara, Romanee, Lal Samarakoon, Rajendra P. Shrestha, and S. L. Ranamukhaarachchi. 2012. "Using GIS and Spatial Statistics to Target Poverty and Improve Poverty Alleviation Programs: A Case Study in Northeast Thailand." *Applied Spatial Analysis and Policy* 5 (2): 157–82. https://doi.org/10.1007/s12061-011-9066-8.

Tokuhata, G. K., P. Newman, E. Digon, L. A. Mann, T. HArtman, and K. Ramaswamy. 1975. "Health Manpower Distribution in Pennsylvania." *American Journal of Public Health* 65 (8): 837–48. https://doi.org/10.2105/AJPH.65.8.837.

Travnikar, T, and L Juvancic. 2015. "*A Winding Road from Investment Support to the Economic Growth of Farms: Evidence from Spatial Econometric Analysis of Agricultural Holdings in Slovenia*" 21 (1): 16–25.

United Nations. 2015. "*Transforming Our World: The 2030 Agenda for Sustainable Development.*" https://doi.org/10.1007/s13398-014-0173-7.2.

Vujicic, Marko, and Pascal Zurn. 2006. "The Dynamics of the Health Labour Market." *International Journal of Health Planning and Management* 21 (2): 101–15. https://doi.org/10.1002/hpm.834.

Wang, Chan, and You Hua Chen. 2017. "Reimbursement and Hospital Competition in China." *Economic Research-Ekonomska Istrazivanja* 30 (1): 1209–23. https://doi.org/10.1080/1331677X.2017.1340177.

Wang, Wei, and David Zakus. 2016. "Healthy China 2030: 'Without National Health, There Will Be No Comprehensive Well-Being.'" *Family Medicine and Community Health* 4 (4): 75–76. https://doi.org/10.15212/FMCH.2016.0126.

Waters, Hugh R. 2000. "Measuring Equity in Access to Health Care." *Social Science & Medicine* 51 (4): 599–612. https://doi.org/10.1016/S0277-9536(00)00003-4.

WHO. 1996. "Equity in Health and Health Care: A WHO/SIDA Initiative." Genova, Switzerland.

WHO. 2004. "*Guidance on Ethics and Equitable Access to HIV Treatment and Care*." Genova: WHO. Genova, Switzerland.

WHO. 2006a. "*Reassessing the Relationship between Human Resources for Health, Intervention Coverage and Health Outcomes.*" Genova, Switherland. https://doi.org/10.1097/00007890-200607152-01424.

WHO. 2006b. "*World Health Report 2006: Working Togehther for Health*." Genova, Switherland. https://doi.org/10.1186/1471-2458-5-67.

WHO. 2008a. "Closing the Gap in a Generation: Health Equity through Action on the Social Determinants of Health." *The Lancet* 372 (9650): 1661–69. https://doi.org/10.1016/S0140-6736(08)61690-6.

WHO. 2008b. "Establishing and Monitoring Benchmarks for Human Resources for Health: The Workforce Density Approach." *Spotlight on Health Workforce Statistics*. Genova, Switzerland. http://www.who.int/hrh/statistics/spotlight/en/index.html.

WHO. 2010a. "*Models and Tools for Health Workforce Planning and Projections.*" World Health Organisation. Genova, Switzerland.

WHO. 2010b. "The World Health Report: Health System Financing." *WHO.* Genova, Switherland. https://doi.org/10.1103/PhysRevD.88.032001.

WHO. 2010c. "*Workload Indicators of Staffing Need (WISN) User's Manual.*" Geneva, Switzerland.

WHO. 2013. "*A Universal Truth: No Health Without a Workforce.*" Genova, Switherland.

WHO. 2015. "*Health in 2015: From MDGs to SDGs.*" Genova, Switherland.

WHO. 2016. "*Global Strategy on Human Resources for Health: Workforce 2030.*" Genova, Switzerland.

Wiseman, Virginia, Mylene Lagarde, Neha Batura, Sophia Lin, Wayne Irava, and Graham Roberts. 2017. "Measuring Inequalities in the Distribution of the Fiji Health Workforce." *International Journal for Equity in Health* 16 (1): 1–8. https://doi.org/10.1186/s12939-017-0575-1.

Wu, Xinrui, Shixiong Hu, Abuaku Benjamin Kwaku, Qi Li, Kaiwei Luo, Ying Zhou, and Hongzhuan Tan. 2017. "Spatio-Temporal Clustering Analysis and Its Determinants of Hand, Foot and Mouth Disease in Hunan, China, 2009-2015." *BMC Infectious Diseases* 17 (1): 1–9. https://doi.org/10.1186/s12879-017-2742-9.

Yajuan, Dong. 2010. "The Spillover Effect of Education on Productivity: Evidence from China." *2010 International Conference on E-Education, e-Business, e-Management and e-Learning*, 420–24. https://doi.org/10.1109/IC4E.2010.64.

Yang, Yang, and Kevin K. F. Wong. 2012. "A Spatial Econometric Approach to Model Spillover Effects in Tourism Flows." *Journal of Travel Research* 51 (6): 768–78. https://doi.org/10.1177/0047287512437855.

Yip, Winnie Chi Man, William C. Hsiao, Wen Chen, Shanlian Hu, Jin Ma, and Alan Maynard. 2012. "Early Appraisal of China's Huge and Complex Health-Care Reforms." *The Lancet* 379 (9818): 833–42. https://doi.org/10.1016/S0140-6736(11)61880-1.

Zaman, Rashid Uz, Isla Gemmell, and Tomas Lievens. 2014. "Factors Affecting Health Worker Density: Evidence from a Quantitative Cross-Country Analysis." *SSRN Electronic Journal*, no. 12: 1–17. https://doi.org/10.2139/ssrn.2541690.

Zhang, Xinyu, Lin Zhao, Zhuang Cui, and Yaogang Wang. 2015. "Study on Equity and Efficiency of Health Resources and Services Based on Key Indicators in China." *PLoS ONE* 10 (12): 1–15. https://doi.org/10.1371/journal.pone.0144809.

Zhang, Yimin, and Xueshan Feng. 2011. "The Relationship between Job Satisfaction, Burnout, and Turnover Intention among Physicians from Urban State-Owned Medical Institutions in Hubei, China: A Cross-Sectional Study." *BMC Health Services Research* 11 (1): 235. https://doi.org/10.1186/1472-6963-11-235.

Zhao, Hongyan, Qiang Zhang, Hong Huo, Jintai Lin, Zhu Liu, Haikun Wang, Dabo Guan, and Kebin He. 2016. "Environment-Economy Tradeoff for Beijing–Tianjin–Hebei's Exports." *Applied Energy* 184: 926–35. https://doi.org/10.1016/j.apenergy.2016.04.038.

Zhao, P. S., F. Dong, D. He, X. J. Zhao, X. L. Zhang, W. Z. Zhang, Q. Yao, and H. Y. Liu. 2013. "Characteristics of Concentrations and Chemical Compositions for PM2.5 in the Region of Beijing, Tianjin, and Hebei, China." *Atmospheric Chemistry and Physics* 13 (9): 4631–44. https://doi.org/10.5194/acp-13-4631-2013.

Zhou, Kaiyuan, Xinyi Zhang, Yi Ding, Duolao Wang, Zhou Lu, and Min Yu. 2015. "Inequality Trends of Health Workforce in Different Stages of Medical System Reform (1985-2011) in China." *Human Resources for Health* 13 (1): 94. https://doi.org/10.1186/s12960-015-0089-0.

Zhou, Zhimin, Xinyue Ye, and Xiangyu Ge. 2017. "The Impacts of Technical Progress on Sulfur Dioxide Kuznets Curve in China: A Spatial Panel Data Approach." *Sustainability.* 9 (4): 674. https://doi.org/10.3390/su9040674.

Zhu, Bin, Yang Fu, Jinlin Liu, Rongxin He, Ning Zhang, and Ying Mao. 2018. "Detecting the Priority Areas for Health Workforce Allocation with LISA Functions : An Empirical Analysis for China." *BMC Health Services Research* 18: 957.

Zhu, Bin, Yang Fu, Jinlin Liu, and Ying Mao. 2017. "Notifiable Sexually Transmitted Infections in China: Epidemiologic Trends and Spatial Changing Patterns." *Sustainability* 9 (10): 1–16. https://doi.org/10.3390/su9101784.

Zhu, Bin, Yang Fu, Jinlin Liu and Ying Mao. 2018. "Modeling the Dynamics and Spillovers of the Health Labor Market: Evidence from China's Provincial Panel Data." *Sustainability* 10 (2): 333. https://doi.org/10.3390/su10020333.

Zhu, Bin, Chih-Wei Hsieh, and Yue Zhang. 2018. "Incorporating Spatial Statistics into Examining Equity in Health Workforce Distribution: An Empirical Analysis in the Chinese Context." *International Journal of Environmental Research and Public Health* 15 (7): 1309. https://doi.org/10.3390/ijerph15071309.

Zhu, Bin, Jinlin Liu, Yang Fu, Bo Zhang, and Ying Mao. 2018. "Spatio-Temporal Epidemiology of Viral Hepatitis in China (2003–2015): Implications for Prevention and Control Policies." *International Journal of Environmental Research and Public Health* 15 (4): 661. https://doi.org/10.3390/ijerph15040661.

Zhu, Jiming, Wenkai Li, and Lincoln Chen. 2016. "Doctors in China: Improving Quality through Modernisation of Residency Education." *The Lancet* 388 (10054): 1922–29. https://doi.org/10.1016/S0140-6736(16)00582-1.

APPENDICES

APPENDIX A. ORIGINAL DATA

- Table A1 Health technicians stock in each provincial unit during 2007–2016.
- Table A2 Licensed doctors stock in each provincial unit during 2007–2016.
- Table A3 Clinicians stock in each provincial unit during 2007–2016.
- Table A4 Traditional Chinese Medicine doctors stock in each provincial unit during 2007–2016.
- Table A5 Dentists stock in each provincial unit during 2007–2016.
- Table A6 Public Health doctors stock in each provincial unit during 2007–2016.
- Table A7 General Practitioners stock in each provincial unit during 2007–2016.
- Table A8 Registered nurses stock in each provincial unit during 2007–2016.
- Table A9 Pharmacists stock in each provincial unit during 2007–2016.
- Table A10 Technologists stock in each provincial unit during 2007–2016.
- Table A11 Interns stock in each provincial unit during 2007–2016.

- Table A12 Number of population in each provincial unit during 2007–2016.
- Table A13 Urban health technicians stock in each provincial unit during 2007–2016.
- Table A14 Urban licensed doctors stock in each provincial unit during 2007–2016.
- Table A15 Urban registered nurses stock in each provincial unit during 2007–2016.
- Table A16 Urban pharmacists stock in each provincial unit during 2007–2016.
- Table A17 Urban technologists stock in each provincial unit during 2007–2016.
- Table A18 Urban interns stock in each provincial unit during 2007–2016.
- Table A19 Urban population in each provincial unit during 2007–2016.
- Table A20 Rural health technicians stock in each provincial unit during 2007–2016.
- Table A21 Rural licensed doctors stock in each provincial unit during 2007–2016.
- Table A22 Rural registered nurses stock in each provincial unit during 2007–2016.
- Table A23 Rural pharmacists stock in each provincial unit during 2007–2016.
- Table A24 Rural technologists stock in each provincial unit during 2007–2016.
- Table A25 Rural interns stock in each provincial unit of China during 2007–2016.
- Table A26 Rural population in each provincial unit during 2007–2016.

- Table A27 Government and social health expenditure in each provincial unit during 2012–2016.
- Table A28 Outpatient and inpatient visits in each provincial unit during 2012–2016.
- Table A29 The number of medical graduates in each provincial unit during 2012–2016.

Table A1. Health technicians stock in each provincial unit during 2007–2016

Region	2007	2008	2009	2010	2011	2012	2013	2014	2015	2016
Beijing	139706	150411	161139	171326	181936	196234	203741	213245	225440	233953
Tianjin	63579	65161	67930	70460	73318	77076	81083	84880	90748	94952
Hebei	243209	247451	268049	292157	301672	314933	333032	351513	372747	393059
Shanxi	145162	159591	186310	193891	191416	199601	203385	209474	213995	225880
Neimenggu	105790	109727	134988	125831	131603	139876	148202	154483	162327	170406
Liaoning	215491	217904	226425	232079	235623	246808	254692	256284	264419	277494
Jilin	125776	127905	132554	138393	139010	144065	145934	151427	158963	166605
Heilongjiang	158726	161939	175319	192048	195029	201155	207601	212207	215264	221362
Shanghai	120903	127471	132826	137131	140740	147807	157109	164054	170125	178196
Jiangsu	286482	291125	308981	328243	350544	395961	428894	458503	487005	516986
Zhejiang	228425	242908	266254	288481	306922	329565	352466	375902	405620	432641
Anhui	174724	187770	208584	211539	217591	236188	253532	268039	280768	293732
Fujian	94563	103341	130809	142916	158791	176074	197545	206516	212931	219557
Jiangxi	126598	139764	150741	158007	165938	179705	190092	201362	210927	220972
Shandong	340519	375817	414971	448861	481738	530082	596987	603785	618192	641701
Henan	297854	309923	359891	372818	396300	428508	468536	494815	519939	547001
Hubei	227116	233823	246985	255793	268122	288695	309343	335583	367902	384532
Hunan	220578	232084	253547	269219	282511	296857	323082	341404	370788	392547
Guangdong	360656	384134	421325	454799	485585	518414	553728	583009	617975	665257
Guangxi	145579	155620	172910	189554	204011	220761	240892	258599	274659	289872
Hainan	32545	33875	37857	39520	43295	45060	48108	50580	54710	57522
Chongqing	83650	88744	100008	111079	120151	131658	142133	154278	166708	179354
Sichuan	255332	267591	303051	325608	352259	389440	426988	451938	472169	495750
Guizhou	85282	89313	96753	103954	113801	129772	155905	169963	187282	204621
Yunnan	123732	126237	135207	143139	150982	166764	193217	208905	227998	249677
Xizang	8069	9435	10115	10083	10782	9336	11638	12882	14341	14829
Shaanxi	141687	148328	171840	181438	197173	216293	239054	252611	265381	288607
Gansu	85348	87633	91255	98865	105908	111609	118089	126396	129454	134641
Qinghai	20337	21745	24044	24909	27520	29311	32431	33936	35422	37010
Ningxia	25521	26415	28428	29962	31983	34250	37288	39800	41497	44700
Xinjiang	104671	106853	116028	124055	130604	136691	145851	153417	161841	170987
SUM	4787610	5030038	5535124	5866158	6192858	6668549	7200578	7579790	7997537	8444403

Unit: Person

Table A2. Licensed doctors stock in each provincial unit during 2007–2016

Region	2007	2008	2009	2010	2011	2012	2013	2014	2015	2016
Beijing	55285	59053	62853	66163	69747	74380	77114	79949	85232	89411
Tianjin	26045	25890	27590	28892	29831	30690	32059	33340	35871	37804
Hebei	108224	109968	124127	133994	136801	142989	150144	157725	166881	177140
Shanxi	64661	72259	84705	88007	84818	87319	88182	89835	90216	91699
Neimenggu	48403	49542	69197	56245	57145	59528	62055	62182	64238	66391
Liaoning	90631	90714	95678	96862	97744	100972	103344	101636	104552	109800
Jilin	56960	57523	60152	62050	59581	61400	61998	63234	67245	69666
Heilongjiang	66984	66771	74178	80282	76780	78589	80475	81371	82708	84422
Shanghai	48855	51047	53024	53009	53751	55797	57944	61202	62983	65386
Jiangsu	118814	119461	125220	128943	134683	157902	169641	178551	189216	204647
Zhejiang	98016	101893	113852	120440	124497	129973	138279	145725	158056	168178
Anhui	69132	73826	84778	86511	84696	92061	98613	103742	107792	112741
Fujian	40114	43013	55066	58630	62484	66740	72642	75324	77984	79685
Jiangxi	51828	55187	59325	61887	62839	67077	70251	74647	76807	79187
Shandong	147162	159809	176193	185164	186034	200465	231754	230883	237118	244900
Henan	115900	119316	150990	154801	156664	167608	180600	189335	198616	206747
Hubei	92242	92037	97869	99542	102094	109149	117191	126123	135997	141741
Hunan	92527	96305	105790	110444	112630	116440	127241	133372	150840	160627
Guangdong	138293	144467	161401	174536	186161	198966	210306	216799	228539	243224
Guangxi	58160	60825	66813	70816	74153	78043	83310	86525	91585	96673
Hainan	12587	12850	14117	14456	15527	15525	16725	17609	19002	19874
Chongqing	38718	39415	44627	47969	49571	51990	55141	58084	60973	64709
Sichuan	117155	121851	138685	145194	153795	162877	173890	179523	181480	185414
Guizhou	37873	38830	41465	43389	45415	49179	55959	57845	63384	69007
Yunnan	56586	57276	60509	63306	64684	68466	74860	75426	79567	85876
Xizang	3853	4376	4552	4469	4175	4043	5176	5609	6213	6542
Shaanxi	59313	58264	69745	66040	65740	69471	74397	76460	79496	85681
Gansu	35144	36176	37646	39331	40870	42956	44887	47681	49610	52791
Qinghai	8713	9414	10221	10564	11396	11918	13239	12953	13791	13670
Ningxia	11185	11444	12088	12267	12258	13011	14317	15023	15860	17070
Xinjiang	43551	43456	46750	49056	49530	50540	53020	54805	57283	60302
SUM	2012914	2082258	2329206	2413259	2466094	2616064	2794754	2892518	3039135	3191005

Unit: Person

Table A3. Clinicians stock in each provincial unit during 2007–2016

Region	2012	2013	2014	2015	2016
Beijing	51810	53519	55570	58701	60897
Tianjin	22747	23537	24308	25607	26895
Hebei	114438	119170	125112	131040	138825
Shanxi	66717	66737	67778	67548	68360
Neimenggu	42683	44095	44073	44328	45960
Liaoning	78648	80474	78870	81223	85248
Jilin	47026	47234	47938	50524	52127
Heilongjiang	61884	63491	63885	64767	66053
Shanghai	42352	44103	46144	47583	49370
Jiangsu	125039	134371	141761	150026	161509
Zhejiang	101142	106192	111008	119086	126150
Anhui	75201	80705	84919	88529	92421
Fujian	49324	53388	55339	57144	57344
Jiangxi	52388	55181	58744	60360	62464
Shandong	159484	184020	181179	183794	189639

Region	2012	2013	2014	2015	2016
Henan	134252	143413	149291	156089	161824
Hubei	87771	94507	101473	109722	114104
Hunan	93313	101351	106590	121079	128589
Guangdong	152754	160446	164123	171728	181339
Guangxi	61154	64762	66765	70323	73871
Hainan	12612	13477	14058	15187	15954
Chongqing	37465	39326	41759	43819	46404
Sichuan	115318	122684	126125	124683	127125
Guizhou	39112	44461	45737	49816	54449
Yunnan	53445	58400	58740	62151	66926
Xizang	2597	3468	3994	4364	4445
Shaanxi	54531	58249	59658	62027	66494
Gansu	29934	30810	32759	33919	36474
Qinghai	9092	10060	9834	10492	10329
Ningxia	9803	10853	11398	11905	12762
Xinjiang	39399	41609	42677	44539	46148
SUM	2023435	2154093	2221609	2322103	2430499

Unit: Person

Table A4. TCM doctor stock in each provincial unit during 2007–2016

Region	2012	2013	2014	2015	2016
Beijing	13196	14073	14652	15947	17010
Tianjin	5345	5642	5977	6863	7341
Hebei	19955	21583	22476	25162	26831
Shanxi	13383	13611	13986	14203	14625
Neimenggu	10669	11204	11474	12926	13367
Liaoning	11499	11549	11666	12136	12906
Jilin	7893	8095	8402	9185	9671
Heilongjiang	9041	9313	9683	10009	10409
Shanghai	6183	6385	7118	7450	7822
Jiangsu	17457	19021	20038	21472	24122
Zhejiang	16696	18641	20321	22874	24687
Anhui	9970	10771	11468	11837	12479
Fujian	10710	11785	12349	12901	13785
Jiangxi	9353	9850	10547	11053	11466
Shandong	22980	27018	28393	31235	32203
Henan	22876	25707	27852	29702	31685
Hubei	13050	13775	14708	15963	16896
Hunan	16255	17947	18604	20744	22449
Guangdong	27868	29668	30903	33401	36079
Guangxi	9986	11029	11883	12874	14191
Hainan	1410	1576	1724	1893	1957
Chongqing	10866	11779	12046	12794	13742
Sichuan	36487	39518	41444	45132	46594
Guizhou	6118	6938	7528	8549	9338
Yunnan	8404	9342	9382	9973	11002
Xizang	999	1126	998	1169	1298
Shaanxi	10019	10841	11182	11533	12593
Gansu	9983	10668	11352	12039	12619
Qinghai	2036	2261	2309	2448	2499
Ningxia	1717	1791	1838	1994	2176
Xinjiang	5860	5777	6270	6729	7748
SUM	368264	398284	418573	452190	481590

Unit: Person

Table A5. Dentists stock in each provincial unit during 2007–2016

Region	2012	2013	2014	2015	2016
Beijing	6223	6482	6832	7603	8327
Tianjin	1553	1779	1936	2168	2360
Hebei	5262	6026	6652	7330	8102
Shanxi	4082	4348	4615	5167	5572
Neimenggu	2703	3044	3165	3628	3879
Liaoning	6150	6760	6828	7088	7568
Jilin	3850	4016	4359	4961	5285
Heilongjiang	4902	4960	5145	5275	5372
Shanghai	3887	4174	4499	4548	4744
Jiangsu	7224	7804	8223	8880	9979
Zhejiang	7354	8540	9386	10972	12073
Anhui	2837	3022	3323	3536	3853
Fujian	3643	4195	4440	4743	5322
Jiangxi	1831	2000	2219	2283	2326
Shandong	8418	10522	11898	13182	14282
Henan	5154	5780	6339	6967	7505
Hubei	4196	4549	5212	5742	6140
Hunan	2579	3243	3493	3996	4511
Guangdong	10413	11488	12646	14010	15726
Guangxi	3434	3781	4172	4719	5036
Hainan	781	852	918	1024	1114
Chongqing	1973	2314	2445	2674	2870
Sichuan	5482	6144	6696	6821	7316
Guizhou	1543	1815	1983	2269	2472
Yunnan	2742	3015	3311	3505	3943
Xizang	105	128	123	143	160
Shaanxi	2840	3152	3540	3925	4381
Gansu	1533	1662	1796	1892	2035
Qinghai	350	370	421	436	416
Ningxia	815	966	1061	1175	1326
Xinjiang	2366	2573	2778	2932	3232
SUM	116225	129504	140454	153594	167227

Unit: Person

Table A6. Public health doctors stock in each provincial unit during 2007–2016

Region	2012	2013	2014	2015	2016
Beijing	3151	3040	2895	2981	3177
Tianjin	1045	1101	1119	1233	1208
Hebei	3334	3365	3485	3349	3382
Shanxi	3137	3486	3456	3298	3142
Neimenggu	3473	3712	3470	3356	3185
Liaoning	4675	4561	4272	4105	4078
Jilin	2631	2653	2535	2575	2583
Heilongjiang	2762	2711	2658	2657	2588
Shanghai	3375	3282	3441	3402	3450
Jiangsu	8182	8445	8529	8838	9037
Zhejiang	4781	4906	5010	5124	5268
Anhui	4053	4115	4032	3890	3988
Fujian	3063	3274	3196	3196	3234
Jiangxi	3505	3220	3137	3111	2931
Shandong	9583	10194	9413	8907	8776

Region	2012	2013	2014	2015	2016
Henan	5326	5700	5853	5858	5733
Hubei	4132	4360	4730	4570	4601
Hunan	4293	4700	4685	5021	5078
Guangdong	7931	8704	9127	9400	10080
Guangxi	3469	3738	3705	3669	3575
Hainan	722	820	909	898	849
Chongqing	1686	1722	1834	1686	1693
Sichuan	5590	5544	5258	4844	4379
Guizhou	2406	2745	2597	2750	2748
Yunnan	3875	4103	3993	3938	4005
Xizang	342	454	494	537	639
Shaanxi	2081	2155	2080	2011	2213
Gansu	1506	1747	1774	1760	1663
Qinghai	440	548	389	415	426
Ningxia	676	707	726	786	806
Xinjiang	2915	3061	3080	3083	3174
SUM	108140	112873	111882	111248	111689

Unit: Person

Table A7. General Practitioners stock in each provincial unit during 2007–2016

Region	2012	2013	2014	2015	2016
Beijing	8137	8458	8221	8269	8402
Tianjin	1095	1427	1622	2144	2403
Hebei	3493	6730	8637	9286	9355
Shanxi	2552	2958	3618	4014	4175
Neimenggu	1679	2374	2937	3085	3178
Liaoning	3304	3513	3777	3624	4195
Jilin	1231	1680	2299	2891	3384
Heilongjiang	2081	2889	3730	4320	4454
Shanghai	5323	5957	6925	7352	7967
Jiangsu	15068	17650	19748	20841	25162
Zhejiang	12251	17041	19640	21627	22571
Anhui	3191	4319	6814	7360	8625
Fujian	2594	3634	4310	5122	5786
Jiangxi	2081	2429	3020	3319	3641
Shandong	6775	7709	8967	9920	11372
Henan	4722	6427	8394	10349	12129
Hubei	3752	5044	6090	6970	7020
Hunan	2582	3928	5055	6121	6516
Guangdong	7940	11765	14404	14955	18338
Guangxi	3087	4039	4527	4671	5104
Hainan	421	580	728	875	986
Chongqing	1632	2187	2527	2872	3127
Sichuan	4665	8983	9819	10394	10360
Guizhou	1032	1511	2416	3147	3714
Yunnan	3212	4261	4106	4289	4737
Xizang	34	67	109	161	202
Shaanxi	1824	1978	2770	2126	2738
Gansu	1389	2106	2710	3312	3773
Qinghai	462	758	881	961	993
Ningxia	260	392	471	565	654
Xinjiang	1925	2717	3325	3707	4022
SUM	109794	145511	172597	188649	209083

Unit: Person

Table A8. Registered nurses stock in each provincial unit during 2007–2016

Region	2007	2008	2009	2010	2011	2012	2013	2014	2015	2016
Beijing	50955	55411	61709	67332	72812	79534	83879	88488	94626	98082
Tianjin	21325	21979	23089	24199	25814	27621	29715	31577	33804	36088
Hebei	65714	69038	74699	87351	93520	101988	111526	121845	132837	143432
Shanxi	44628	48765	57260	62628	64810	70337	74849	79055	83344	92112
Neimenggu	29732	31459	35414	38251	42494	46774	52358	56723	61223	66445
Liaoning	78172	80470	84498	88882	91912	98036	103409	105828	110976	119147
Jilin	40615	41066	42406	45776	47938	50975	52715	57433	60719	65749
Heilongjiang	48629	51353	55853	62759	66144	70073	73974	77720	80955	85418
Shanghai	46771	48758	52271	55866	58885	63245	67939	71929	75436	79373
Jiangsu	94630	100736	111039	122509	135602	155247	174158	188767	203998	221168
Zhejiang	71944	78284	88144	99610	109275	121313	132705	145141	159945	174523
Anhui	55081	60856	69959	77317	84454	95046	103404	111497	119303	126350
Fujian	33833	37760	47860	53511	62463	71124	79929	85664	90450	95641
Jiangxi	42508	48241	53653	58405	64440	72055	78209	84140	89579	95519
Shandong	109596	122866	139610	156692	170968	191721	240078	245711	254170	268379
Henan	90187	96571	112181	121384	137124	156041	176534	191117	205366	222123
Hubei	76868	80614	87334	93844	102114	115745	127871	144109	165077	174918
Hunan	66543	72551	83159	92346	101867	112906	125696	136247	149345	161531
Guangdong	128037	135922	153391	167882	182660	199534	217629	233483	254098	283793
Guangxi	51704	55992	62798	70243	76506	85515	94814	103955	113202	122602
Hainan	12444	13212	15225	16319	18200	19432	20892	22383	24662	26495
Chongqing	23933	26799	31881	37611	42765	49823	55460	62739	69954	77463
Sichuan	73456	77892	91164	104886	121266	139810	158457	175520	190602	207633
Guizhou	26503	28642	31984	36165	41589	48646	58666	67204	76032	85993
Yunnan	41040	42011	46329	49408	52315	60755	73305	82823	93278	105966
Xizang	1798	1920	2007	1988	2140	1732	2397	2715	3190	3833
Shaanxi	42515	46918	54836	61816	70225	79390	89551	97221	104317	116803
Gansu	24014	24950	26578	29868	33673	37202	40954	45472	47782	50530
Qinghai	6841	7280	7833	8339	9660	10026	11492	12750	13194	14364
Ningxia	8579	8897	9856	10341	11625	12504	13978	15096	16135	18069
Xinjiang	34662	36084	40798	44543	48760	52449	56578	59792	63870	67624
SUM	1543257	1653297	1854818	2048071	2244020	2496599	2783121	3004144	3241469	3507166

Unit: Person

Table A9. Pharmacists stock in each provincial unit during 2007–2016

Region	2007	2008	2009	2010	2011	2012	2013	2014	2015	2016
Beijing	8890	9195	9600	10250	10871	11578	12125	12744	13206	13682
Tianjin	4455	4341	4512	4561	4699	4843	5059	5193	5376	5579
Hebei	13708	13533	13532	14067	13888	14040	14415	14975	15657	16418
Shanxi	8716	9388	10052	10173	9934	9973	9942	10045	9840	10385
Neimenggu	7530	7695	8543	8919	9276	9496	9546	9668	10271	10429
Liaoning	13669	13686	13520	13607	13329	13273	13427	13214	13272	13463
Jilin	7755	7824	7934	8077	8094	7964	7924	7794	7903	7933
Heilongjiang	10128	9956	10303	11086	11145	11141	11455	11390	11479	11550
Shanghai	7037	7236	7495	7577	7929	8281	8780	9225	9498	9779
Jiangsu	20143	20042	20501	21352	22122	23308	24226	25521	26454	27757
Zhejiang	17086	17212	17998	19167	20339	21613	23036	24451	25763	26872
Anhui	10375	10778	11005	10919	11002	11817	12276	12909	13456	13875
Fujian	7380	7947	9415	9954	10727	11767	13323	13794	13866	14336
Jiangxi	10916	11676	11683	12207	12407	13013	13418	13700	14021	14246
Shandong	25789	26105	26700	27853	28827	30315	31038	31741	32304	33395

Region	2007	2008	2009	2010	2011	2012	2013	2014	2015	2016
Henan	19300	19472	20241	20488	20721	21401	22882	23963	24950	25904
Hubei	17873	17852	17717	17698	17689	17377	17652	17837	18222	18508
Hunan	19694	19679	19944	20071	20359	19639	20126	20321	20388	20684
Guangdong	28416	29256	30426	31520	32608	33910	35570	36548	37621	39311
Guangxi	8988	9067	9573	10326	10998	11893	13154	14353	15730	16693
Hainan	1786	1828	1928	2000	2161	2354	2539	2685	2831	2931
Chongqing	5550	5643	5911	6267	6437	6884	7209	7628	8181	8574
Sichuan	16543	16990	17870	18547	19417	20421	21637	22642	23275	23998
Guizhou	4216	4401	4633	4679	4898	5448	6336	6912	7600	8128
Yunnan	5905	6011	6217	6426	6783	7285	8136	8790	9569	10377
Xizang	350	394	412	451	495	428	540	593	636	654
Shaanxi	9353	9526	10167	10781	11522	12133	13095	13544	13979	14815
Gansu	4972	4859	4771	5082	5301	5588	5814	6056	6107	6222
Qinghai	1291	1378	1425	1457	1478	1550	1675	1729	1753	1915
Ningxia	1751	1834	1893	1990	2054	2108	2300	2376	2543	2722
Xinjiang	5647	5721	5989	6364	6483	6557	6923	7254	7543	8111
SUM	325212	330525	341910	353916	363993	377398	395578	409595	423294	439246

Unit: Person

Table A10. Technologists stock in each provincial unit during 2007–2016

Region	2007	2008	2009	2010	2011	2012	2013	2014	2015	2016
Beijing	8124	8752	9176	9507	10123	10318	10763	11291	11538	12150
Tianjin	3983	3944	4097	4139	4293	4298	4489	4697	4901	5250
Hebei	15127	15700	16035	17179	16762	16442	17394	17831	19084	20006
Shanxi	7924	8460	9622	10097	10204	10313	10510	11127	11126	11650
Neimenggu	5969	6295	6683	7028	7020	7407	7830	8235	8474	8743
Liaoning	13286	13602	13779	13924	13964	14047	14217	14297	14720	15383
Jilin	7256	7275	7588	7907	7786	7925	8004	7845	7956	8421
Heilongjiang	10320	10549	11062	12127	11904	12218	12474	12465	12807	12793
Shanghai	7779	8176	8202	8319	8104	8607	9091	9497	9966	10338
Jiangsu	17720	18128	18602	19261	19966	20868	21721	23063	24241	25685
Zhejiang	12912	13837	14440	15614	16126	16950	18047	19372	20477	21979
Anhui	11190	12196	13287	13426	13572	14362	15040	15908	16573	17111
Fujian	5565	5952	7126	7521	8197	9055	10007	10496	10917	11418
Jiangxi	8201	9392	9879	10578	10900	11653	12556	13212	14197	15095
Shandong	20942	22698	23846	25310	26348	27754	29582	30441	31567	33137
Henan	20387	21051	22638	23343	24399	24924	27411	29346	30631	32713
Hubei	14370	15003	15398	15532	15826	16017	16765	17520	18641	19038
Hunan	13119	14172	15155	15729	16432	16829	17997	19030	19983	20843
Guangdong	22028	23923	25250	26479	25994	27272	29158	29433	30899	32662
Guangxi	7793	8132	8767	9651	10168	11056	12297	13542	14759	15740
Hainan	2001	2005	2222	2278	2329	2398	2602	2649	2914	3120
Chongqing	4548	4715	5052	5433	5792	6288	6658	7210	7868	8748
Sichuan	13517	14058	15383	16090	17280	19193	21075	22093	23376	24932
Guizhou	4820	5179	5568	5927	6279	7263	8693	9562	10979	11883
Yunnan	6617	6928	7236	7670	8132	8987	10086	11130	12538	13625
Xizang	481	522	514	491	513	455	567	583	627	695
Shaanxi	9296	9679	10603	11490	12220	13334	14743	15734	16690	18539
Gansu	4747	5148	5329	5560	5779	5804	6029	6423	6698	7005
Qinghai	1200	1351	1531	1566	1612	1760	1905	2119	2025	2104
Ningxia	1481	1594	1670	1837	1857	1861	2051	2179	2307	2440
Xinjiang	6701	6876	7164	7742	7726	7984	8659	8966	9450	9939
SUM	289404	305292	322904	338755	347607	363642	388421	407296	428929	453185

Unit: Person

Table A11. Interns stock in each provincial unit during 2007–2016

Region	2007	2008	2009	2010	2011	2012	2013	2014	2015	2016
Beijing	16452	18000	17801	18074	18383	20424	19860	20773	20838	20628
Tianjin	7771	9007	8642	8669	8681	9624	9761	10073	10796	10231
Hebei	40436	39212	39656	39566	40701	39474	39553	39137	38288	36063
Shanxi	19233	20719	24671	22986	21650	21659	19902	19412	19469	20034
Neimenggu	14156	14736	15151	15388	15668	16671	16413	17675	18121	18398
Liaoning	19733	19432	18950	18804	18674	20480	20295	21309	20899	19701
Jilin	13190	14217	14474	14583	15611	15801	15293	15121	15140	14836
Heilongjiang	22665	23310	23923	25794	29056	29134	29223	29261	27315	27179
Shanghai	10461	12254	11834	12360	12071	11877	13355	12201	12242	13320
Jiangsu	35175	32758	33619	36178	38171	38636	39148	42601	43096	37729
Zhejiang	28467	31682	31820	33650	36685	39716	40399	41213	41379	41089
Anhui	28946	30114	29555	23366	23867	22902	24199	23983	23644	23655
Fujian	7671	8669	11342	13300	14920	17388	21644	21238	19714	18477
Jiangxi	13145	15268	16201	14930	15352	15907	15658	15663	16323	16925
Shandong	37030	44339	48622	53842	69561	79827	64535	65009	63033	61890
Henan	52080	53513	53841	52802	57392	58534	61109	61054	60376	59514
Hubei	25763	28317	28667	29177	30399	30407	29864	29994	29965	30327
Hunan	28695	29377	29499	30629	31223	31043	32022	32434	30232	28862
Guangdong	43882	50566	50857	54382	58162	58732	61065	66746	66818	66267
Guangxi	18934	21604	24959	28518	32186	34254	37317	40224	39383	38164
Hainan	3727	3980	4365	4467	5078	5351	5350	5254	5301	5102
Chongqing	10901	12172	12537	13799	15586	16673	17665	18617	19732	19860
Sichuan	34661	36800	39949	40891	40501	47139	51929	52160	53436	53773
Guizhou	11870	12261	13103	13794	15620	19236	26251	28440	29287	29610
Yunnan	13584	14011	14916	16329	19068	21271	26830	30736	33046	33833
Xizang	1587	2223	2630	2684	3459	2678	2958	3382	3675	3105
Shaanxi	21210	23941	26489	31311	37466	41965	47268	49652	50899	52769
Gansu	16471	16500	16931	19024	20285	20059	20405	20764	19257	18093
Qinghai	2292	2322	3034	2983	3374	4057	4120	4385	4659	4957
Ningxia	2525	2646	2921	3527	4189	4766	4642	5126	4652	4399
Xinjiang	14110	14716	15327	16350	18105	19161	20671	22600	23695	25011
SUM	616823	658666	686286	712157	771144	814846	838704	866237	864710	853801

Unit: Person

Table A12. Number of population in each provincial unit during 2007–2016

Region	2007	2008	2009	2010	2011	2012	2013	2014	2015	2016
Beijing	1633	1695	1755	1961	2019	2069	2115	2152	2171	2173
Tianjin	1115	1176	1228	1299	1355	1413	1472	1517	1547	1562
Hebei	6943	6988.82	7034	7194	7241	7288	7333	7384	7425	7470
Shanxi	3393	3410.61	3427	3574	3593	3611	3630	3648	3664	3682
Neimenggu	2405	2413.73	2458	2472	2482	2490	2498	2505	2511	2520
Liaoning	4298	4314.7	4341	4375	4383	4389	4390	4391	4382	4378
Jilin	2730	2734	2740	2747	2749	2750	2751	2752	2753	2733
Heilongjiang	3824	3825.39	3826	3833	3834	3834	3835	3833	3812	3799
Shanghai	1858	1888.46	2210	2303	2347	2380	2415	2426	2415	2420
Jiangsu	7625	7677.3	7810	7869	7899	7920	7939	7960	7976	7999
Zhejiang	5060	5120	5276	5447	5463	5477	5498	5508	5539	5590
Anhui	6118	6135	6131	5957	5968	5988	6030	6083	6144	6196
Fujian	3581	3604	3666	3693	3720	3748	3774	3806	3839	3874
Jiangxi	4368	4400	4432	4462	4488	4504	4522	4542	4566	4592
Shandong	9367	9417.23	9470	9588	9637	9685	9733	9789	9847	9947

Region	2007	2008	2009	2010	2011	2012	2013	2014	2015	2016
Henan	9360	9429	9487	9405	9388	9406	9413	9436	9480	9532
Hubei	5699	5711	5720	5728	5758	5779	5799	5816	5852	5885
Hunan	6355	6380	6406	6570	6596	6639	6691	6737	6783	6822
Guangdong	9449	9544	10130	10441	10505	10594	10644	10724	10849	10999
Guangxi	4768	4816	4856	4610	4645	4682	4719	4754	4796	4838
Hainan	845	854	864	869	877	887	895	903	911	917
Chongqing	2816	2839	2859	2885	2919	2945	2970	2991	3017	3048
Sichuan	8127	8138	8185	8045	8050	8076	8107	8140	8204	8262
Guizhou	3762	3792.73	3537	3479	3469	3484	3502	3508	3530	3555
Yunnan	4514	4543	4571	4602	4631	4659	4687	4714	4742	4771
Xizang	284	287	297	301	303	308	312	318	324	331
Shaanxi	3748	3762	3727	3735	3743	3753	3764	3775	3793	3813
Gansu	2617	2628.12	2555	2560	2564	2578	2582	2591	2600	2610
Qinghai	552	554.3	557	563	568	573	578	583	588	593
Ningxia	610	617.69	625	633	639	647	654	662	668	675
Xinjiang	2095	2130.8	2159	2185	2209	2233	2264	2298	2360	2398
SUM	132129	132802	133450	134091	134735	135404	136072	136782	137462	138271

Unit: 10 thousands

Table A13. Urban health technicians stock in each provincial unit during 2007–2016

Region	2007	2008	2009	2010	2011	2012	2013	2014	2015	2016
Beijing	135454	145803	156343	166064	176466	190692	197948	207455	219248	233627
Tianjin	56819	58520	60768	60796	63797	67270	71451	74720	80569	87682
Hebei	144909	146362	157373	119034	122161	128145	136657	149065	164119	181354
Shanxi	89929	99461	115302	98179	97816	103687	107714	111876	116539	125427
Neimenggu	63856	66138	72525	58571	61954	67126	72873	76121	81500	86863
Liaoning	184230	185892	192388	155139	158203	166586	173309	177254	182863	197368
Jilin	98305	100052	103713	62468	61454	63770	65284	69605	77564	82569
Heilongjiang	118306	120657	131953	107948	110362	113492	117111	121203	123390	126899
Shanghai	117838	124290	129081	131843	135439	142618	151885	158915	164975	173076
Jiangsu	237157	242098	256375	167494	178875	202987	230959	247730	268031	286054
Zhejiang	178485	189617	207590	132646	144955	154643	173817	188343	208265	224095
Anhui	95908	103850	114448	103172	105216	114904	122927	131305	137649	144949
Fujian	65954	73239	93058	70172	80246	88539	97174	104209	109608	113533
Jiangxi	68015	73663	79397	61328	63608	69859	75315	80855	86621	91987
Shandong	245088	273371	299481	180744	195157	213576	256781	276794	294842	314660
Henan	168151	173602	196006	147082	159744	174680	191010	204605	217357	231944
Hubei	171075	176077	186382	126326	134600	145829	145906	158141	179612	189786
Hunan	119977	127781	141471	104605	109332	116922	128144	137163	147459	157667
Guangdong	308745	331054	363257	306290	330386	356426	387564	410041	446653	481604
Guangxi	82320	88741	97313	82269	88101	96421	106701	115562	127204	134482
Hainan	23838	24797	28087	16917	19368	20105	21693	22483	28727	30917
Chongqing	55047	58822	66409	61225	67296	78602	86407	97092	106245	114805
Sichuan	148227	157284	177445	139034	150934	169192	189655	202665	215391	233624
Guizhou	47137	49616	53447	38418	40588	48889	53893	57474	64807	72786
Yunnan	61529	62286	66820	47313	49242	55024	63404	68507	76861	87644
Xizang	2921	2977	2982	2483	2444	2031	2883	2938	5647	7250
Shaanxi	80261	84714	95315	92098	101008	110360	119633	128389	138689	152096
Gansu	47749	48611	50927	45496	48666	52103	55020	60470	62012	64857
Qinghai	10385	11237	12568	11495	12533	12818	15242	16501	18062	19218
Ningxia	19686	20281	22082	20307	21421	23010	25108	27220	28434	30308
Xinjiang	68546	69292	75253	37957	40040	42987	36808	37752	41167	48577
SUM	3315847	3490185	3805559	2954913	3131412	3393293	3680276	3922453	4220110	4527708

Unit: Person

Table A14. Urban licensed doctors stock in each provincial unit during 2007–2016

Region	2007	2008	2009	2010	2011	2012	2013	2014	2015	2016
Beijing	53497	57150	56971	63847	67276	71848	74503	77268	82461	89129
Tianjin	23016	22922	22688	24120	24850	25644	27153	28264	30839	34158
Hebei	63689	64017	58703	50241	50744	52827	55419	60548	65536	73134
Shanxi	38199	43869	44131	40880	40161	42212	43415	44530	45249	47562
Neimenggu	27949	28730	27760	24116	25044	26313	28475	28341	30100	31737
Liaoning	76314	76267	71588	61373	62289	64909	67094	67871	69994	75594
Jilin	44446	44694	41996	27270	26438	27524	27598	28449	32662	34295
Heilongjiang	49206	48825	47548	42621	40662	41583	42572	43957	45136	46311
Shanghai	47503	49694	47166	49823	50622	52835	55027	58355	60234	62735
Jiangsu	97949	98767	93477	63013	65656	74169	84081	88969	95675	104107
Zhejiang	75994	79271	73586	51993	55408	57517	64691	69682	77743	83538
Anhui	38444	41342	38296	39277	38104	41535	43716	46311	48319	50999
Fujian	27635	30107	33986	28042	31293	33237	35797	37863	40457	41539
Jiangxi	27019	28498	27330	23165	22782	24358	25818	27799	29180	31050
Shandong	106313	116932	108006	73737	76496	83556	97786	104005	111656	117967
Henan	66975	67949	65087	57017	58724	60984	65710	70403	75159	79779
Hubei	68866	69361	64319	47929	50319	53148	52728	56116	62566	65779
Hunan	49358	52172	47537	38752	39339	41594	45485	48390	52826	56934
Guangdong	118069	124015	116565	112046	120100	129523	140414	146287	158968	171107
Guangxi	31930	33982	32036	30490	32140	34144	36898	39377	43759	46150
Hainan	8983	9298	8468	6008	6729	6633	7404	7705	9770	10583
Chongqing	24595	25125	22083	24477	26005	28986	31771	34798	37259	39928
Sichuan	65373	68749	65024	55631	59136	63873	70095	74098	77408	83251
Guizhou	19738	20518	19290	15000	15509	18410	20157	20572	23338	26570
Yunnan	27713	27730	26040	20625	21356	23200	25267	26043	28080	31351
Xizang	1350	1371	1213	1093	1085	904	1231	1293	2513	3265
Shaanxi	32842	32724	31870	33641	34937	37121	39242	41158	44554	47916
Gansu	19994	20507	18383	18657	19567	20744	21506	23041	23707	25229
Qinghai	4113	4550	4564	4280	4621	4599	5657	5982	6643	6601
Ningxia	8221	8337	8171	7706	7473	8154	9200	9898	10502	11276
Xinjiang	28896	28215	26829	15233	15742	16266	14208	14318	15337	18102
SUM	1374189	1425688	1350711	1152103	1190607	1268350	1360118	1431691	1537630	1647676

Unit: Person

Table A15. Urban registered nurses stock in each provincial unit during 2007–2016

Region	2007	2008	2009	2010	2011	2012	2013	2014	2015	2016
Beijing	49731	54099	60274	65735	71133	77862	81913	86629	92502	98038
Tianjin	20009	20688	21610	22229	23537	25217	27232	28888	31072	34179
Hebei	46677	48492	52408	47458	49227	53533	58140	64890	72327	79954
Shanxi	32142	34643	41430	38873	39824	43366	46465	48808	52238	57848
Neimenggu	21518	22412	25414	21991	24273	26873	30472	32559	35213	38666
Liaoning	70013	71994	75949	66310	68295	72651	77147	79162	82639	90271
Jilin	33491	33860	35047	23716	24071	25413	26554	29804	32702	35879
Heilongjiang	39074	41292	45374	42142	44518	46519	49168	51996	53729	56522
Shanghai	45727	47684	51076	54571	57460	61748	66374	70352	73785	77729
Jiangsu	79989	85528	94084	68710	75609	87943	102616	110834	121384	132383
Zhejiang	57909	63164	71337	52298	57266	63157	71533	79107	87943	96236
Anhui	35403	39635	45524	45467	47761	53261	58016	62857	66684	70375
Fujian	24348	27683	35592	28615	33733	38405	42028	46076	48878	52049
Jiangxi	25285	27852	31277	26396	28839	32515	35787	38888	41735	44604

Region	2007	2008	2009	2010	2011	2012	2013	2014	2015	2016
Shandong	83702	94971	108083	73239	80707	89399	114039	124046	132804	143337
Henan	59000	62739	71578	60372	68704	79626	88801	95734	102292	111477
Hubei	61538	64508	69859	53059	58414	65794	67407	74932	88565	94382
Hunan	41677	45746	53544	46543	50096	54997	60999	65979	71401	77181
Guangdong	112846	120362	136383	122216	134304	148056	162759	174865	193102	214189
Guangxi	30687	33454	37448	34564	37370	42307	46903	51396	57803	62217
Hainan	9310	9956	11738	7547	8772	9376	10253	10788	13746	15085
Chongqing	17573	19714	23230	24237	27745	33670	37501	43528	48630	53493
Sichuan	48439	51644	61588	56475	63913	72889	83233	91191	99239	109792
Guizhou	17199	18602	20840	16757	18178	21867	23674	26239	29635	33664
Yunnan	21978	22231	25180	17830	18316	21527	26351	29565	34681	40708
Xizang	943	1003	1021	869	854	618	1006	1005	1824	2495
Shaanxi	27813	30457	35665	37292	41861	46997	52071	56605	61733	68837
Gansu	16065	16524	17731	17457	19284	20948	22768	25568	26626	28221
Qinghai	4104	4416	4862	4733	5275	5486	6769	7630	8154	8857
Ningxia	7092	7365	8189	7638	8585	9274	10373	11247	12032	13282
Xinjiang	24174	24976	28347	15004	16278	18219	15561	16199	17737	21069
SUM	1165456	1247694	1401682	1200343	1304202	1449513	1603913	1737367	1892835	2063019

Unit: Person

Table A16. Urban pharmacists stock in each provincial unit during 2007-2016

Region	2007	2008	2009	2010	2011	2012	2013	2014	2015	2016
Beijing	8500	8823	9191	9823	10436	11099	11651	12267	12726	13682
Tianjin	4092	4100	4231	4100	4179	4328	4559	4687	4862	5172
Hebei	7672	7641	7614	5609	5466	5569	5806	6267	6804	7337
Shanxi	5044	5404	6067	4973	4725	4852	4852	4993	4916	5456
Neimenggu	4296	4482	5011	4317	4511	4668	4741	4743	5074	5114
Liaoning	11253	11192	11122	8550	8479	8609	8801	8778	8866	9219
Jilin	5864	5889	5994	3350	3290	3185	3242	3259	3547	3568
Heilongjiang	7060	6967	7320	5513	5554	5473	5488	5486	5744	5821
Shanghai	6852	7045	7281	7367	7703	8053	8532	8971	9240	9513
Jiangsu	16144	16133	16567	9826	10150	11227	12412	13355	14182	14959
Zhejiang	12920	13057	13780	8193	8995	9466	10685	11624	12640	13264
Anhui	5482	5803	5923	4964	4968	5371	5543	5782	6033	6332
Fujian	4681	5162	6227	4518	4795	5424	6372	6678	6763	6952
Jiangxi	5207	5563	5575	3837	3789	4072	4393	4602	4882	5099
Shandong	17588	17879	18326	10556	11003	11735	12956	13780	14324	15438
Henan	10168	10226	10809	7666	7880	8310	8765	9276	9766	10369
Hubei	12407	12345	12306	7799	7839	7801	7476	7790	8394	8627
Hunan	9102	9233	9651	5838	5928	5977	6316	6562	6839	7030
Guangdong	23371	24229	25368	20536	21751	23147	24609	25303	26739	27859
Guangxi	4950	5028	5317	4195	4391	4799	5450	6104	6949	7310
Hainan	1390	1427	1508	850	917	1011	1112	1174	1450	1532
Chongqing	3834	3924	4162	3673	3829	4346	4551	4947	5324	5567
Sichuan	9554	10008	10505	7674	7954	8514	9288	9902	10103	10812
Guizhou	2430	2504	2622	1781	1780	2167	2262	2359	2621	2804
Yunnan	3140	3089	3206	2206	2290	2595	2873	3055	3457	3910
Xizang	158	159	159	125	126	114	158	149	267	292
Shaanxi	4884	4876	5353	5049	5354	5657	6016	6252	6687	7113
Gansu	2932	2828	2837	2538	2555	2765	2849	2945	2978	2994
Qinghai	614	667	730	622	647	702	795	822	835	975
Ningxia	1304	1347	1426	1229	1267	1274	1432	1466	1594	1730
Xinjiang	3813	3812	3978	1913	1964	1990	1790	1828	1862	2311
SUM	216706	220842	230166	169190	174515	184300	195775	205206	216468	228161

Unit: Person

Table A17. Urban technologists stock in each provincial unit during 2007–2016

Region	2007	2008	2009	2010	2011	2012	2013	2014	2015	2016
Beijing	7815	8449	8888	9203	9810	9972	10432	10958	11157	12150
Tianjin	3642	3678	3789	3731	3853	3890	4085	4260	4482	4935
Hebei	8926	9304	9529	7350	6939	6912	7178	7679	8521	9606
Shanxi	4899	5149	6111	5435	5411	5463	5752	6062	6112	6473
Neimenggu	3624	3858	4161	3387	3338	3582	3820	4140	4317	4475
Liaoning	11542	11756	11835	9630	9780	9791	9847	9969	10345	11057
Jilin	5635	5688	5951	3734	3599	3749	3822	3679	4003	4417
Heilongjiang	7744	7880	8280	6788	6556	6655	6743	6710	7085	6973
Shanghai	7536	7941	7973	8091	7868	8370	8854	9256	9728	10093
Jiangsu	14404	14771	15141	9954	10264	11149	12235	13103	14116	14817
Zhejiang	10103	10895	11378	7627	8300	8570	9479	10322	11252	12376
Anhui	6034	6617	7208	6261	6390	6754	6946	7367	7746	8059
Fujian	3968	4353	5150	3896	4266	4685	5154	5497	5773	5907
Jiangxi	4348	4899	5181	4136	4143	4460	4803	5057	5324	5797
Shandong	14643	16207	16889	10229	10645	10970	12980	13885	14824	15807
Henan	10856	11148	12056	8988	9242	9558	10522	11391	11640	12638
Hubei	10924	11416	11691	7687	7996	8231	8081	8593	9453	9542
Hunan	6851	7385	7984	5914	6139	6303	6850	7354	7838	8339
Guangdong	19002	20855	22055	18973	18760	20005	21607	21840	23488	24667
Guangxi	4380	4645	4938	4307	4486	4814	5361	6012	6673	7070
Hainan	1564	1560	1767	1121	1167	1208	1288	1236	1621	1773
Chongqing	3239	3330	3577	3457	3630	4213	4451	4862	5315	5931
Sichuan	8043	8442	9324	7397	7945	9180	10158	10378	11174	12107
Guizhou	2794	2918	3128	2140	2199	2765	2919	3060	3570	3835
Yunnan	3540	3622	3767	2774	2807	3134	3446	3751	4233	4716
Xizang	209	202	194	115	123	115	156	150	315	447
Shaanxi	5290	5610	6002	5809	6026	6537	7060	7486	8191	9079
Gansu	3053	3353	3445	3097	3104	3014	3072	3352	3552	3701
Qinghai	635	743	870	769	788	844	932	1099	957	986
Ningxia	1162	1250	1313	1262	1232	1236	1332	1489	1519	1582
Xinjiang	4477	4542	4696	2213	2190	2237	1920	1916	2031	2394
SUM	200882	212466	224271	175475	178996	188366	201285	211913	226355	241749

Unit: Person

Table A18. Urban interns stock in each provincial unit during 2007–2016

Region	2007	2008	2009	2010	2011	2012	2013	2014	2015	2016
Beijing	15911	17282	17105	17456	17811	19911	19449	20333	20402	20628
Tianjin	6060	7132	6778	6616	7378	8191	8422	8621	9314	9238
Hebei	17945	16908	17216	8376	9785	9304	10114	9681	10931	11323
Shanxi	9645	10396	11472	8018	7695	7794	7230	7483	8024	8088
Neimenggu	6469	6656	6919	4760	4788	5690	5365	6338	6796	6871
Liaoning	15108	14683	14085	9276	9360	10626	10420	11474	11019	11227
Jilin	8869	9921	10027	4398	4056	3899	4068	4414	4650	4410
Heilongjiang	15222	15693	16381	10884	13072	13262	13140	13054	11696	11272
Shanghai	10220	11926	11490	11991	11786	11612	13098	11981	11988	13006
Jiangsu	28671	26899	27320	15991	17196	18499	19615	21469	22674	19788
Zhejiang	21559	23230	23348	12535	14986	15933	17429	17608	18687	18681

Region	2007	2008	2009	2010	2011	2012	2013	2014	2015	2016
Anhui	10545	10453	10097	7203	7993	7983	8706	8988	8867	9184
Fujian	5322	5934	7629	5101	6159	6788	7823	8095	7737	7086
Jiangxi	6156	6851	7064	3794	4055	4454	4514	4509	5500	5437
Shandong	22842	27382	29028	12983	16306	17916	19020	21078	21234	22111
Henan	21152	21540	22221	13039	15194	16202	17212	17801	18500	17681
Hubei	17340	18447	18564	9852	10032	10855	10214	10710	10634	11456
Hunan	12989	13245	12890	7558	7830	8051	8494	8878	8555	8183
Guangdong	35457	41593	41514	32519	35471	35695	38175	41746	44356	43782
Guangxi	10373	11632	12415	8713	9714	10357	12089	12673	12020	11735
Hainan	2591	2556	2792	1391	1783	1877	1636	1580	2140	1944
Chongqing	5806	6729	7268	5381	6087	7387	8133	8957	9717	9886
Sichuan	16818	18441	19104	11857	11986	14736	16881	17096	17467	17662
Guizhou	4976	5074	5066	2740	2922	3680	4881	5244	5643	5913
Yunnan	5158	5614	5677	3878	4473	4568	5467	6093	6410	6959
Xizang	261	242	223	281	256	280	332	341	728	751
Shaanxi	9432	11047	11634	10307	12830	14048	15244	16888	17524	19151
Gansu	5705	5399	5600	3747	4156	4632	4825	5564	5149	4712
Qinghai	919	861	1171	1091	1202	1187	1089	968	1473	1799
Ningxia	1907	1982	2238	2472	2864	3072	2771	3120	2787	2438
Xinjiang	7186	7747	7652	3594	3866	4275	3329	3491	4200	4701
SUM	358614	383495	391988	257802	283092	302764	319185	336276	346822	347103

Unit: Person

Table A19. Urban population in each provincial unit during 2007–2016

Region	2007	2008	2009	2010	2011	2012	2013	2014	2015	2016
Beijing	1145.00	1160.85	1176.40	1191.28	1210.33	1229.48	1246.52	1266.51	1289.69	1358.30
Tianjin	791.35	799.45	808.09	811.70	820.01	815.39	824.12	833.00	848.09	963.54
Hebei	2578.45	2608.95	2636.06	1295.26	1303.75	1319.72	1329.35	1361.32	1578.07	1850.55
Shanxi	1342.22	1360.62	1374.28	972.07	977.18	978.18	990.93	987.43	987.62	995.45
Neimenggu	859.43	870.24	876.96	604.45	666.17	614.14	620.72	680.26	684.87	683.96
Liaoning	2995.61	3012.84	3024.97	1878.20	1894.65	1908.20	2274.40	1918.33	1924.87	1916.19
Jilin	1858.32	1866.64	1872.08	868.82	870.45	866.44	496.83	831.60	834.02	842.54
Heilongjiang	2283.90	2289.51	2294.83	1369.90	1350.82	1362.45	1358.60	1340.74	1326.77	1321.86
Shanghai	1309.31	1322.23	1332.11	1343.97	1350.34	1358.27	1364.65	1372.32	1374.79	1384.61
Jiangsu	4961.44	4991.71	5017.12	2533.95	2760.42	2569.46	2595.04	2758.69	2680.31	2918.92
Zhejiang	3131.32	3155.02	3174.16	1500.52	1513.10	1525.08	1687.54	1625.05	1652.90	1836.84
Anhui	2194.69	2219.02	2239.69	1961.44	1895.78	2074.08	1957.44	1977.48	1994.91	2100.71
Fujian	1754.10	1777.65	1789.58	912.51	923.43	935.93	951.75	1008.80	1118.45	1146.80
Jiangxi	1518.19	1531.46	1566.02	899.24	908.69	921.62	926.38	912.58	931.41	948.32
Shandong	5316.44	5328.87	5347.88	2759.45	2808.01	2813.91	2837.36	2976.28	3008.59	3084.90
Henan	3510.46	3557.42	3616.35	1917.63	2061.21	2012.44	2045.07	2058.40	2089.97	2108.58
Hubei	3932.76	3947.91	3974.03	1949.48	1942.28	1841.28	1844.58	1834.58	1851.67	1917.03
Hunan	2338.73	2375.11	2393.76	1278.79	1353.12	1353.26	1360.34	1318.88	1340.54	1371.02
Guangdong	5533.06	5601.59	5684.77	3332.86	3388.57	3417.32	3290.02	3628.68	3952.68	4187.86
Guangxi	1785.68	1814.74	1843.05	1368.87	1378.73	1391.36	1411.39	1460.96	1479.12	1563.74
Hainan	522.76	532.12	541.18	217.44	220.59	218.77	220.91	230.36	231.67	237.82
Chongqing	1524.85	1535.82	1544.40	1561.86	1576.02	1778.33	1785.27	1602.18	1609.77	1616.97
Sichuan	3286.63	3311.24	3335.43	2397.14	2414.94	2434.42	2469.47	2533.31	2534.01	2849.07
Guizhou	1011.52	1023.01	1041.85	513.61	556.76	615.73	726.32	522.97	535.60	555.62
Yunnan	1007.02	1022.76	1037.58	605.03	610.94	613.42	636.59	624.49	630.01	658.98
Xizang	28.50	31.27	32.41	18.20	18.77	19.53	20.17	21.05	48.68	61.44
Shaanxi	1322.26	1395.62	1414.17	1297.15	1308.39	1315.38	1327.78	1322.23	1333.55	1421.46

Table A19. (Continued).

Region	2007	2008	2009	2010	2011	2012	2013	2014	2015	2016
Gansu	857.25	864.96	872.04	815.34	799.11	811.57	813.91	814.96	815.95	831.50
Qinghai	105.75	107.22	108.34	90.30	90.95	91.75	92.71	94.29	94.57	97.06
Ningxia	302.86	304.06	308.84	263.04	284.85	272.63	276.82	280.62	296.19	303.08
Xinjiang	821.89	838.89	856.12	261.41	378.45	280.41	285.78	243.56	247.99	321.70
SUM	6193.18	6255.88	6313.45	3879.09	3963.68	3975.99	4006.88	4044.19	4132.73	4345.64

Unit: 10 thousands

Table A20. Rural health technicians stock in each provincial unit during 2007–2016

Region	2007	2008	2009	2010	2011	2012	2013	2014	2015	2016
Beijing	4252	4608	4796	5262	5470	5542	5793	5790	6192	326
Tianjin	6760	6641	7162	9664	9521	9806	9632	10160	10179	7270
Hebei	98300	101089	110676	173123	179511	186788	196375	202448	208628	211705
Shanxi	55233	60130	71008	95712	93600	95914	95671	97598	97456	100453
Neimenggu	41934	43589	62463	67260	69649	72750	75329	78362	80827	83543
Liaoning	31261	32012	34037	76940	77420	80222	81383	79030	81556	80126
Jilin	27471	27853	28841	75925	77556	80295	80650	81822	81399	84036
Heilongjiang	40420	41282	43366	84100	84667	87663	90490	91004	91874	94463
Shanghai	3065	3181	3745	5288	5301	5189	5224	5139	5150	5120
Jiangsu	49325	49027	52606	160749	171669	192974	197935	210773	218974	230932
Zhejiang	49940	53291	58664	155835	161967	174922	178649	187559	197355	208546
Anhui	78816	83920	94136	108367	112375	121284	130605	136734	143119	148783
Fujian	28609	30102	37751	72744	78545	87535	100371	102307	103323	106024
Jiangxi	58583	66101	71344	96679	102330	109846	114777	120507	124306	128985
Shandong	95431	102446	115490	268117	286581	316506	340206	326991	323350	327041
Henan	129703	136321	163885	225736	236556	253828	277526	290210	302582	315057
Hubei	56041	57746	60603	129467	133522	142866	163437	177442	188290	194746
Hunan	100601	104303	112076	164614	173179	179935	194938	204241	223329	234880
Guangdong	51911	53080	58068	148509	155199	161988	166164	172968	171322	183653
Guangxi	63259	66879	75597	107285	115910	124340	134191	143037	147455	155390
Hainan	8707	9078	9770	22603	23927	24955	26415	28097	25983	26605
Chongqing	28603	29922	33599	49854	52855	53056	55726	57186	60463	64549
Sichuan	107105	110307	125606	186574	201325	220248	237333	249273	256778	262126
Guizhou	38145	39697	43306	65536	73213	80883	102012	112489	122475	131835
Yunnan	62203	63951	68387	95826	101740	111740	129813	140398	151137	162033
Xizang	5148	6458	7133	7600	8338	7305	8755	9944	8694	7579
Shaanxi	61426	63614	76525	89340	96165	105933	119421	124222	126692	136511
Gansu	37599	39022	40328	53369	57242	59506	63069	65926	67442	69784
Qinghai	9952	10508	11476	13414	14987	16493	17189	17435	17360	17792
Ningxia	5835	6134	6346	9655	10562	11240	12180	12580	13063	14392
Xinjiang	36125	37561	40775	86098	90564	93704	109043	115665	120674	122410
SUM	1471763	1539853	1729565	2911245	3061446	3275256	3520302	3657337	3777427	3916695

Unit: Person

Table A21. Rural licensed doctors stock in each provincial unit during 2007–2016

Region	2007	2008	2009	2010	2011	2012	2013	2014	2015	2016
Beijing	1788	1903	1968	2316	2471	2532	2611	2681	2771	282
Tianjin	3029	2968	3230	4772	4981	5046	4906	5076	5032	3646
Hebei	44535	45951	53521	83753	86057	90162	94725	97177	101345	104006
Shanxi	26462	28390	34483	47127	44657	45107	44767	45305	44967	44137
Neimenggu	20454	20812	38177	32129	32101	33215	33580	33841	34138	34654
Liaoning	14317	14447	16281	35489	35455	36063	36250	33765	34558	34206
Jilin	12514	12829	13458	34780	33143	33876	34400	34785	34583	35371
Heilongjiang	17778	17946	19580	37661	36118	37006	37903	37414	37572	38111
Shanghai	1352	1353	1763	3186	3129	2962	2917	2847	2749	2651
Jiangsu	20865	20694	21957	65930	69027	83733	85560	89582	93541	100540
Zhejiang	22022	22622	26105	68447	69089	72456	73588	76043	80313	84640
Anhui	30688	32484	39082	47234	46592	50526	54897	57431	59473	61742
Fujian	12479	12906	16606	30588	31191	33503	36845	37461	37527	38146
Jiangxi	24809	26689	29025	38722	40057	42719	44433	46848	47627	48137
Shandong	40849	42877	49038	111427	109538	116909	133968	126878	125462	126933
Henan	48925	51367	71648	97784	97940	106624	114890	118932	123457	126968
Hubei	23376	22676	23907	51613	51775	56001	64463	70007	73431	75962
Hunan	43169	44133	48388	71692	73291	74846	81756	84982	98014	103693
Guangdong	20224	20452	23464	62490	66061	69443	69892	70512	69571	72117
Guangxi	26230	26843	29618	40326	42013	43899	46412	47148	47826	50523
Hainan	3604	3552	3835	8448	8798	8892	9321	9904	9232	9291
Chongqing	14123	14290	16455	23492	23566	23004	23370	23286	23714	24781
Sichuan	51782	53102	61761	89563	94659	99004	103795	105425	104072	102163
Guizhou	18135	18312	19674	28389	29906	30769	35802	37273	40046	42437
Yunnan	28873	29546	31519	42681	43328	45266	49593	49383	51487	54525
Xizang	2503	3005	3167	3376	3090	3139	3945	4316	3700	3277
Shaanxi	26471	25540	33084	32399	30803	32350	35155	35302	34942	37765
Gansu	15150	15669	16332	20674	21303	22212	23381	24640	25903	27562
Qinghai	4600	4864	5286	6284	6775	7319	7582	6971	7148	7069
Ningxia	2964	3107	3172	4561	4785	4857	5117	5125	5358	5794
Xinjiang	14655	15241	16170	33823	33788	34274	38812	40487	41946	42200
SUM	638725	656570	771754	1261156	1275487	1347714	1434636	1460827	1501505	1543329

Unit: Person

Table A22. Rural registered nurses stock in each provincial unit during 2007–2016

Region	2007	2008	2009	2010	2011	2012	2013	2014	2015	2016
Beijing	1224	1312	1435	1597	1679	1672	1966	1859	2124	44
Tianjin	1316	1291	1479	1970	2277	2404	2483	2689	2732	1909
Hebei	19037	20546	22291	39893	44293	48455	53386	56955	60510	63478
Shanxi	12486	14122	15830	23755	24986	26971	28384	30247	31106	34264
Neimenggu	8214	9047	10000	16260	18221	19901	21886	24164	26010	27779
Liaoning	8159	8476	8549	22572	23617	25385	26262	26666	28337	28876
Jilin	7124	7206	7359	22060	23867	25562	26161	27629	28017	29870
Heilongjiang	9555	10061	10479	20617	21626	23554	24806	25724	27226	28896
Shanghai	1044	1074	1195	1295	1425	1497	1565	1577	1651	1644
Jiangsu	14641	15208	16955	53799	59993	67304	71542	77933	82614	88785
Zhejiang	14035	15120	16807	47312	52009	58156	61172	66034	72002	78287
Anhui	19678	21221	24435	31850	36693	41785	45388	48640	52619	55975
Fujian	9485	10077	12268	24896	28730	32719	37901	39588	41572	43592

Table A22. (Continued).

Region	2007	2008	2009	2010	2011	2012	2013	2014	2015	2016
Jiangxi	17223	20389	22376	32009	35601	39540	42422	45252	47844	50915
Shandong	25894	27895	31527	83453	90261	102322	126039	121665	121366	125042
Henan	31187	33832	40603	61012	68420	76415	87733	95383	103074	110646
Hubei	15330	16106	17475	40785	43700	49951	60464	69177	76512	80536
Hunan	24866	26805	29615	45803	51771	57909	64697	70268	77944	84350
Guangdong	15191	15560	17008	45666	48356	51478	54870	58618	60996	69604
Guangxi	21017	22538	25350	35679	39136	43208	47911	52559	55399	60385
Hainan	3134	3256	3487	8772	9428	10056	10639	11595	10916	11410
Chongqing	6360	7085	8651	13374	15020	16153	17959	19211	21324	23970
Sichuan	25017	26248	29576	48411	57353	66921	75224	84329	91363	97841
Guizhou	9304	10040	11144	19408	23411	26779	34992	40965	46397	52329
Yunnan	19062	19780	21149	31578	33999	39228	46954	53258	58597	65258
Xizang	855	917	986	1119	1286	1114	1391	1710	1366	1338
Shaanxi	14702	16461	19171	24524	28364	32393	37480	40616	42584	47966
Gansu	7949	8426	8847	12411	14389	16254	18186	19904	21156	22309
Qinghai	2737	2864	2971	3606	4385	4540	4723	5120	5040	5507
Ningxia	1487	1532	1667	2703	3040	3230	3605	3849	4103	4787
Xinjiang	10488	11108	12451	29539	32482	34230	41017	43593	46133	46555
SUM	377801	405603	453136	847728	939818	1047086	1179208	1266777	1348634	1444147

Unit: Person

Table A23. Rural pharmacists stock in each provincial unit during 2007–2016

Region	2007	2008	2009	2010	2011	2012	2013	2014	2015	2016
Beijing	390	372	409	427	435	479	474	477	480	0
Tianjin	363	241	281	461	520	515	500	506	514	407
Hebei	6036	5892	5918	8458	8422	8471	8609	8708	8853	9081
Shanxi	3672	3984	3985	5200	5209	5121	5090	5052	4924	4929
Neimenggu	3234	3213	3532	4602	4765	4828	4805	4925	5197	5315
Liaoning	2416	2494	2398	5057	4850	4664	4626	4436	4406	4244
Jilin	1891	1935	1940	4727	4804	4779	4682	4535	4356	4365
Heilongjiang	3068	2989	2983	5573	5591	5668	5967	5904	5735	5729
Shanghai	185	191	214	210	226	228	248	254	258	266
Jiangsu	3999	3909	3934	11526	11972	12081	11814	12166	12272	12798
Zhejiang	4166	4155	4218	10974	11344	12147	12351	12827	13123	13608
Anhui	4893	4975	5082	5955	6034	6446	6733	7127	7423	7543
Fujian	2699	2785	3188	5436	5932	6343	6951	7116	7103	7384
Jiangxi	5709	6113	6108	8370	8618	8941	9025	9098	9139	9147
Shandong	8201	8226	8374	17297	17824	18580	18082	17961	17980	17957
Henan	9132	9246	9432	12822	12841	13091	14117	14687	15184	15535
Hubei	5466	5507	5411	9899	9850	9576	10176	10047	9828	9881
Hunan	10592	10446	10293	14233	14431	13662	13810	13759	13549	13654
Guangdong	5045	5027	5058	10984	10857	10763	10961	11245	10882	11452
Guangxi	4038	4039	4256	6131	6607	7094	7704	8249	8781	9383
Hainan	396	401	420	1150	1244	1343	1427	1511	1381	1399
Chongqing	1716	1719	1749	2594	2608	2538	2658	2681	2857	3007
Sichuan	6989	6982	7365	10873	11463	11907	12349	12740	13172	13186

Region	2007	2008	2009	2010	2011	2012	2013	2014	2015	2016
Guizhou	1786	1897	2011	2898	3118	3281	4074	4553	4979	5324
Yunnan	2765	2922	3011	4220	4493	4690	5263	5735	6112	6467
Xizang	192	235	253	326	369	314	382	444	369	362
Shaanxi	4469	4650	4814	5732	6168	6476	7079	7292	7292	7702
Gansu	2040	2031	1934	2544	2746	2823	2965	3111	3129	3228
Qinghai	677	711	695	835	831	848	880	907	918	940
Ningxia	447	487	467	761	787	834	868	910	949	992
Xinjiang	1834	1909	2011	4451	4519	4567	5133	5426	5681	5800
SUM	108506	109683	111744	184726	189478	193098	199803	204389	206826	211085

Unit: Person

Table A24. Rural technologists stock in each provincial unit during 2007–2016

Region	2007	2008	2009	2010	2011	2012	2013	2014	2015	2016
Beijing	309	303	288	304	313	346	331	333	381	0
Tianjin	341	266	308	408	440	408	404	437	419	315
Hebei	6201	6396	6506	9829	9823	9530	10216	10152	10563	10400
Shanxi	3025	3311	3511	4662	4793	4850	4758	5065	5014	5177
Neimenggu	2345	2437	2522	3641	3682	3825	4010	4095	4157	4268
Liaoning	1744	1846	1944	4294	4184	4256	4370	4328	4375	4326
Jilin	1621	1587	1637	4173	4187	4176	4182	4166	3953	4004
Heilongjiang	2576	2669	2782	5339	5348	5563	5731	5755	5722	5820
Shanghai	243	235	229	228	236	237	237	241	238	245
Jiangsu	3316	3357	3461	9307	9702	9719	9486	9960	10125	10868
Zhejiang	2809	2942	3062	7987	7826	8380	8568	9050	9225	9603
Anhui	5156	5579	6079	7165	7182	7608	8094	8541	8827	9052
Fujian	1597	1599	1976	3625	3931	4370	4853	4999	5144	5511
Jiangxi	3853	4493	4698	6442	6757	7193	7753	8155	8873	9298
Shandong	6299	6491	6957	15081	15703	16784	16602	16556	16743	17330
Henan	9531	9903	10582	14355	15157	15366	16889	17955	18991	20075
Hubei	3446	3587	3707	7845	7830	7786	8684	8927	9188	9496
Hunan	6268	6787	7171	9815	10293	10526	11147	11676	12145	12504
Guangdong	3026	3068	3195	7506	7234	7267	7551	7593	7411	7995
Guangxi	3413	3487	3829	5344	5682	6242	6936	7530	8086	8670
Hainan	437	445	455	1157	1162	1190	1314	1413	1293	1347
Chongqing	1309	1385	1475	1976	2162	2075	2207	2348	2553	2817
Sichuan	5474	5616	6059	8693	9335	10013	10917	11715	12202	12825
Guizhou	2026	2261	2440	3787	4080	4498	5774	6502	7409	8048
Yunnan	3077	3306	3469	4896	5325	5853	6640	7379	8305	8909
Xizang	272	320	320	376	390	340	411	433	312	248
Shaanxi	4006	4069	4601	5681	6194	6797	7683	8248	8499	9460
Gansu	1694	1795	1884	2463	2675	2790	2957	3071	3146	3304
Qinghai	565	608	661	797	824	916	973	1020	1068	1118
Ningxia	319	344	357	575	625	625	719	690	788	858
Xinjiang	2224	2334	2468	5529	5536	5747	6739	7050	7419	7545
SUM	88522	92826	98633	163280	168611	175276	187136	195383	202574	211436

Unit: Person

Table A25. Rural interns stock in each provincial unit of China during 2007–2016

Region	2007	2008	2009	2010	2011	2012	2013	2014	2015	2016
Beijing	541	718	696	618	572	513	411	246	436	0
Tianjin	1711	1875	1864	2053	1303	1433	1339	328	1482	993
Hebei	22491	22304	22440	31190	30916	30170	29439	6406	27357	24740
Shanxi	9588	10323	13199	14968	13955	13865	12672	3466	11445	11946
Neimenggu	7687	8080	8232	10628	10880	10981	11048	2626	11325	11527
Liaoning	4625	4749	4865	9528	9314	9854	9875	2844	9880	8474
Jilin	4321	4296	4447	10185	11555	11902	11225	2713	10490	10426
Heilongjiang	7443	7617	7542	14910	15984	15872	16083	3766	15619	15907
Shanghai	241	328	344	369	285	265	257	181	254	314
Jiangsu	6504	5859	6299	20187	20975	20137	19533	7495	20422	17941
Zhejiang	6908	8452	8472	21115	21699	23783	22970	6994	22692	22408
Anhui	18401	19661	19458	16163	15874	14919	15493	5431	14777	14471
Fujian	2349	2735	3713	8199	8761	10600	13821	3511	11977	11391
Jiangxi	6989	8417	9137	11136	11297	11453	11144	5491	10823	11488
Shandong	14188	16957	19594	40859	53255	61911	45515	10346	41799	39779
Henan	30928	31973	31620	39763	42198	42332	43897	10123	41876	41833
Hubei	8423	9870	10103	19325	20367	19552	19650	6095	19331	18871
Hunan	15706	16132	16609	23071	23393	22992	23528	7330	21677	20679
Guangdong	8425	8973	9343	21863	22691	23037	22890	5494	22462	22485
Guangxi	8561	9972	12544	19805	22472	23897	25228	5431	27363	26429
Hainan	1136	1424	1573	3076	3295	3474	3714	1029	3161	3158
Chongqing	5095	5443	5269	8418	9499	9286	9532	1588	10015	9974
Sichuan	17843	18359	20845	29034	28515	32403	35048	7786	35969	36111
Guizhou	6894	7187	8037	11054	12698	15556	21370	4035	23644	23697
Yunnan	8426	8397	9239	12451	14595	16703	21363	5076	26636	26874
Xizang	1326	1981	2407	2403	3203	2398	2626	232	2947	2354
Shaanxi	11778	12894	14855	21004	24636	27917	32024	4852	33375	33618
Gansu	10766	11101	11331	15277	16129	15427	15580	1708	14108	13381
Qinghai	1373	1461	1863	1892	2172	2870	3031	649	3186	3158
Ningxia	618	664	683	1055	1325	1694	1871	453	1865	1961
Xinjiang	6924	6969	7675	12756	14239	14886	17342	4795	19495	20310
SUM	258209	275171	294298	454355	488052	512082	519519	128520	517888	506698

Unit: Person

Table A26. Rural population in each provincial unit during 2007–2016

Region	2007	2008	2009	2010	2011	2012	2013	2014	2015	2016
Beijing	70.87	71.11	71.26	70.73	70.85	70.96	71.17	71.57	72.00	0.00
Tianjin	172.89	175.22	176.84	177.97	180.32	180.92	182.42	184.06	185.07	86.55
Hebei	4447.96	4533.14	4573.39	6011.22	6044.14	6104.18	6175.31	6229.17	6136.12	5880.69
Shanxi	2053.27	2066.32	2088.47	2499.01	2522.91	2524.05	2530.98	2535.01	2498.87	2511.33
Neimenggu	1553.11	1567.95	1577.35	1847.80	1799.72	1846.45	1846.30	1780.95	1757.11	1740.48
Liaoning	1235.61	1231.23	1233.22	2374.69	2360.37	2338.83	1965.77	2324.41	2330.17	2289.31
Jilin	840.09	844.03	848.26	1856.36	1855.41	1837.41	2179.73	1838.70	1808.87	1788.00
Heilongjiang	1536.88	1540.37	1548.79	2473.53	2482.90	2448.69	2419.52	2382.30	2355.74	2303.98
Shanghai	69.66	69.30	68.97	68.94	68.75	68.55	68.20	67.80	66.88	67.37

Region	2007	2008	2009	2010	2011	2012	2013	2014	2015	2016
Jiangsu	2394.42	2391.56	2402.10	4930.95	4755.37	4986.41	5023.73	4913.12	5092.42	4913.45
Zhejiang	1527.22	1535.76	1543.79	3246.56	3265.46	3275.69	3139.70	3222.66	3235.33	3112.63
Anhui	4478.18	4511.83	4547.63	4859.51	4994.44	4832.03	4965.97	4918.49	4935.14	4959.43
Fujian	1682.88	1700.68	1708.19	2616.69	2626.92	2644.56	2683.72	2685.22	2583.08	2650.60
Jiangxi	3004.26	3046.13	3061.97	3791.33	3846.99	3881.48	3890.75	4003.55	4009.87	4030.78
Shandong	4026.62	4065.32	4095.39	6770.63	6774.96	6762.95	6777.01	6770.00	6879.79	6958.32
Henan	6862.59	6955.15	7033.69	8887.24	8859.78	8906.25	8981.42	9097.49	9169.15	9266.38
Hubei	2155.42	2162.77	2164.39	4203.47	4225.38	4329.27	4323.73	4255.20	4279.32	4233.61
Hunan	4531.58	4574.69	4612.18	5796.27	5772.63	5785.69	5784.51	5868.99	5877.08	6022.56
Guangdong	2621.77	2667.34	2675.94	5192.62	5243.21	5225.42	5465.92	5225.62	5038.88	5101.47
Guangxi	3277.67	3327.31	3359.87	3958.86	3983.16	3985.26	4005.70	3995.45	4095.97	3984.36
Hainan	326.10	332.53	338.06	678.77	687.56	683.70	687.89	683.63	666.23	665.13
Chongqing	1712.75	1719.66	1731.91	1743.15	1750.17	1565.07	1569.75	1770.46	1778.32	1793.03
Sichuan	5520.88	5599.34	5657.93	6592.72	6644.39	6674.18	6666.66	6629.60	6584.05	6241.10
Guizhou	2980.08	3007.35	3049.72	3681.80	3679.05	3516.65	3554.43	3762.17	3827.34	3877.50
Yunnan	3362.32	3401.65	3436.53	3927.30	3943.41	3962.41	3969.82	4022.87	3977.29	4050.83
Xizang	245.14	250.31	257.51	275.36	283.61	289.88	296.78	302.25	263.45	261.34
Shaanxi	2457.04	2418.78	2437.10	2574.64	2599.05	2609.19	2630.42	2598.79	2585.55	2575.68
Gansu	1790.43	1814.98	1833.09	1899.25	1927.34	1901.15	1916.99	1916.45	1926.91	1938.44
Qinghai	416.40	423.71	434.70	459.38	466.88	473.94	480.14	487.01	482.22	480.86
Ningxia	310.37	321.15	325.44	380.12	366.74	386.25	391.64	391.90	362.86	369.03
Xinjiang	1220.44	1243.74	1266.30	1904.82	1825.89	1944.07	1982.60	1987.37	1978.26	1943.02
SUM	6888.49	6957.04	7016.00	9575.17	9590.78	9604.16	9662.87	9692.23	9683.94	9609.72

Unit: 10 thousands

Table A27. Government and social health expenditure in each provincial unit during 2012–2016

Region	Government health expenditure					Social health expenditure				
	2012	2013	2014	2015	2016	2012	2013	2014	2015	2016
Beijing	320.4	356.42	394.38	445.81	467.99	600.96	708.36	890.57	1069.88	1247.23
Tianjin	120.9	145.31	171.18	202.24	211.76	184.37	212.38	266.71	317.37	361.64
Hebei	368.32	429.83	458.64	552.58	567.79	353.03	440.62	558.25	622.13	720.65
Shanxi	206.68	229.62	250.19	298.09	309.73	222.7	235.75	266.84	319.43	363.03
Neimenggu	204.46	223	240.81	271.46	303.94	175.21	208.31	190.85	255.6	299.7
Liaoning	233.02	263.26	289.38	292.79	316.59	382.73	471.8	561.3	610.7	626.64
Jilin	174.02	197.68	212.13	252.11	280.02	177.75	223.02	244.42	274.95	352.48
Heilongjiang	191	206.55	242.6	284.34	287.45	279.84	359.48	353.75	383.51	486.94
Shanghai	232.49	250.82	275.29	319.94	430.73	646.51	740.42	791.87	882.39	1061.73
Jiangsu	483.75	549.23	581.99	674.73	753.25	863.51	1010.36	1289.48	1496	1754.96
Zhejiang	342.67	393.16	443.89	500.08	557.81	689.32	750.8	910.59	1086.54	1295.37
Anhui	365.75	415.45	434.77	497.29	550.55	300.83	381.54	440.5	527.68	597.92
Fujian	222.81	268.01	296.48	357.42	388.46	263.37	330.72	407.52	478.01	547.97
Jiangxi	269.45	325.75	358.98	421.78	468.18	175.06	191.81	240.42	287.37	325.37
Shandong	498.38	571.45	619.7	722.22	813.19	726.42	874.71	1039.5	1212.98	1536.92
Henan	489.46	561.33	612.55	729.7	794.42	381.86	443.38	533.89	734.65	859.06
Hubei	305.89	368.37	415.91	530.67	611.23	335.88	397.23	465.85	565.72	669.42
Hunan	338.82	392.91	434.09	506.82	560.26	305.35	380.71	471.1	573.11	743.41
Guangdong	587.32	667.69	803.78	956	1158.7	858.11	1049.98	1236.96	1485.88	2009.16
Guangxi	286.69	322.49	359.27	386.97	475.69	235.55	267.91	294.79	353.17	437.5

Table A27. (Continued).

Region	Government health expenditure					Social health expenditure				
	2012	2013	2014	2015	2016	2012	2013	2014	2015	2016
Hainan	66.82	77.4	88.92	102.7	116.54	59.45	59.92	75.22	93.61	118.75
Chongqing	195.56	226.79	255.09	323.69	339.75	204.8	253.79	320.2	393.8	411.82
Sichuan	473.89	546.11	592.32	696.24	784.42	467.31	556.02	688.86	825.99	1111.62
Guizhou	242.62	278	310.36	371.7	403.29	97.97	124.77	161.37	206.1	270.34
Yunnan	288.23	322.14	359.63	425.76	473.34	211.84	241.43	271.81	338.2	463.17
Xizang	43.49	47.56	57.53	72.39	85.54	15.78	20.75	19.11	25.62	32.6
Shaanxi	257.49	293.96	317.92	377.76	391.7	276.12	327.87	423.52	465.24	527.58
Gansu	168.88	188.17	212.32	259.1	283.95	113.94	141.28	164.19	199.6	250.6
Qinghai	61.72	78.1	87.25	107.08	111.83	42.26	43.06	46.67	57.17	61.95
Ningxia	51.8	60.44	67.56	77.14	85.59	36.51	48.91	71.22	75.9	93.1
Xinjiang	190	208.68	232.5	262.92	299.05	224.26	269.55	325.41	390.81	415.58
SUM	8282.78	9465.68	10477.41	12279.5	13682.7	9908.6	11766.64	14022.74	16609.11	20054.21

Unit: 100 million Yuan

Table A28. Outpatient and inpatient visits in each provincial unit during 2012–2016

Region	Outpatient visits					Inpatient visits				
	2012	2013	2014	2015	2016	2012	2013	2014	2015	2016
Beijing	18530	20466	21360	21780	23205	225	246	270	276	312
Tianjin	9608	10533	11578	11881	12004	132	136	149	151	162
Hebei	36792	39309	41289	42134	43494	870	923	981	991	1118
Shanxi	11901	12486	12767	12521	12942	349	367	391	381	430
Neimenggu	9334	9883	10034	10025	10340	259	284	300	296	329
Liaoning	17526	17838	18451	18551	19294	550	595	635	646	693
Jilin	9743	10205	10635	10469	10761	302	308	336	341	369
Heilongjiang	11529	12094	12084	11475	11891	420	471	490	515	564
Shanghai	22086	23407	25060	25616	25932	277	291	319	335	367
Jiangsu	45055	49440	52579	54579	55195	953	1054	1152	1218	1309
Zhejiang	45191	47526	50425	52973	55521	626	690	756	791	871
Anhui	23492	25474	26282	26124	26300	712	763	821	843	897
Fujian	19203	20396	21212	21190	21927	510	528	534	523	535
Jiangxi	18972	19853	21087	20838	21341	658	689	697	712	745
Shandong	58265	62208	63127	61521	62163	1397	1415	1502	1522	1692
Henan	49655	51860	54963	55553	57777	1273	1327	1447	1502	1602
Hubei	30579	32060	34475	34839	35479	862	952	1053	1108	1198
Hunan	22900	24438	25051	25696	26431	1053	1161	1227	1304	1401
Guangdong	71492	75779	78095	78526	81201	1216	1298	1393	1441	1547
Guangxi	23189	24970	24933	25188	25423	700	819	833	831	860
Hainan	3904	4248	4531	4641	4866	84	91	97	105	110
Chongqing	13305	13910	13798	14500	14906	450	507	551	591	631
Sichuan	42439	43549	44521	45082	46425	1383	1452	1509	1547	1656
Guizhou	11515	12662	13016	13201	13844	563	654	640	634	662
Yunnan	20009	21120	21890	22837	24460	621	675	729	749	819
Xizang	1012	1178	1313	1376	1394	15	19	23	29	34
Shaanxi	16052	17192	17508	17501	18500	498	547	596	625	681
Gansu	11921	12393	12329	12531	13042	293	319	339	352	400
Qinghai	2134	2204	2253	2282	2357	76	82	86	84	91
Ningxia	3115	3339	3562	3577	3832	82	91	96	98	107
Xinjiang	8387	9382	9979	10333	10923	448	464	491	512	535
SUM	688833	731401	760187	769343	793170	17857	19215	20441	21054	22728

Unit: 10 thousands times

Table A29. The number of medical graduates in each provincial unit during 2012–2016

Region	Medical graduates				
	2012	2013	2014	2015	2016
Beijing	3022	3021	2722	3138	3324
Tianjin	6595	7071	7427	8208	8482
Hebei	23202	29653	30660	28744	31230
Shanxi	9703	9593	10136	10293	10605
Neimenggu	3114	4016	4146	4531	4380
Liaoning	14968	16402	16965	18272	20638
Jilin	7695	8051	8214	8772	8847
Heilongjiang	11628	12909	12933	13793	14786
Shanghai	2600	2937	3377	5203	5698
Jiangsu	15649	15416	17072	18032	18096
Zhejiang	12442	12323	12041	12933	13281
Anhui	19977	20878	21528	20990	23913
Fujian	9984	11383	12181	13221	14594
Jiangxi	9798	11116	12192	12645	13716
Shandong	35255	38835	41301	45722	50080
Henan	23160	28378	29374	32433	32790
Hubei	8387	9682	10259	10428	10650
Hunan	15482	16526	18315	20730	22045
Guangdong	19783	21139	21945	22687	22566
Guangxi	12131	11803	12695	14191	14014
Hainan	2223	2136	2417	2432	2603
Chongqing	8842	10145	10770	11874	12411
Sichuan	15060	17025	16523	18352	19221
Guizhou	11358	12468	14234	15577	15973
Yunnan	6582	8649	9846	11397	12650
Xizang	174	216	270	159	175
Shaanxi	7127	7462	9776	10234	9836
Gansu	4310	5296	3824	3941	3888
Qinghai	692	1133	951	898	645
Ningxia	1136	1282	1304	1984	2091
Xinjiang	4730	4904	4533	4529	4344
SUM	326809	361848	379931	406343	427572

Unit: Person

APPENDIX B. CHARACTERISTICS OF THE HEALTH MANPOWER DISTRIBUTION (2007–2016)

- Figure B1 Boxplots of the density of total health manpower during 2007–2016
- Figure B2 Boxplots of the density of urban health manpower during 2007–2016

- Figure B3 Boxplots of the density of rural health manpower during 2007–2016
- Figure B4 Space–scan for units with higher change rates of health technician density during 2007–2016
- Figure B5 Space–scan for units with lower change rates of health technician density during 2007–2016
- Figure B6 Space–scan for units with higher change rates of urban health technician density during 2007–2016
- Figure B7 Space–scan for units with lower change rates of urban health technician density during 2007–2016
- Figure B8 Space–scan for units with higher change rates of rural health technician density during 2007–2016
- Figure B9 Space–scan for units with lower change rates of rural health technician density during 2007–2016
- Table B1 Detailed information of space–time clusters of higher and lower rates of change of health technician densities from 2007 to 2016
- Figure B10 Hierarchical maps and univariate LISA cluster maps of the density of health technicians in 2007, 2010, 2013, and 2016.
- Figure B11 Hierarchical maps and univariate LISA cluster maps of the density of licensed doctors in 2007, 2010, 2013, and 2016.
- Figure B12 Hierarchical maps and univariate LISA cluster maps of the density of registered nurses in 2007, 2010, 2013, and 2016.
- Figure B13 Hierarchical maps and univariate LISA cluster maps of the density of pharmacists in 2007, 2010, 2013, and 2016.
- Figure B14 Hierarchical maps and univariate LISA cluster maps of the density of technologists in 2007, 2010, 2013, and 2016.
- Figure B15 Hierarchical maps and univariate LISA cluster maps of the density of interns in 2007, 2010, 2013, and 2016.
- Figure B16 Hierarchical maps and univariate LISA cluster maps of the density of urban health technicians in 2007, 2010, 2013, and 2016.

- Figure B17 Hierarchical maps and univariate LISA cluster maps of the density of urban licensed doctors in 2007, 2010, 2013, and 2016.
- Figure B18 Hierarchical maps and univariate LISA cluster maps of the density of urban registered nurses in 2007, 2010, 2013, and 2016.
- Figure B19 Hierarchical maps and univariate LISA cluster maps of the density of urban pharmacists in 2007, 2010, 2013, and 2016.
- Figure B20 Hierarchical maps and univariate LISA cluster maps of the density of urban technologists in 2007, 2010, 2013, and 2016.
- Figure B21 Hierarchical maps and univariate LISA cluster maps of the density of urban interns in 2007, 2010, 2013, and 2016.
- Figure B22 Hierarchical maps and univariate LISA cluster maps of the density of rural health technicians in 2007, 2010, 2013, and 2016.
- Figure B23 Hierarchical maps and univariate LISA cluster maps of the density of rural licensed doctors in 2007, 2010, 2013, and 2016.
- Figure B24 Hierarchical maps and univariate LISA cluster maps of the density of rural registered nurses in 2007, 2010, 2013, and 2016.
- Figure B25 Hierarchical maps and univariate LISA cluster maps of the density of rural pharmacists in 2007, 2010, 2013, and 2016.
- Figure B26 Hierarchical maps and univariate LISA cluster maps of the density of rural technologists in 2007, 2010, 2013, and 2016.
- Figure B27 Hierarchical maps and univariate LISA cluster maps of the density of rural interns in 2007, 2010, 2013, and 2016.

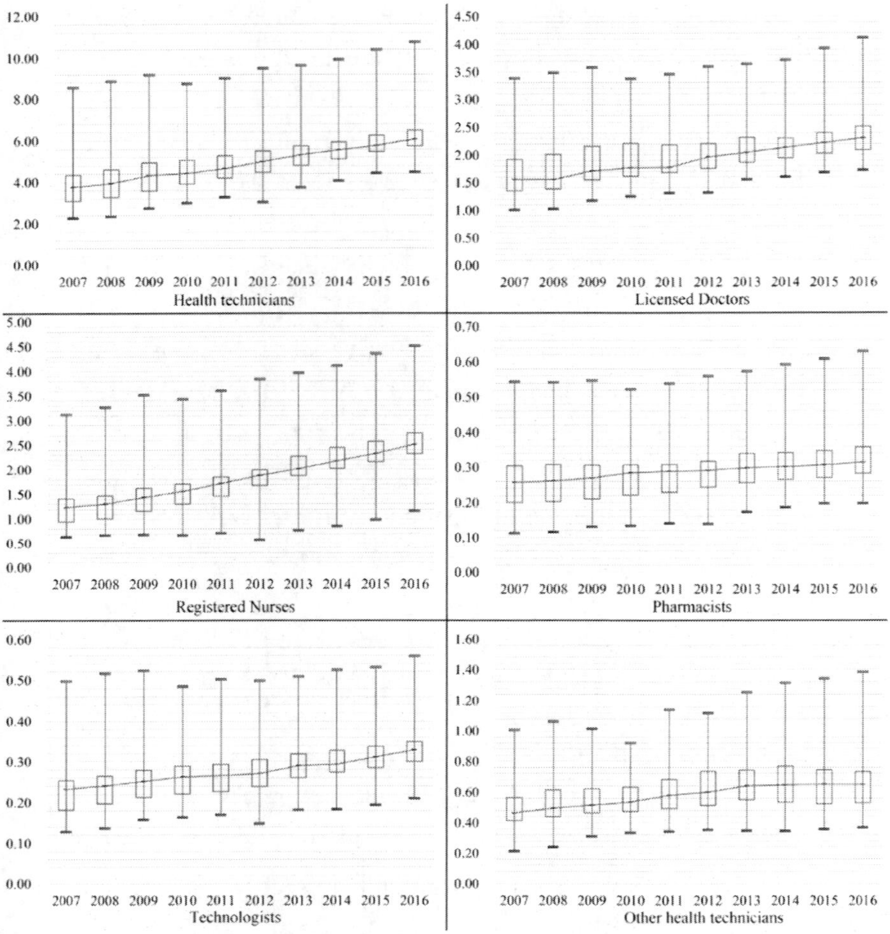

Figure B1. Boxplots of the density of total health manpower during 2007–2016.

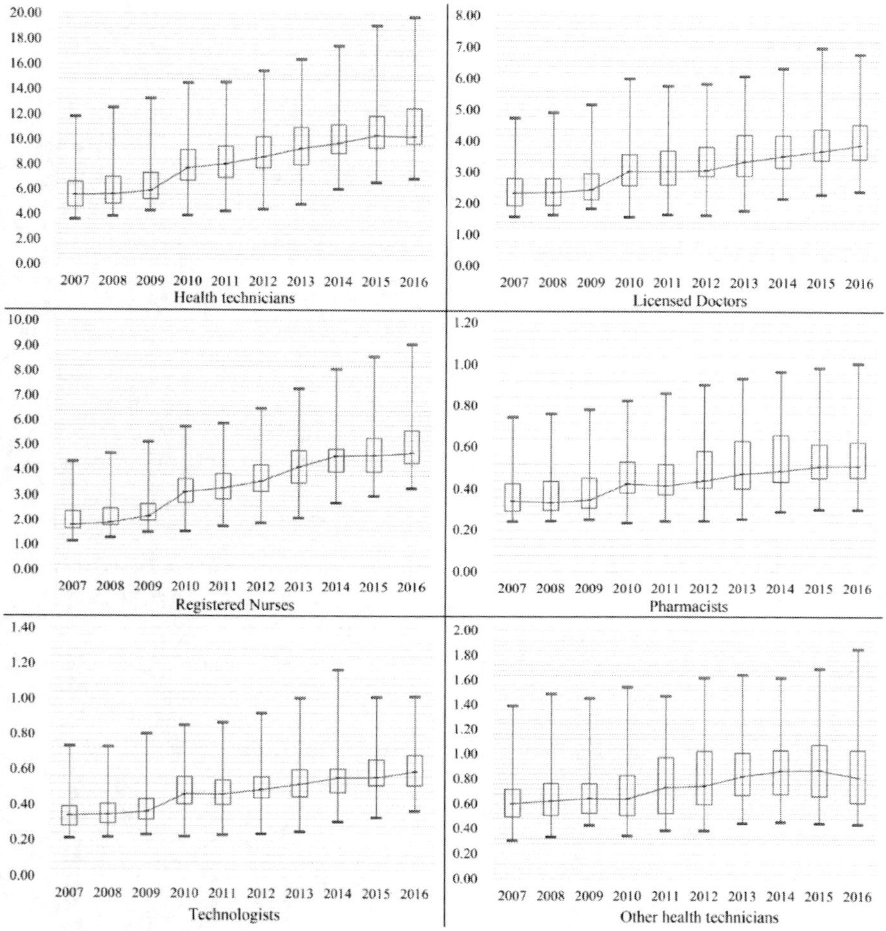

Figure B2. Boxplots of the density of urban health manpower during 2007–2016.

Table B1. Detailed information of space–time clusters of higher and lower rate of health technicians from 2007 to 2016

Type	Cluster type	Location IDs included	Coordinates of cluster center	Radius (Km)	Average density	Inside time trend (annual)	Outside time trend (annual)	LLR	P–value
Health technicians	Higher	Sichuan (center), Chongqing, Guizhou, Gansu, Shaanxi, Yunnan, Ningxia, Qinghai, Hunan, Hubei, Guangxi, Henan	30.28 N, 102.90 E	1079.52	4.522	7.316%	5.085%	27120.45	0.001
Health technicians	Higher	Fujian (center)	26.00 N, 118.02 E	0	4.404	8.687%	5.854%	4449.19	0.001
Health technicians	Lower	Heilongjiang (center), Jilin, Liaoning, Beijing, Tianjin, Hebei	46.77 N, 127.89 E	1392.77	5.375	3.473%	6.454%	31084.49	0.001
Health technicians	Lower	Shanghai	31.21 N, 121.68 E	0	6.513	1.651%	6.009%	9954.27	0.001
Licensed doctors	Higher	Guangdong (center), Guangxi, Jiangxi, Hunan, Fujian, Hainan, Guizhou, Hubei, Chongqing, Zhejiang, Anhui, Henan	23.28 N, 113.36 E	1169.60	1.766	5.419%	3.793%	6243.40	0.001
Licensed doctors	Lower	Heilongjiang (center), Jilin, Liaoning, Beijing, Tianjin	46.77 N, 127.89 E	1196.92	2.389	2.106%	4.868%	8585.82	0.001
Licensed doctors	Lower	Ningxia (center), Gansu, Shaanxi, Shanxi, Neimenggu	37.37 N, 105.99E	624.63	2.074	3.000%	4.685%	2607.95	0.001
Licensed doctors	Lower	Xizang (center), Qinghai, Xinjiang	31.10 N, 89.12 E	1249.86	2.164	2.692%	4.552%	864.76	0.001
Registered nurses	Higher	Sichuan (center), Chongqing, Guizhou, Gansu, Shaanxi, Yunnan, Ningxia, Qinghai, Hunan, Hubei, Guangxi, Henan	30.28 N, 102.90 E	1079.52	1.674	11.065%	7.934%	18231.14	0.001
Registered nurses	Lower	Jilin (center), Liaoning, Heilongjiang, Tianjin, Beijing	43.50 N, 126.45 E	904.01	2.218	5.157%	9.688%	19565.81	0.001
Registered nurses	Lower	Shanghai	31.21 N, 121.68 E	0	2.737	3.582%	9.216%	6546.90	0.001
Pharmacists	Higher	Xizang (center), Qinghai, Xinjiang, Sichuan, Yunnan, Gansu, Ningxia, Guizhou, Chongqing, Shaanxi, Guangxi	31.10 N, 89.12 E	2106.09	0.236	5.249%	2.214%	2221.83	0.001
Pharmacists	Higher	Fujian (center)	26.00 N, 118.02 E	0	0.302	6.834%	2.759%	667.65	0.001

Type	Cluster type	Location IDs included	Coordinates of cluster center	Radius (Km)	Average density	Inside time trend (annual)	Outside time trend (annual)	LLR	P–value
Pharmacists	Higher	Jiangsu (center), Shanghai, Anhui, Zhejiang	32.47 N, 119.97 E	374.35	0.299	3.667%	2.714%	186.04	0.001
Pharmacists	Lower	Hunan, Hubei	28.02 N, 111.58 E	349.86	0.307	0.229%	3.234%	1635.32	0.001
Pharmacists	Lower	Heilongjiang (center), Jilin, Liaoning, Beijing, Tianjin, Hebei, Shandong, Neimenggu, Shanxi	46.77 N, 127.89 E	1620.87	0.299	1.433%	3.484%	1285.71	0.001
Technologists	Higher	Yunnan (center), Guizhou, Sichuan, Guangxi, Chongqing	24.14 N, 101.30 E	896.95	0.221	8.259%	3.665%	3455.16	0.001
Technologists	Higher	Fujian (center), Jiangxi	26.00 N, 118.02 E	305.25	0.246	6.547%	4.212%	378.80	0.001
Technologists	Higher	Ningxia (center), Gansu, Shaanxi	37.37 N, 105.96 E	439.66	0.300	6.468%	4.212%	369.52	0.001
Technologists	Lower	Jilin (center), Liaoning, Heilongjiang, Tianjin, Beijing, Shandong, Hebei, Neimenggu, Shanxi, Jiangsu, Shanghai	43.50 N, 126.45 E	1428.28	0.296	2.618%	5.410%	2528.41	0.001
Interns	Higher	Xizang (center), Qinghai, Xinjiang, Sichuan, Yunnan, Gansu, Ningxia, Guizhou, Chongqing, Shaanxi, Guangxi	31.10 N, 89.12 E	2106.09	0.648	7.777%	1.553%	22693.92	0.001
Interns	Lower	Shandong (center), Tianjin, Hebei, Jiangsu, Anhui, Beijing, Henan, Shanxi, Shanghai, Liaoning, Hubei	36.18 N, 118.43 E	770.54	0.552	0.864%	5.152%	13339.34	0.001
Urban health techncians	Higher	Guangdong (center), Guangxi, Jiangxi, Hunan, Fujian, Hainan, Guizhou, Hubei	23.28 N, 113.36 E	847.67	7.578	9.870%	7.604%	14246.52	0.001
Urban health techncians	Lower	Beijing (center), Tianjin	40.22 N, 116.44 E	135.55	12.195	4.010%	8.367%	16485.81	0.001
Urban health techncians	Lower	Shanghai (center)	31.21 N, 121.68 E	0	10.581	3.731%	8.358%	10675.00	0.001
Urban health techncians	Lower	Xinjiang (center), Qinghai, Xizang, Gansu, Ningxia, Sichuan, Neimenggu, Shaanxi, Shanxi, Chongqing	42.00 N, 85.66 E	2396.49	7.474	6.466%	8.682%	10238.73	0.001
Urban licensed doctors	Higher	Guangdong (center), Guangxi, Jiangxi, Hunan, Fujian, Hainan, Guizhou, Hubei	23.28 N, 113.36 E	847.67	2.750	8.911%	6.273%	7281.99	0.001
Urban licensed doctors	Lower	Xinjiang (center), Qinghai, Xizang, Gansu, Ningxia, Sichuan, Neimenggu, Shaanxi, Shanxi, Chongqing	42.00 N, 85.66 E	2396.49	2.842	4.598%	7.584%	7284.33	0.001

Table B1. (Continued).

Type	Cluster type	Location IDs included	Coordinates of cluster center	Radius (Km)	Average density	Inside time trend (annual)	Outside time trend (annual)	LLR	P–value
Urban licensed doctors	Lower	Beijing (center), Tianjin	40.22 N, 116.44 E	135.55	4.650	3.696%	7.058%	3878.20	0.001
Urban licensed doctors	Lower	Shanghai (center)	31.21 N, 121.68 E	0	3.951	2.689%	7.111%	3743.29	0.001
Urban registered nurses	Higher	Shandong (center)	36.18 N, 118.43 E	0	2.747	8.203%	6.897%	625.38	0.001
Urban registered nurses	Higher	Hubei (center), Henan, Hunan	30.90 N, 113.03 E	349.86	3.109	14.537%	10.931%	8169.98	0.001
Urban registered nurses	Lower	Beijing (center), Tianjin	40.22 N, 116.44 E	135.55	4.820	5.523%	11.681%	12142.97	0.001
Urban registered nurses	Lower	Shanghai (center)	31.21 N, 121.68 E	0	4.488	5.679%	11.598%	6942.10	0.001
Urban registered nurses	Lower	Xinjiang (center), Qinghai, Xizang, Gansu, Ningxia	42.00 N, 85.66 E	1808.12	3.387	7.650%	11.580%	3105.86	0.001
Urban pharmacists	Higher	Fujian (center), Jiangxi, Zhejiang, Guangdong	26.00 N, 118.02 E	560.26	0.536	7.028%	4.740%	764.30	0.001
Urban pharmacists	Higher	Yunnan (center), Guizhou	24.14 N, 101.30 E	602.35	0.365	8.676%	5.135%	252.57	0.001
Urban pharmacists	Lower	Shaanxi (center), Ningxia, Henan, Chongqing, Gansu, Shanxi, Hubei, Sichuan, Hunan, Hebei, Anhui	34.12 N, 108.76 E	818.20	0.363	3.832%	6.040%	892.56	0.001
Urban pharmacists	Lower	Liaoning (center), Jilin, Tianjin	41.47 N, 123.52 E	579.04	0.427	3.222%	5.427%	326.11	0.001
Urban technologists	Higher	Jiangxi (center), Fujian, Hunan, Hubei, Zhejiang	27.73 N, 115.63 E	462.58	0.422	8.811%	6.020%	919.78	0.001
Urban technologists	Lower	Beijing (center), Tianjin	40.22 N, 116.44 E	1808.12	0.502	2.308%	6.709%	638.44	0.001
Urban technologists	Lower	Shanghai (center)	31.21 N, 121.68 E	0	0.634	2.619%	6.619%	495.07	0.001
Urban interns	Higher	Guangxi (center), Hainan, Guizhou, Guangdong, Hunan, Yunnan, Chongqing, Jiangxi, Sichuan, Hubei, Fujian, Shaanxi, Henan	23.02 N, 108.41 E	1300.28	0.685	5.585%	3.342%	1704.08	0.001
Urban interns	Higher	Zhejiang (center)	29.10 N, 120.10 E	0	0.885	5.657%	4.319%	132.64	0.001
Urban interns	Lower	Shanxi (center), Hebei	37.70 N, 112.38 E	270.94	0.720	0.247%	4.647%	1636.02	0.001
Urban interns	Lower	Anhui (center)	32.01 N, 117.19 E	0	0.437	0.593%	4.568%	958.18	0.001
Urban interns	Lower	Shanghai (center)	31.21 N, 121.68 E	0	0.881	1.003%	4.439%	530.46	0.001

Type	Cluster type	Location IDs included	Coordinates of cluster center	Radius (Km)	Average density	Inside time trend (annual)	Outside time trend (annual)	LLR	P–value
Rural health technicians	Higher	Xizang (center), Qinghai, Xinjiang, Sichuan, Yunnan, Gansu, Ningxia, Guizhou, Chongqing, Shaanxi, Guangxi	31.10 N, 89.12 E	2106.09	3.113	9.005%	6.552%	11469.52	0.001
Rural health technicians	Higher	Zhejiang (center), Shanghai, Jiangsu, Fujian, Anhui	29.10 N, 120.10 E	426.92	3.479	8.441%	7.065%	2375.94	0.001
Rural health technicians	Lower	Heilongjiang (center), Jilin, Liaoning, Beijing, Tianjin, Hebei, Shandong, Neimenggu, Shanxi	46.77 N, 127.89 E	1620.87	3.647	5.405%	7.981%	12226.53	0.001
Rural health technicians	Lower	Jiangxi (center)	27.73 N, 115.63 E	0	2.716	5.171%	7.380%	1584.23	0.001
Rural licensed doctors	Higher	Anhui (center), Jiangsu, Henan, Hubei, Zhejiang, Shanghai, Shandong, Jiangxi, Fujian, Hunan	32.01 N, 117.19 E	698.79	1.359	7.077%	4.979%	4317.82	0.001
Rural licensed doctors	Lower	Ningxia (center), Gansu, Shaanxi, Shanxi, Neimenggu	37.37 N, 105.99 E	624.63	1.459	3.441%	6.315%	3426.64	0.001
Rural licensed doctors	Lower	Guangxi (center), Hainan	23.02 N, 108.41 E	444.53	1.088	4.960%	5.983%	164.58	0.001
Rural registered nruses	Higher	Sichuan (center), Chongqing, Guizhou, Gansu, Shaanxi, Yunnan	30.28 N, 102.90 E	699.87	0.947	14.604%	10.930%	5753.29	0.001
Rural registered nruses	Higher	Anhui (center), Jiangsu, Henan, Hubei, Zhejiang	32.01 N, 117.19 E	426.92	1.090	12.180%	11.571%	192.30	0.001
Rural registered nruses	Lower	Heilongjiang (center), Jilin, Liaoning, Beijing, Tianjin	46.77 N, 127.89 E	1196.92	1.097	7.620%	12.040%	3306.90	0.001
Rural registered nruses	Lower	Guangdong (center), Guangxi, Jiangxi	23.28 N, 113.36 E	545.34	1.003	9.295%	12.114%	2380.85	0.001
Rural registered nruses	Lower	Shanxi (center), Hebei	37.70 N, 112.38 E	270.94	0.839	9.760%	11.888%	829.49	0.001
Rural registered nruses	Lower	Shanghai (center)	31.21 N, 121.68 E	0	2.040	5.901%	11.758%	162.29	0.001
Rural pharmacists	Higher	Xizang (center), Qinghai, Xinjiang, Sichuan, Yunnan, Gansu, Ningxia, Guizhou, Chongqing, Shaanxi, Guangxi	31.10 N, 89.12 E	2106.09	0.161	6.953%	2.709%	2037.96	0.001
Rural pharmacists	Higher	Zhejiang (center), Shanghai, Jiangsu, Fujian, Anhui	29.10 N, 120.10 E	426.92	0.223	5.907%	3.459%	516.99	0.001
Rural pharmacists	Lower	Hunan (center), Hubei, Jiangxi	28.02 N, 111.58 E	399.45	0.231	0.279%	4.671%	1712.27	0.001

Table B1. (Continued).

Type	Cluster type	Location IDs included	Coordinates of cluster center	Radius (Km)	Average density	Inside time trend (annual)	Outside time trend (annual)	LLR	P–value
Rural pharmacists	Lower	Beijing (center), Tianjin, Hebei, Shanxi, Neimenggu, Shandong, Liaoning, Henan, Jilin	40.22 N, 116.44 E	904.01	0.191	2.314%	4.649%	709.16	0.001
Rural technologists	Higher	Xizang (center), Qinghai, Xinjiang, Sichuan, Yunnan, Gansu, Ningxia, Guizhou, Chongqing, Shaanxi, Guangxi	31.10 N, 89.12 E	2106.09	0.166	9.593%	4.620%	2587.57	0.001
Rural technologists	Lower	Heilongjiang (center), Jilin, Liaoning, Beijing, Tianjin, Hebei, Shandong, Neimenggu, Shanxi, Jiangsu, Shanghai, Anhui, Henan	46.77 N, 127.89 E	1877.24	0.187	4.377%	7.517%	1288.47	0.001
Rural technologists	Lower	Guangdong (center)	23.28 N, 113.36 E	0	0.139	2.960%	6.229%	200.02	0.001
Rural technologists	Lower	Hunan (center), Hubei	28.02 N, 111.58 E	349.86	0.186	4.351%	6.271%	185.48	0.001
Rural interns	Higher	Xizang (center), Qinghai, Xinjiang, Sichuan, Yunnan, Gansu, Ningxia, Guizhou, Chongqing, Shaanxi, Guangxi	31.10 N, 89.12 E	2106.09	0.503	6.359%	1.092%	18091.34	0.001
Rural interns	Lower	Shandong (center), Tianjin, Hebei, Jiangsu, Anhui, Beijing, Henan, Shanxi, Shanghai, Liaoning, Hubei	36.18 N, 118.43 E	770.54	0.432	2.213%	3.813%	13117.52	0.001

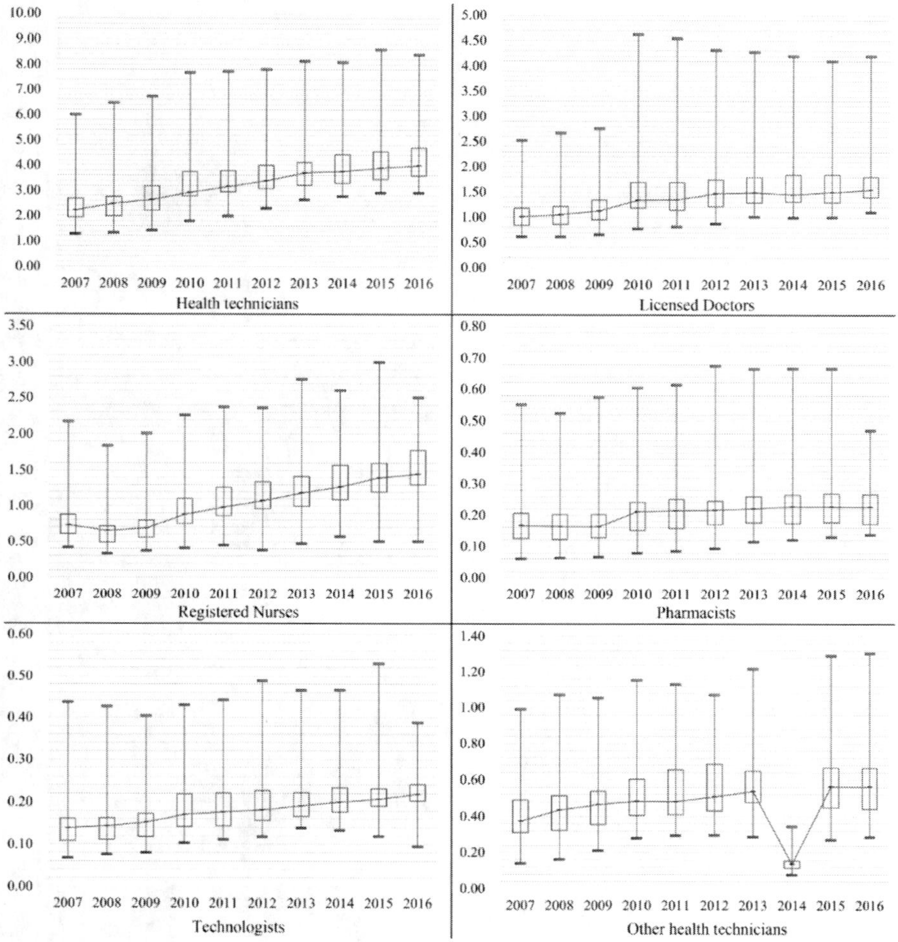

Figure B3. Boxplots of the density of rural health manpower during 2007–2016.

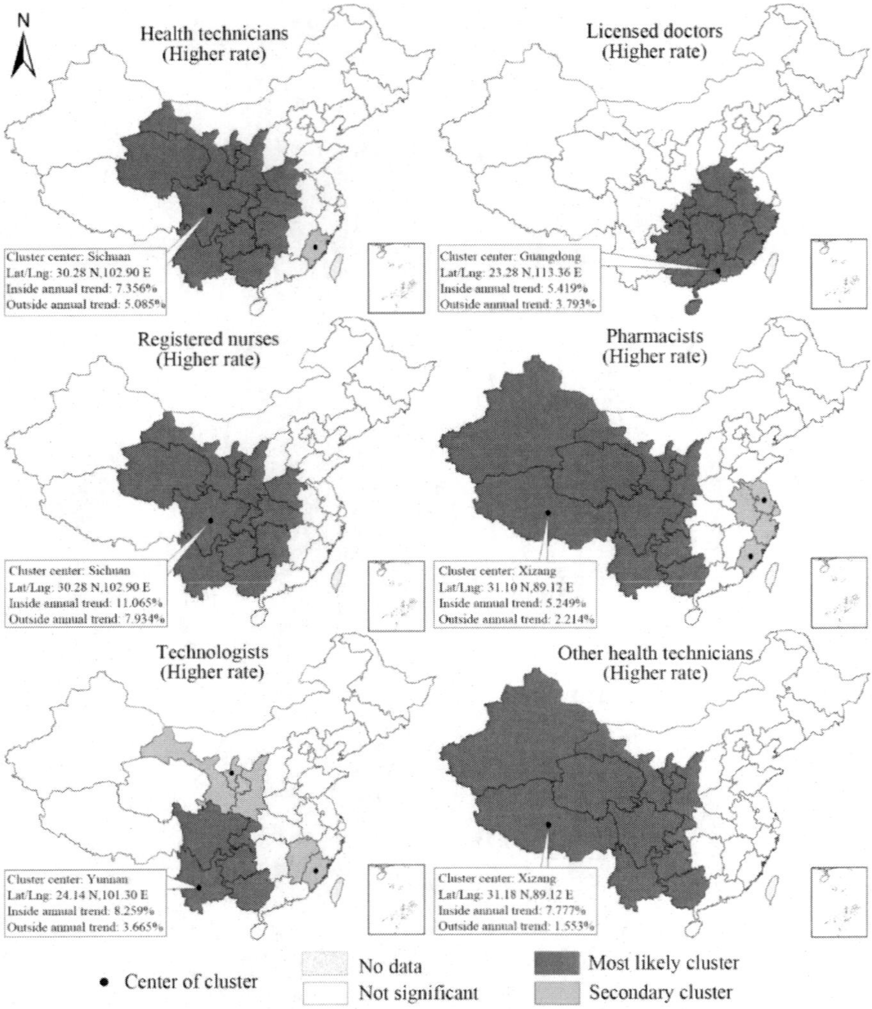

Figure B4. Space–scan for units with higher change rates of health technician density during 2007–2016.

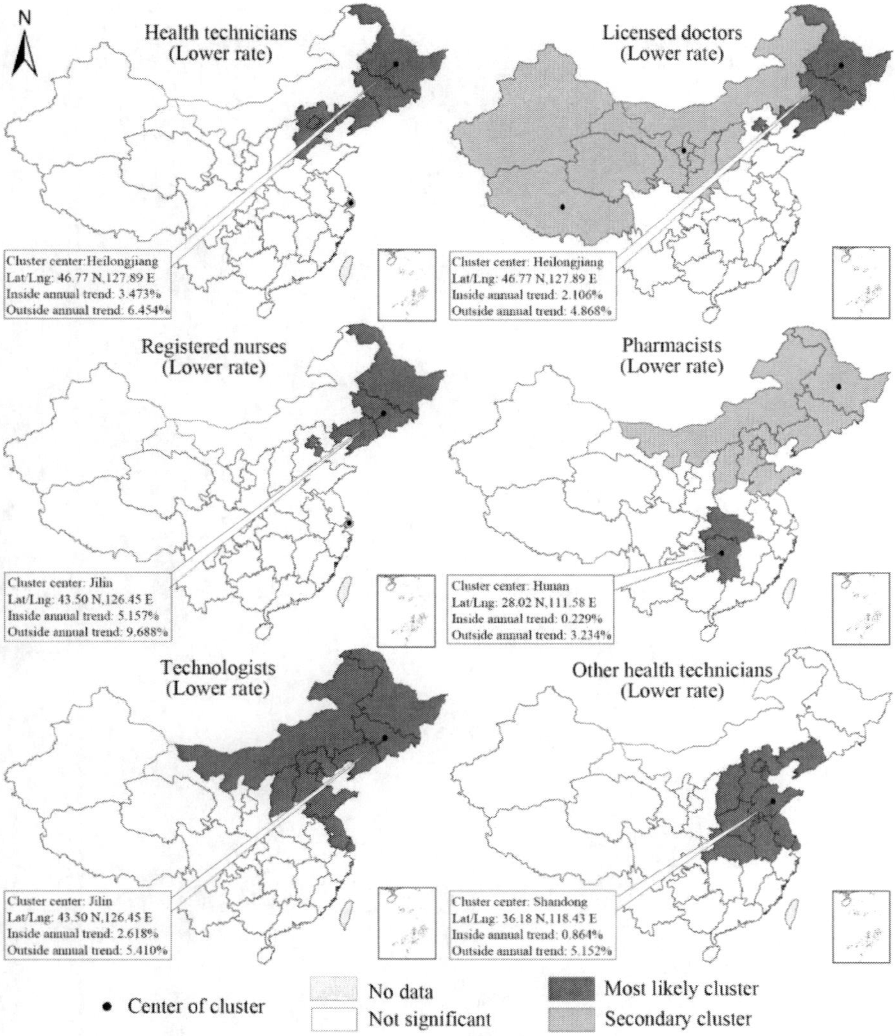

Figure B5. Space–scan for units with lower change rates of health technician density during 2007–2016.

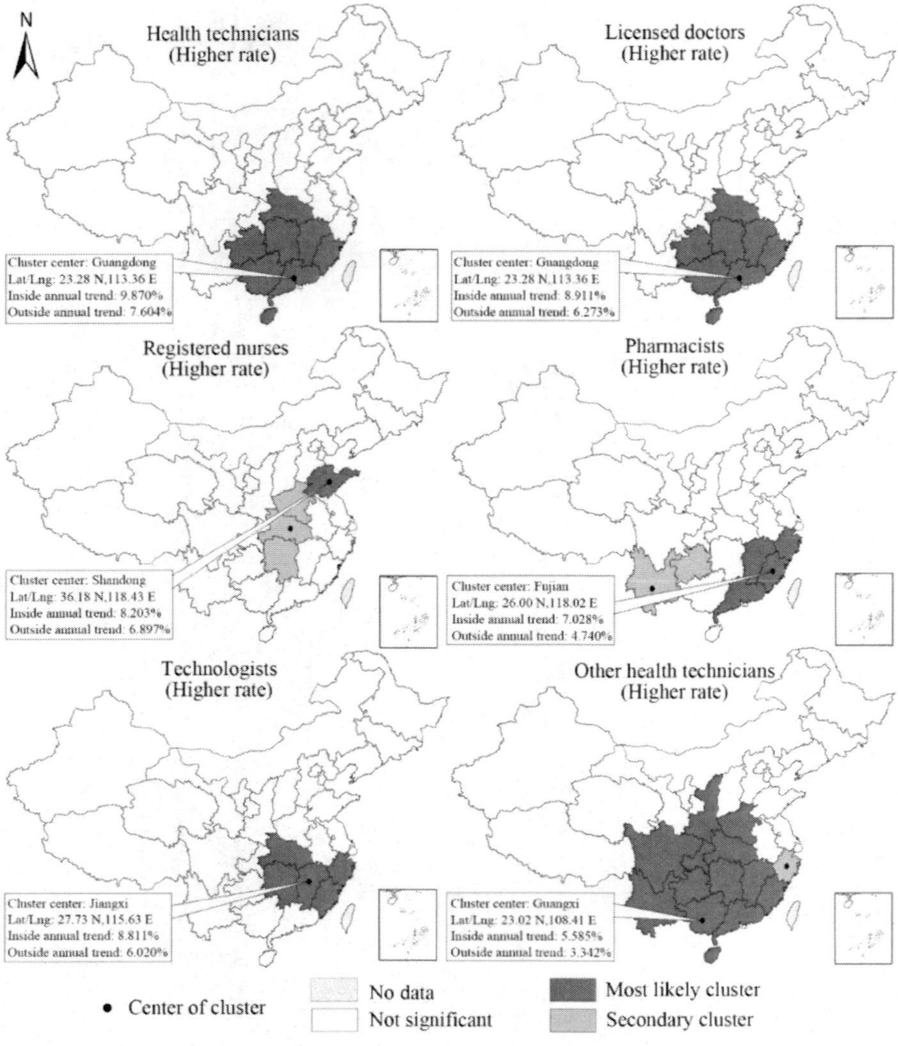

Figure B6. Space–scan for units with higher change rates of urban health technician density during 2007–2016.

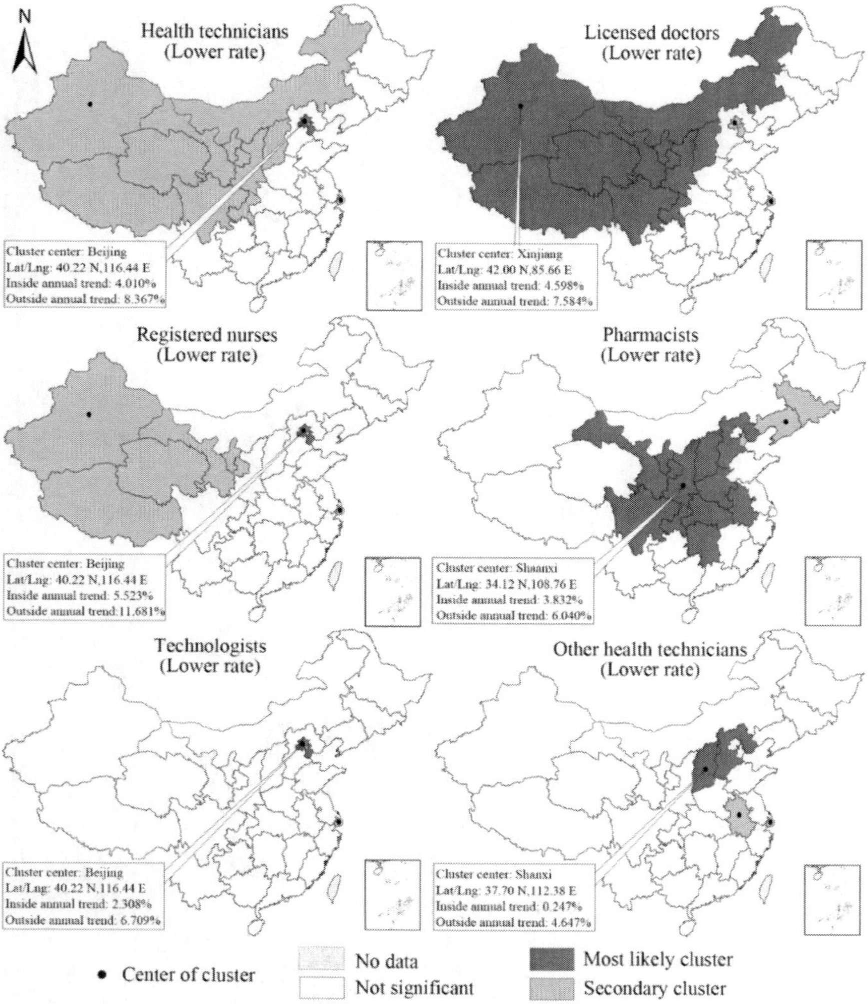

Figure B7. Space–scan for units with lower change rates of urban health technician density during 2007–2016.

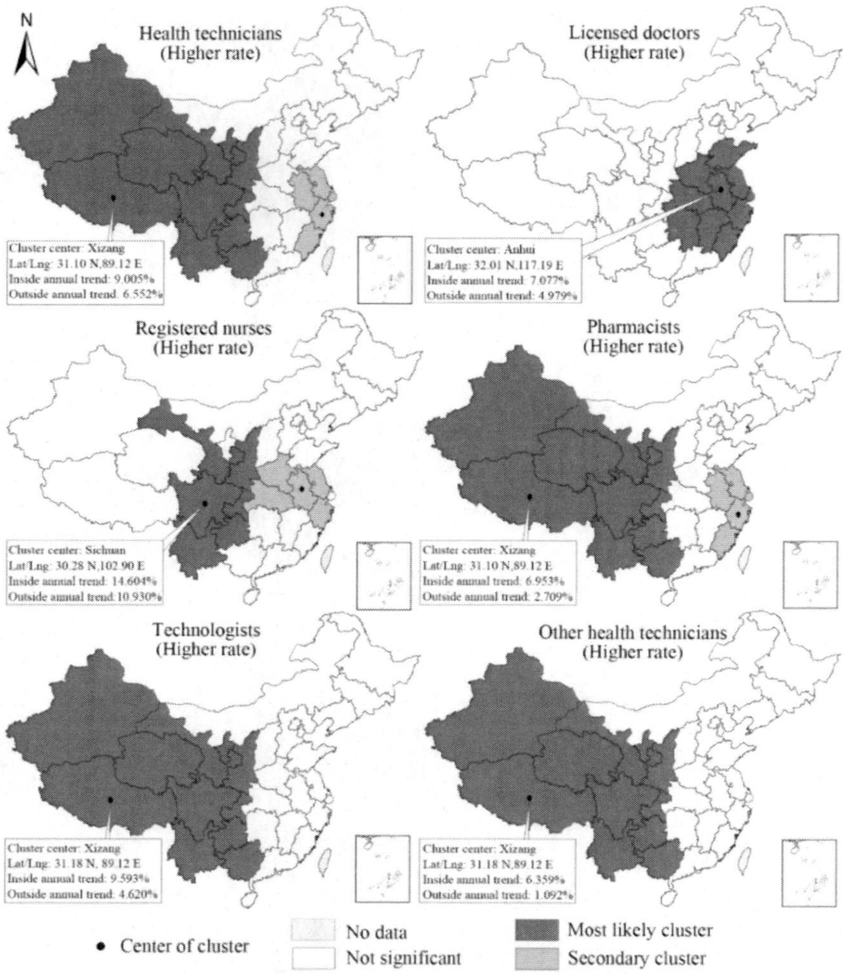

Figure B8. Space–scan for units with higher change rates of rural health technician density during 2007–2016.

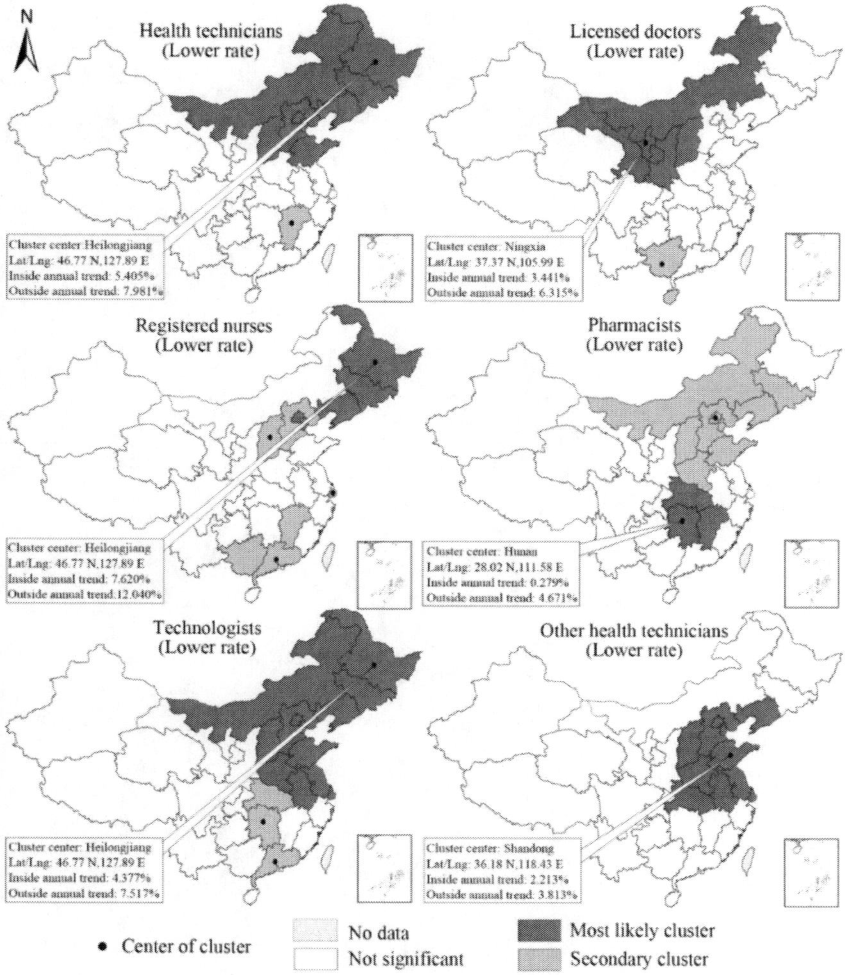

Figure B9. Space–scan for units with lower change rates of rural health technician density during 2007–2016.

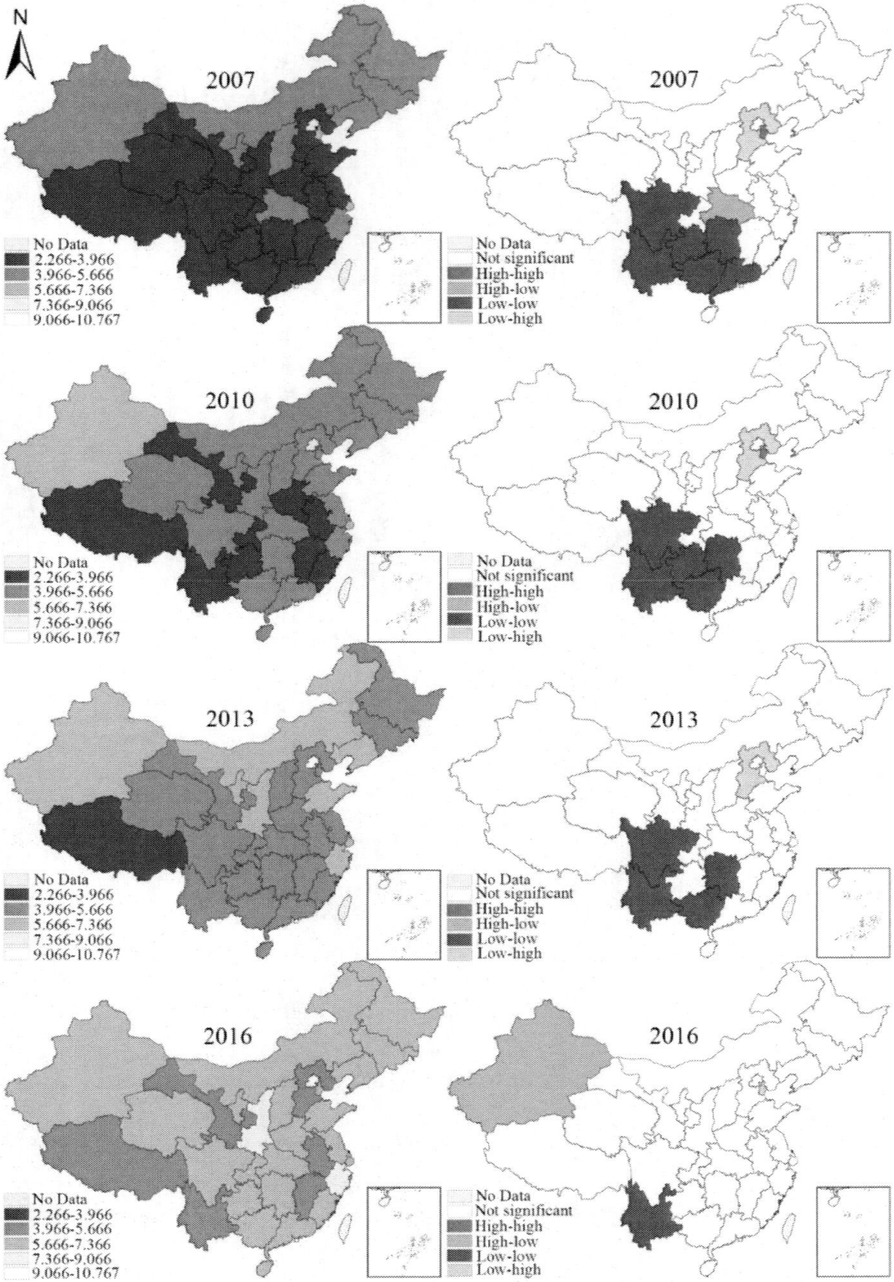

Figure B10. Hierarchical maps and univariate LISA cluster maps of the density of health technicians in 2007, 2010, 2013, and 2016.

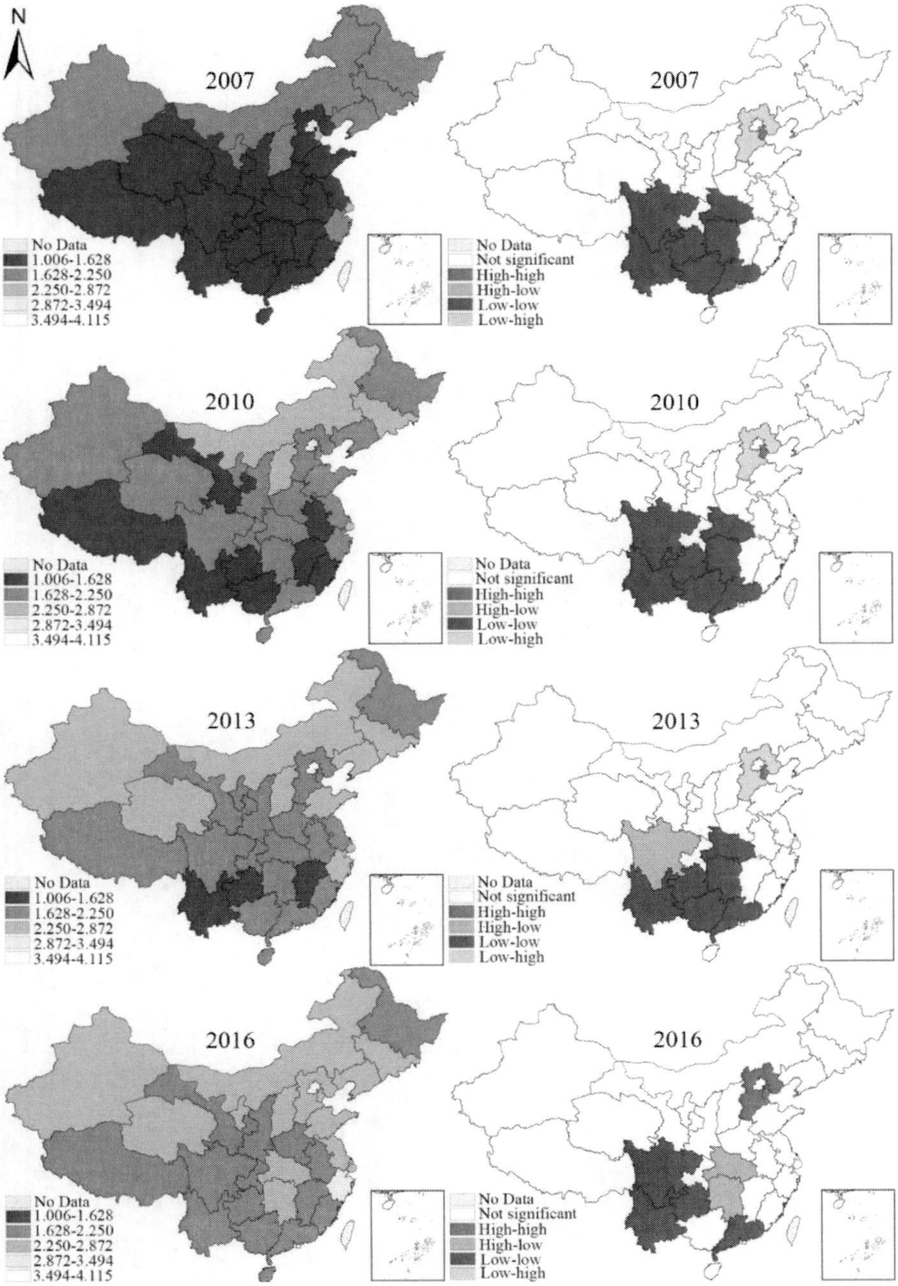

Figure B11. Hierarchical maps and univariate LISA cluster maps of the density of licensed doctors in 2007, 2010, 2013, and 2016.

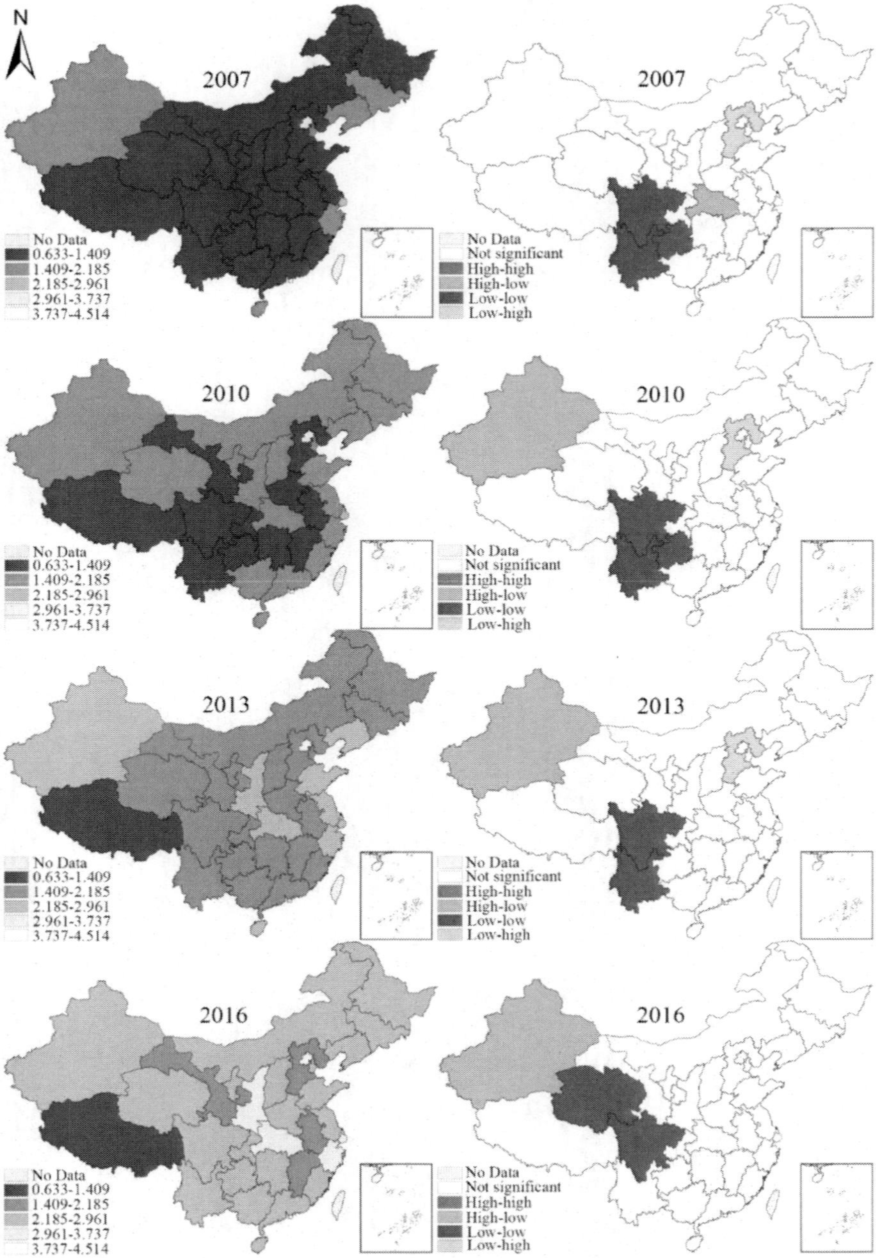

Figure B12. Hierarchical maps and univariate LISA cluster maps of the density of registered nurses in 2007, 2010, 2013, and 2016.

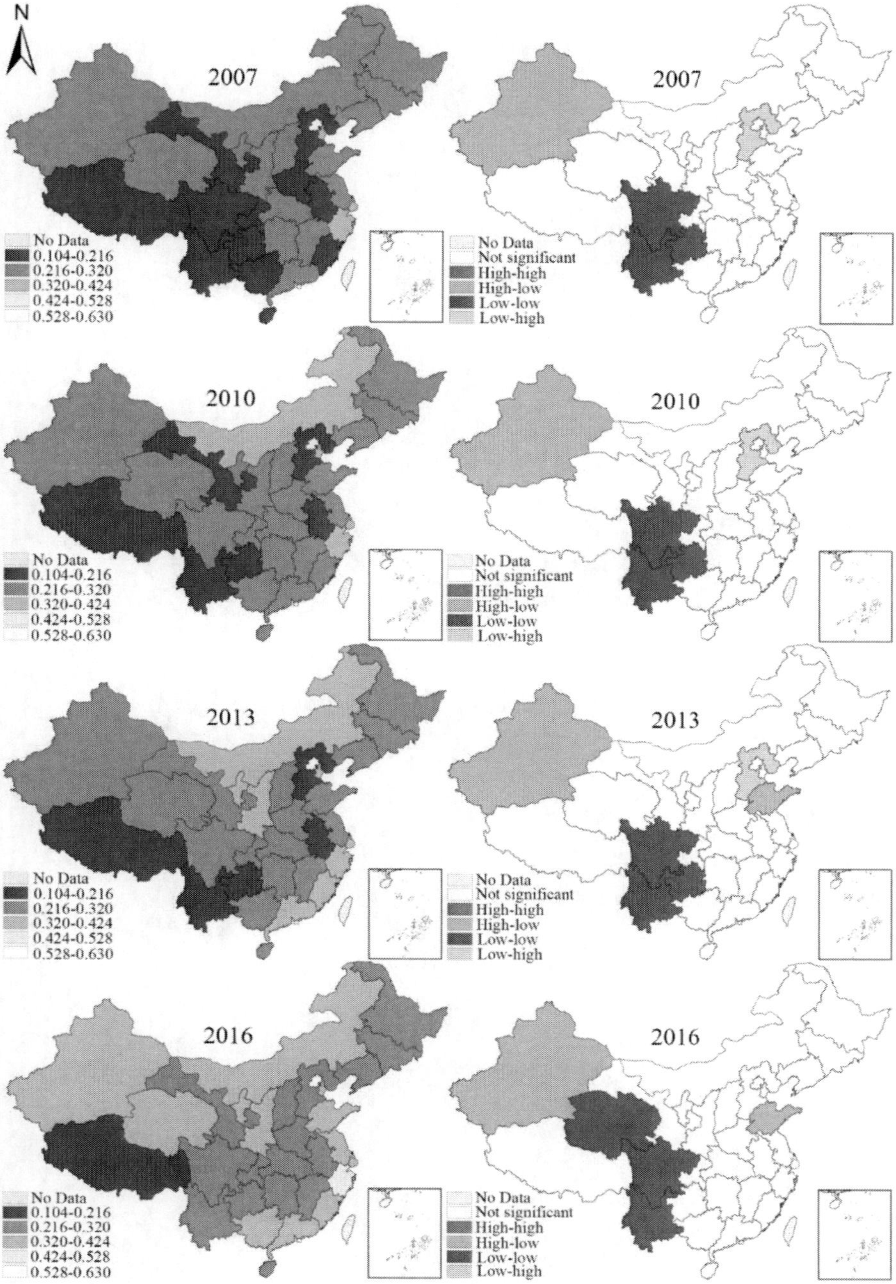

Figure B13. Hierarchical maps and univariate LISA cluster maps of the density of pharmacists in 2007, 2010, 2013, and 2016.

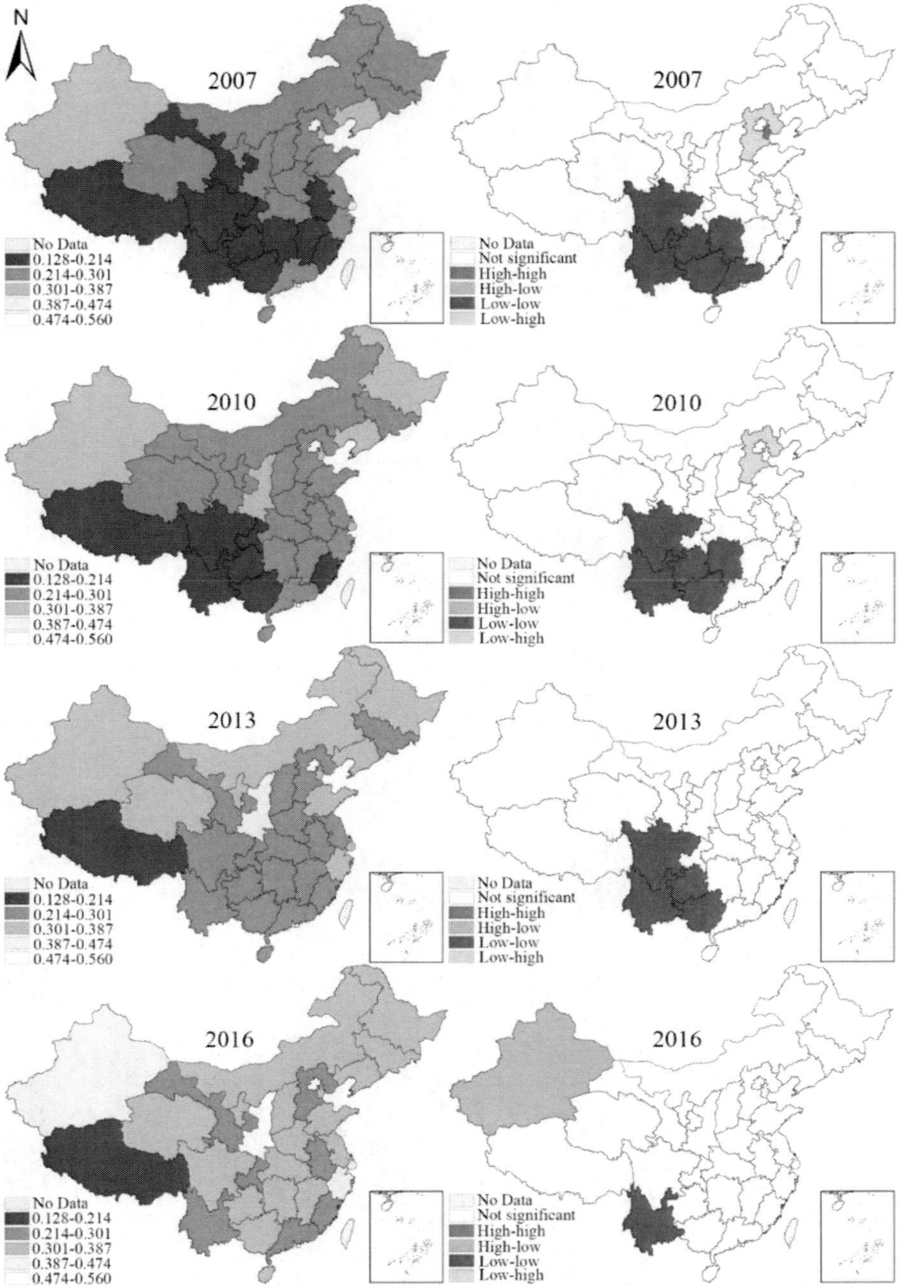

Figure B14. Hierarchical maps and univariate LISA cluster maps of the density of technologists in 2007, 2010, 2013, and 2016.

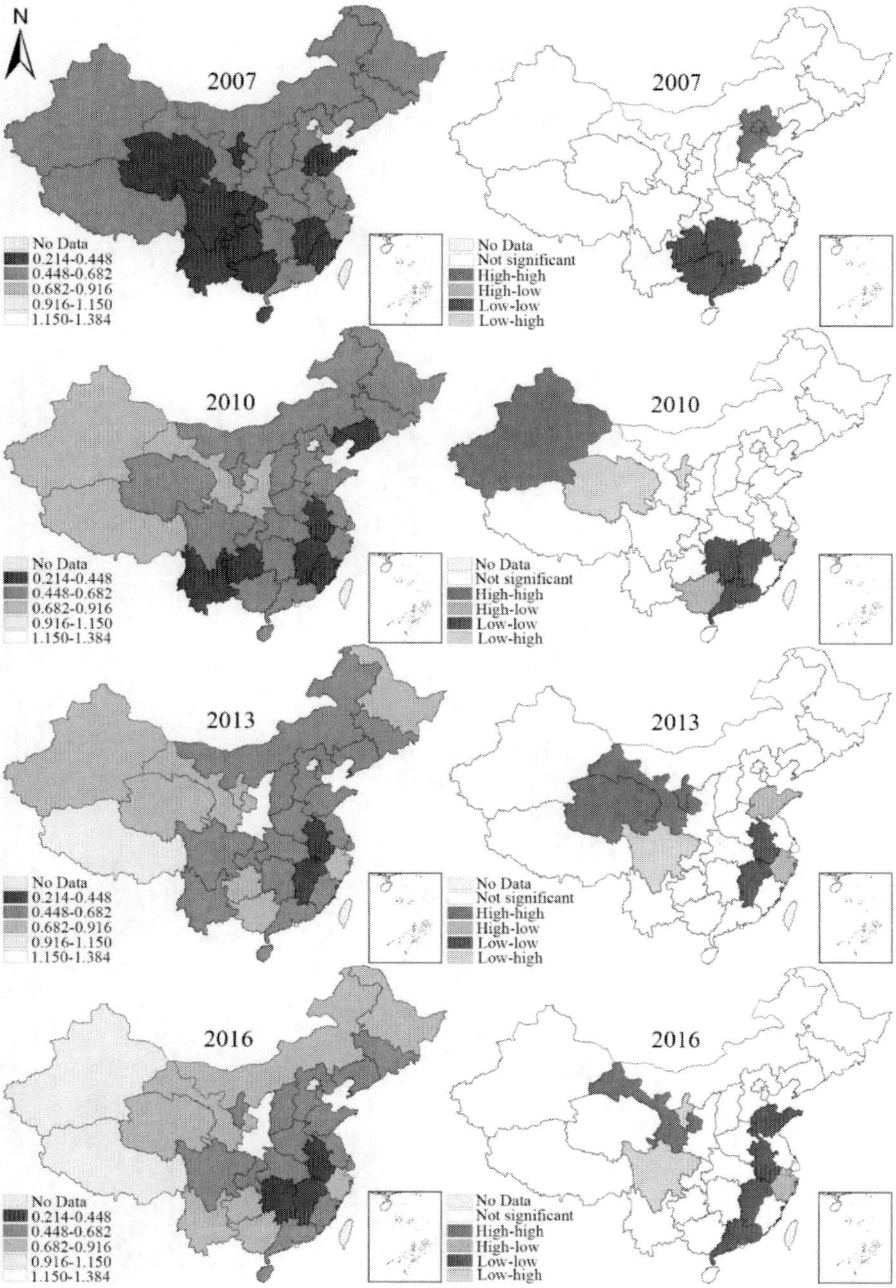

Figure B15. Hierarchical maps and univariate LISA cluster maps of the density of interns in 2007, 2010, 2013, and 2016.

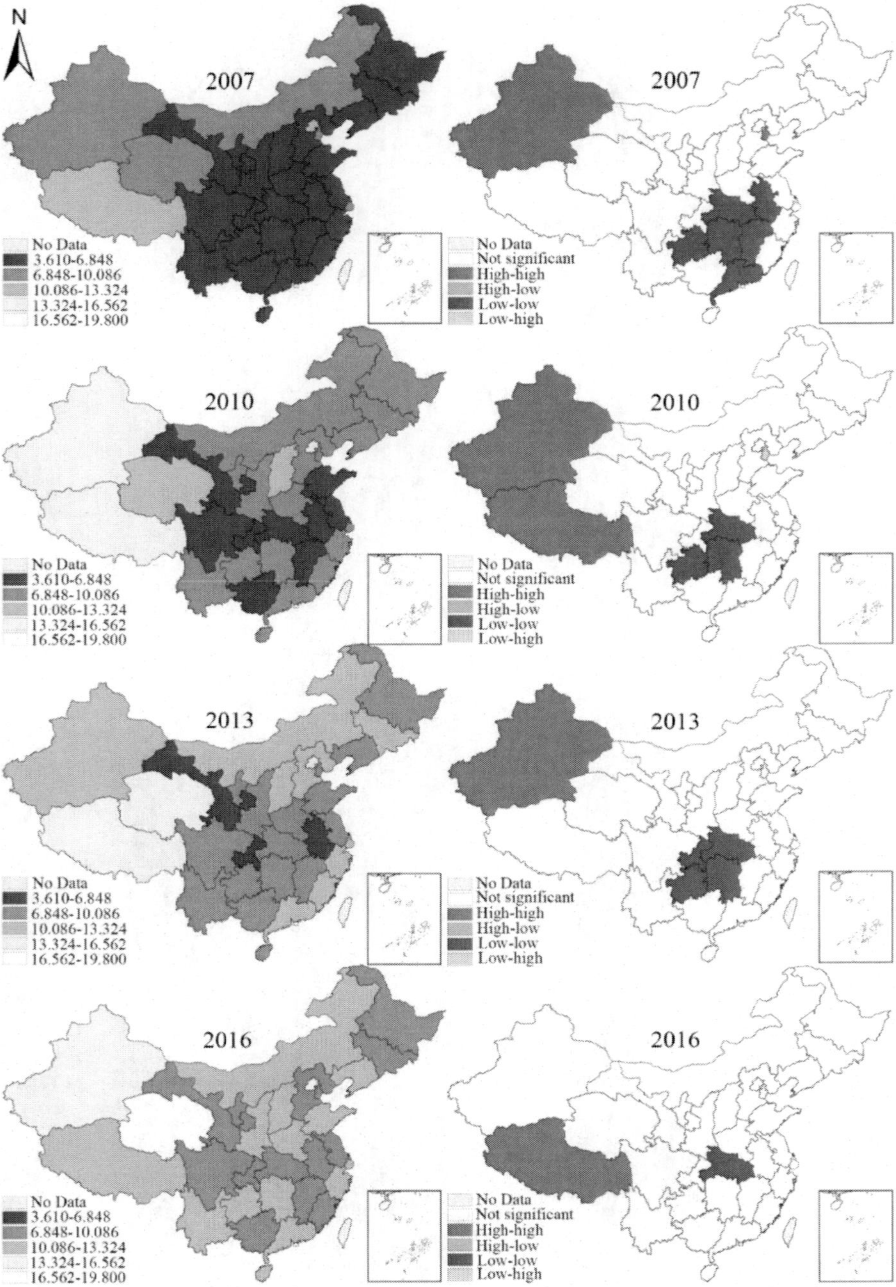

Figure B16. Hierarchical maps and univariate LISA cluster maps of the density of urban health technicians in 2007, 2010, 2013, and 2016.

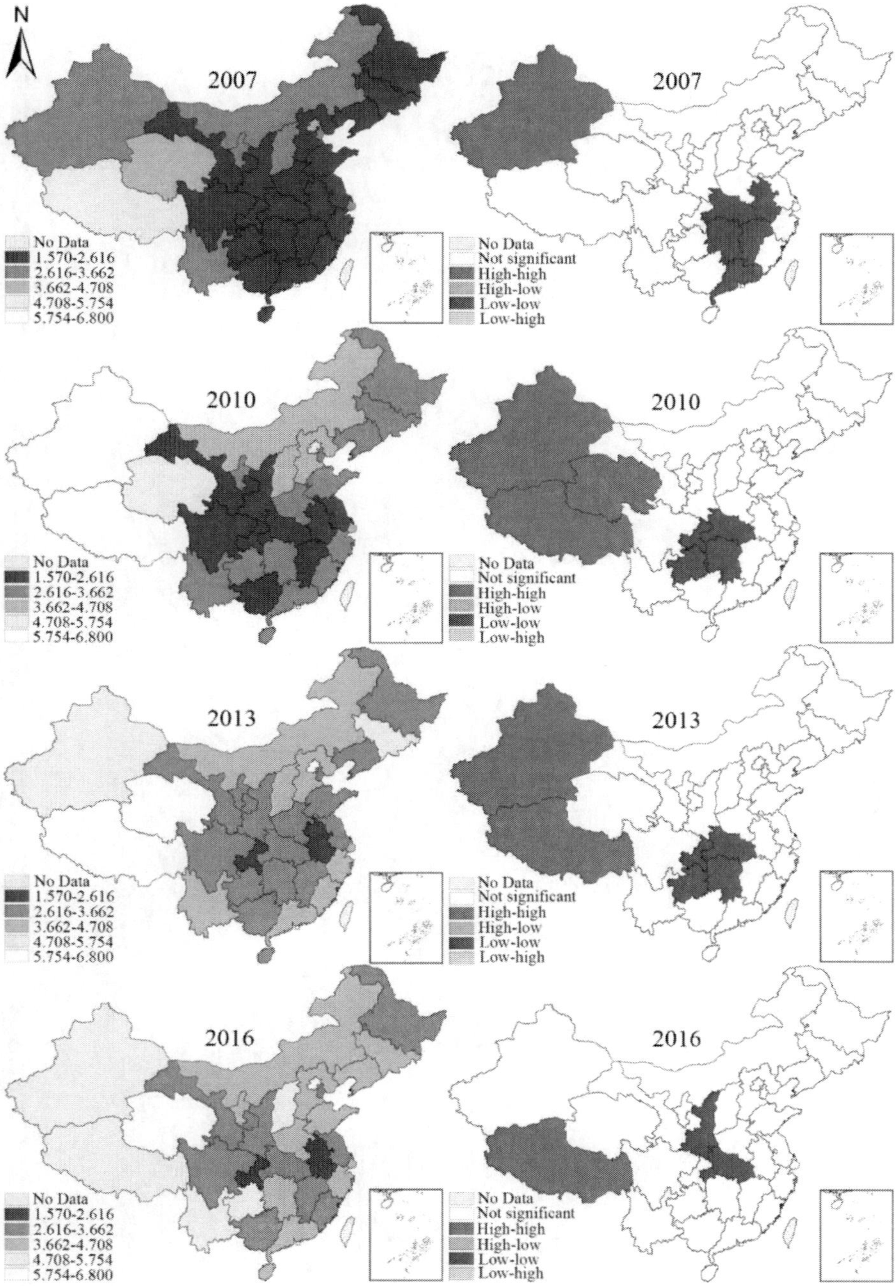

Figure B17. Hierarchical maps and univariate LISA cluster maps of the density of urban licensed doctors in 2007, 2010, 2013, and 2016.

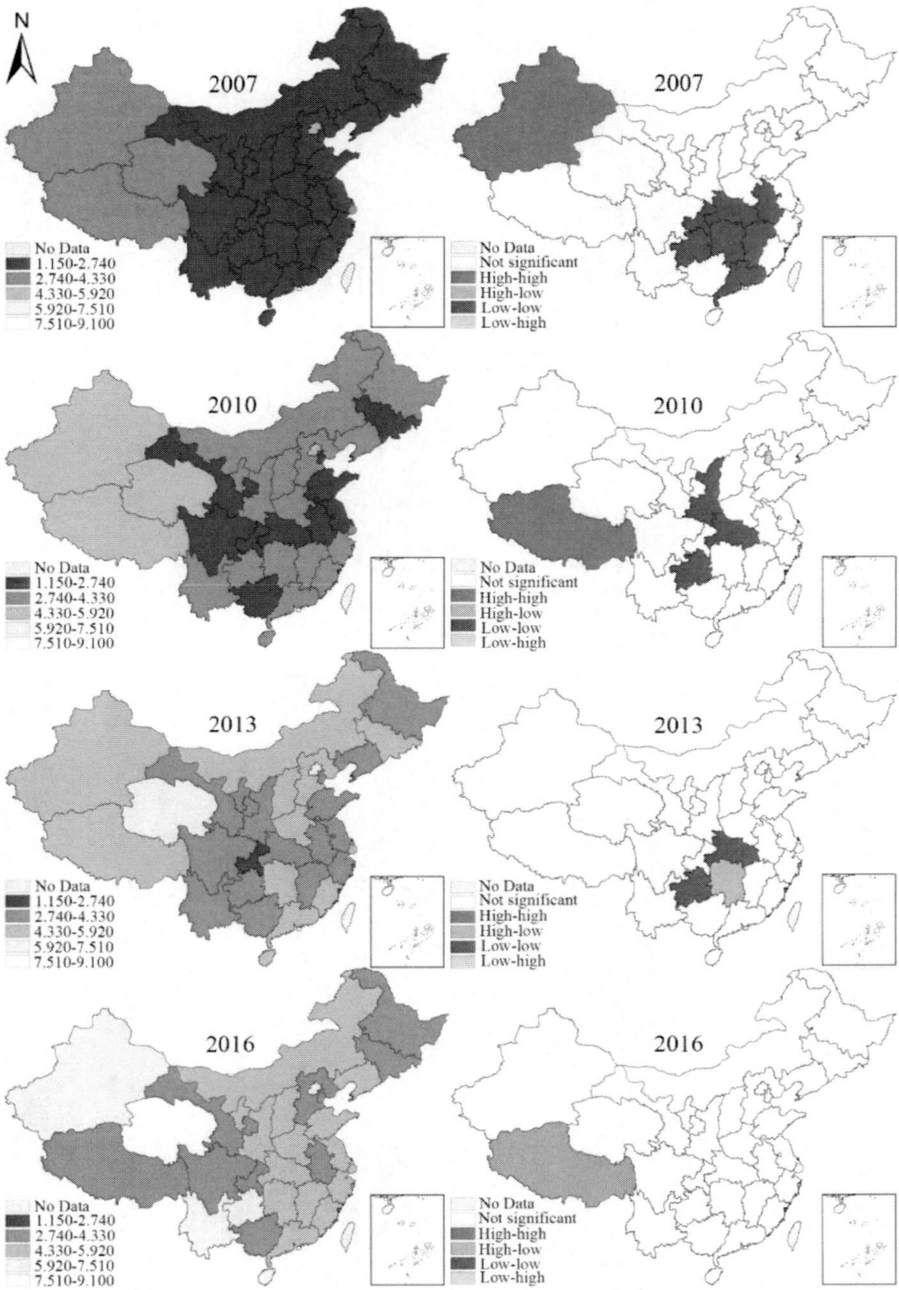

Figure B18. Hierarchical maps and univariate LISA cluster maps of the density of urban registered nurses in 2007, 2010, 2013, and 2016.

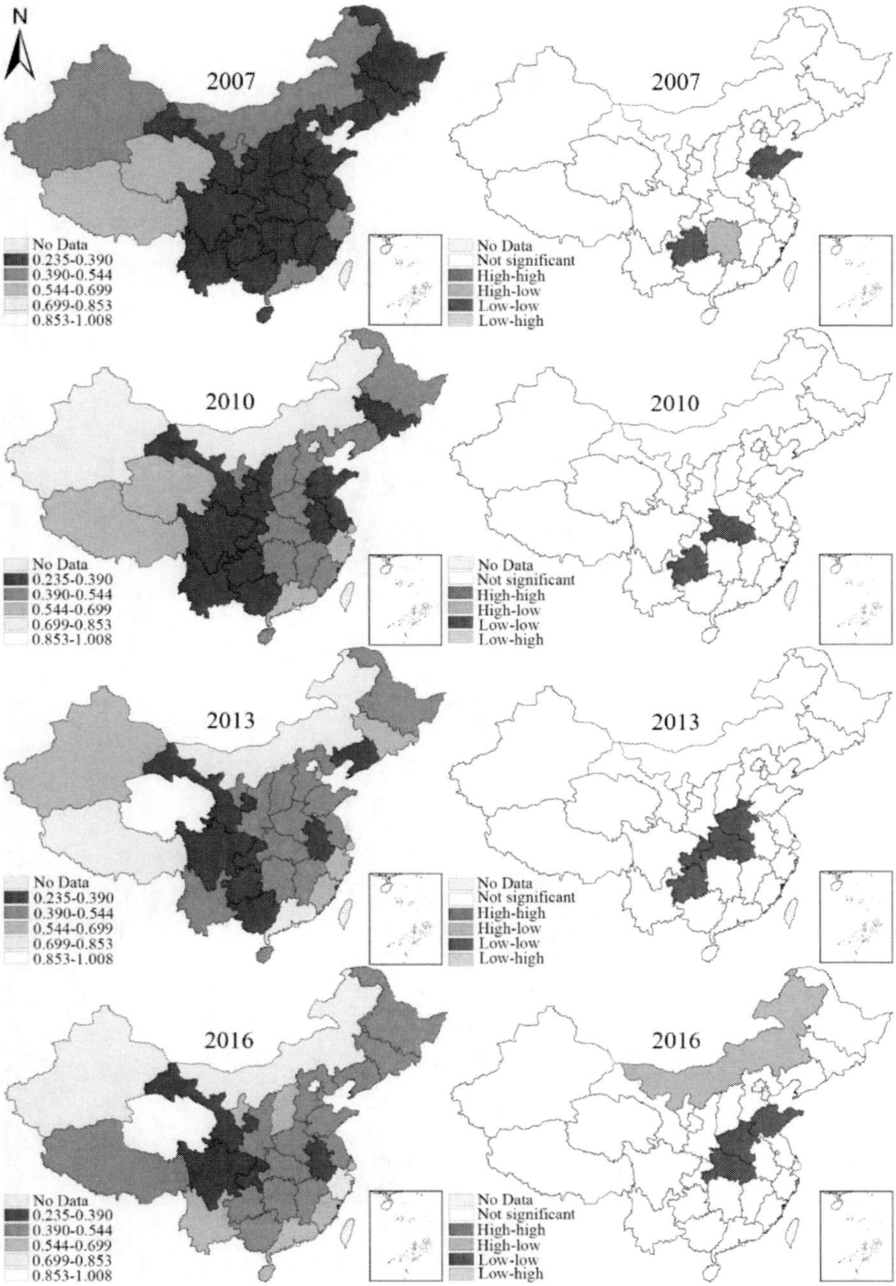

Figure B19. Hierarchical maps and univariate LISA cluster maps of the density of urban pharmacists in 2007, 2010, 2013, and 2016.

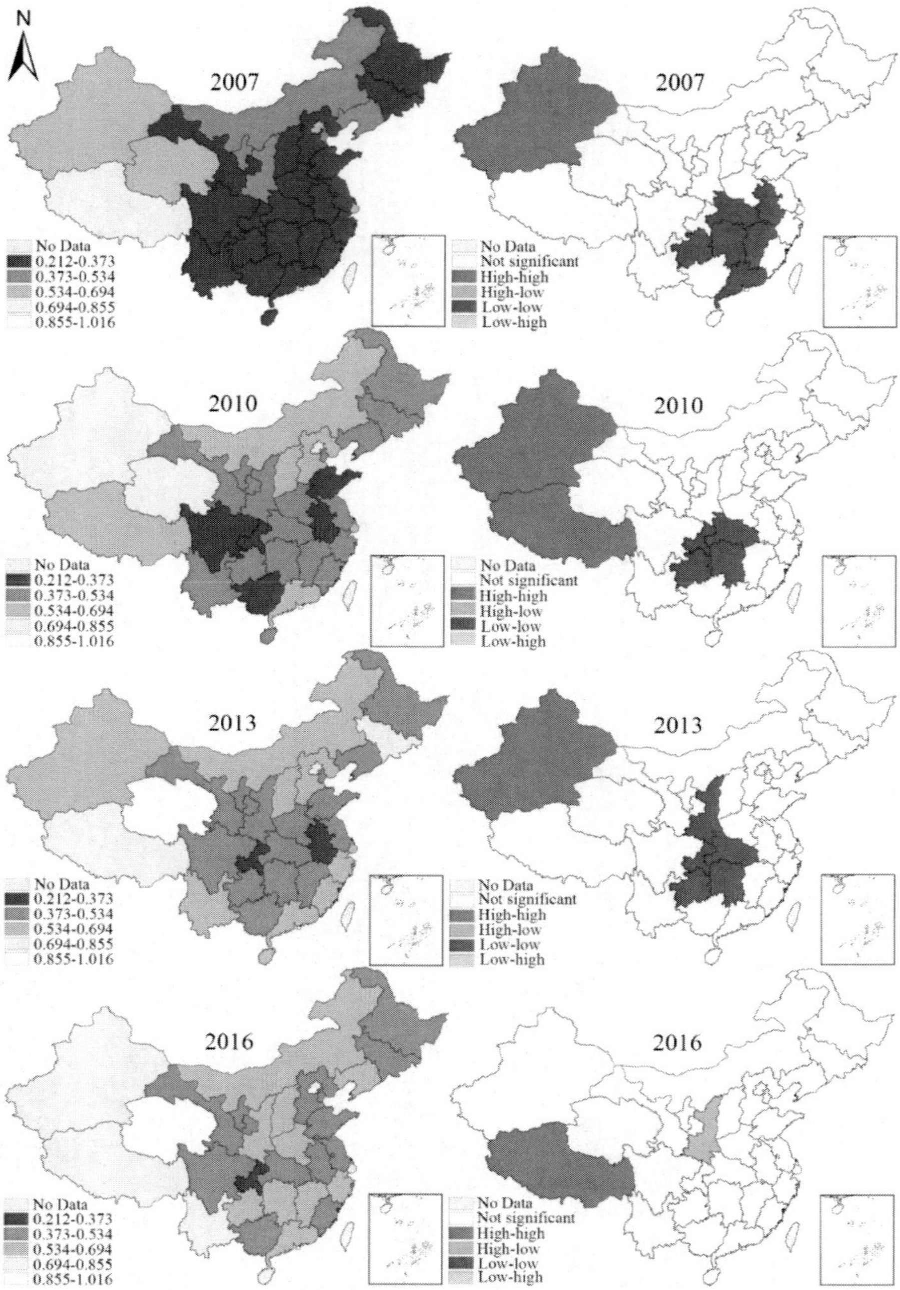

Figure B20. Hierarchical maps and univariate LISA cluster maps of the density of urban technologists in 2007, 2010, 2013, and 2016.

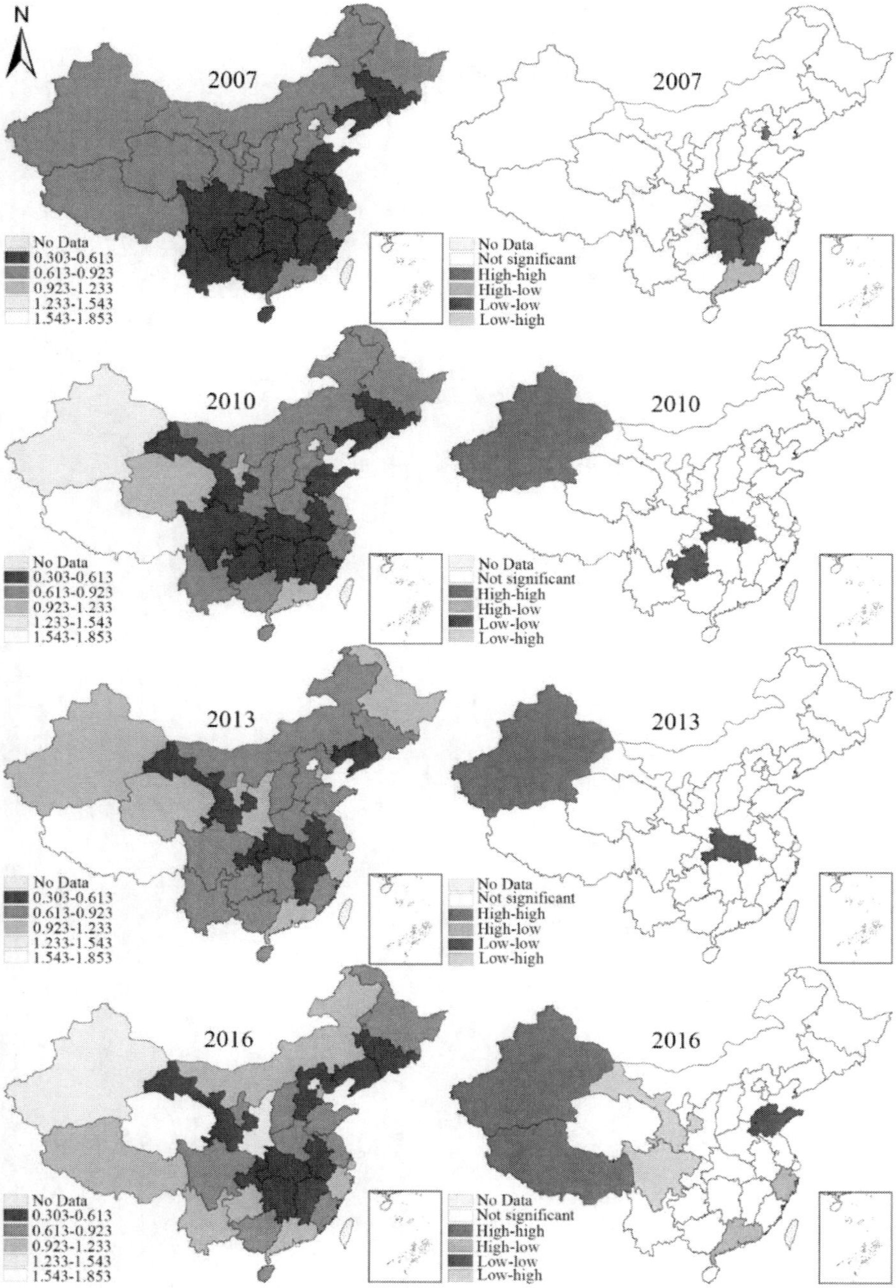

Figure B21. Hierarchical maps and univariate LISA cluster maps of the density of urban interns in 2007, 2010, 2013, and 2016.

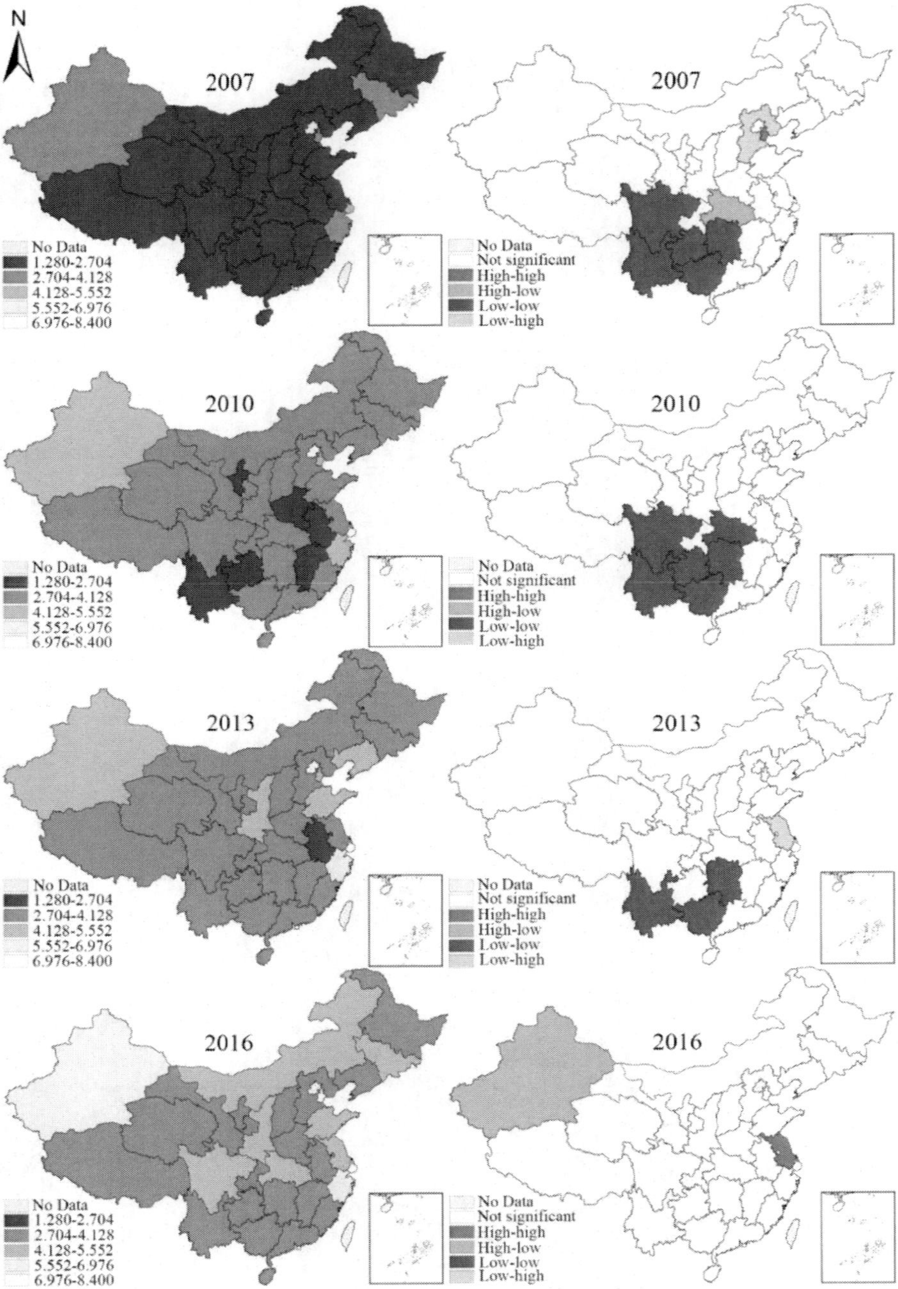

Figure B22. Hierarchical maps and univariate LISA cluster maps of the density of rural health technicians in 2007, 2010, 2013, and 2016.

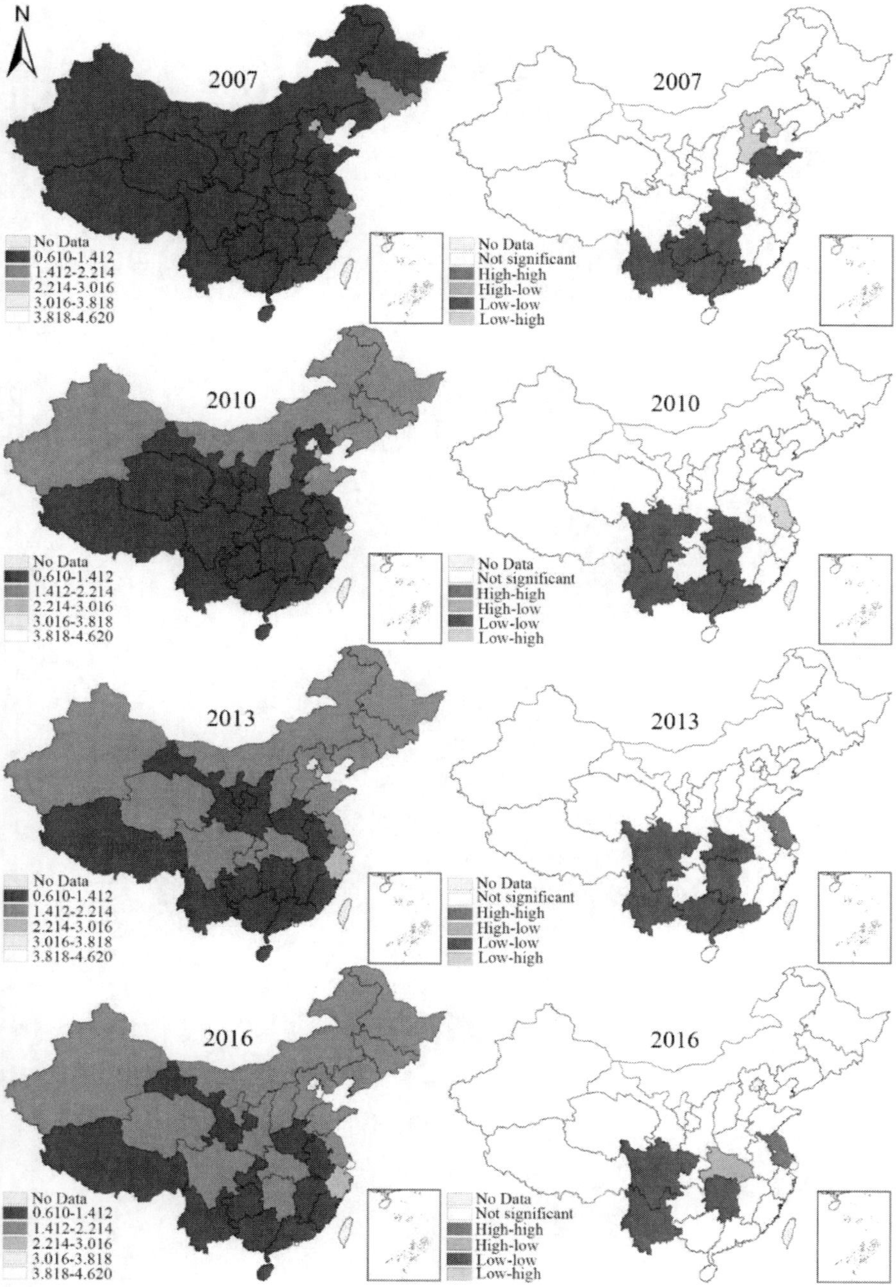

Figure B23. Hierarchical maps and univariate LISA cluster maps of the density of rural licensed doctors in 2007, 2010, 2013, and 2016.

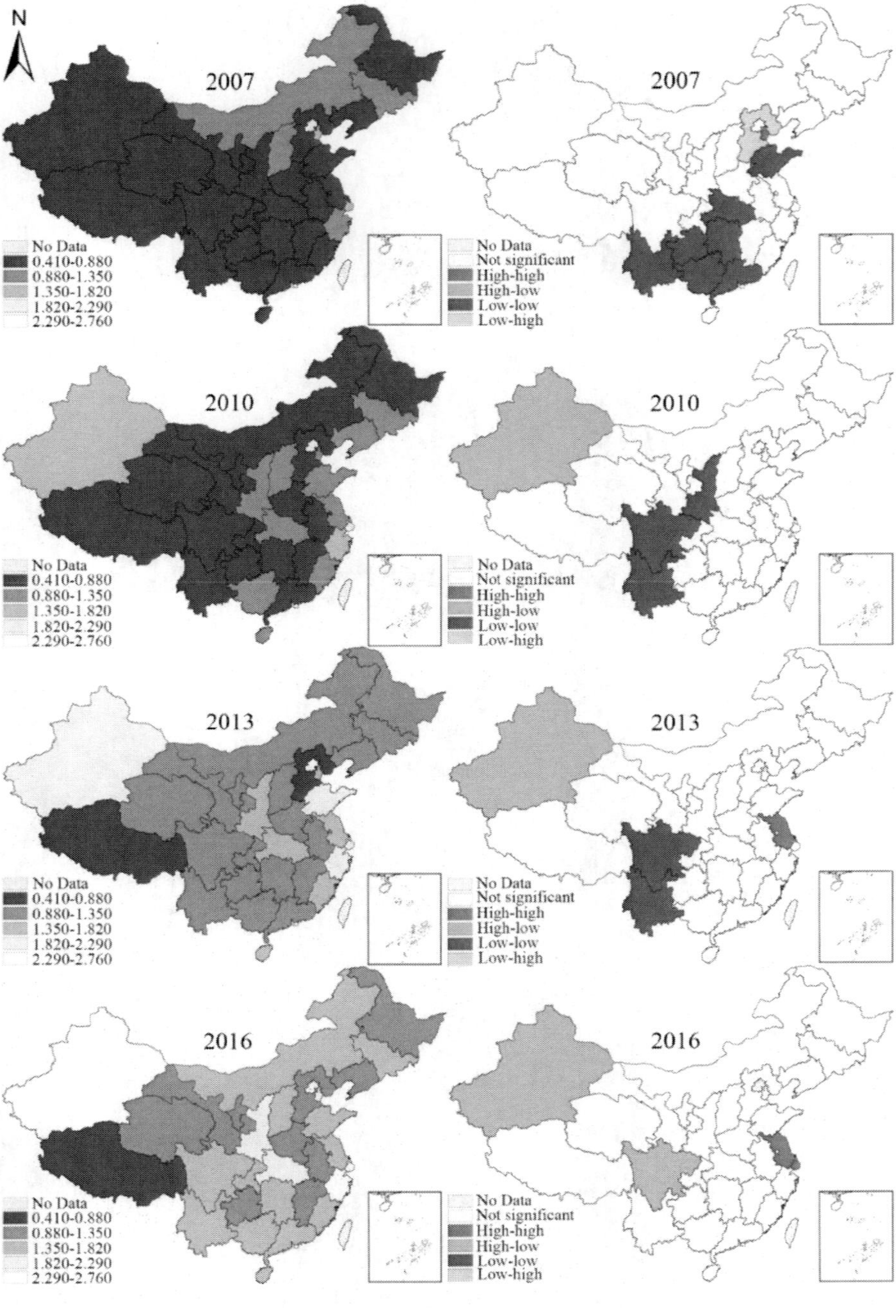

Figure B24. Hierarchical maps and univariate LISA cluster maps of the density of rural registered nurses in 2007, 2010, 2013, and 2016.

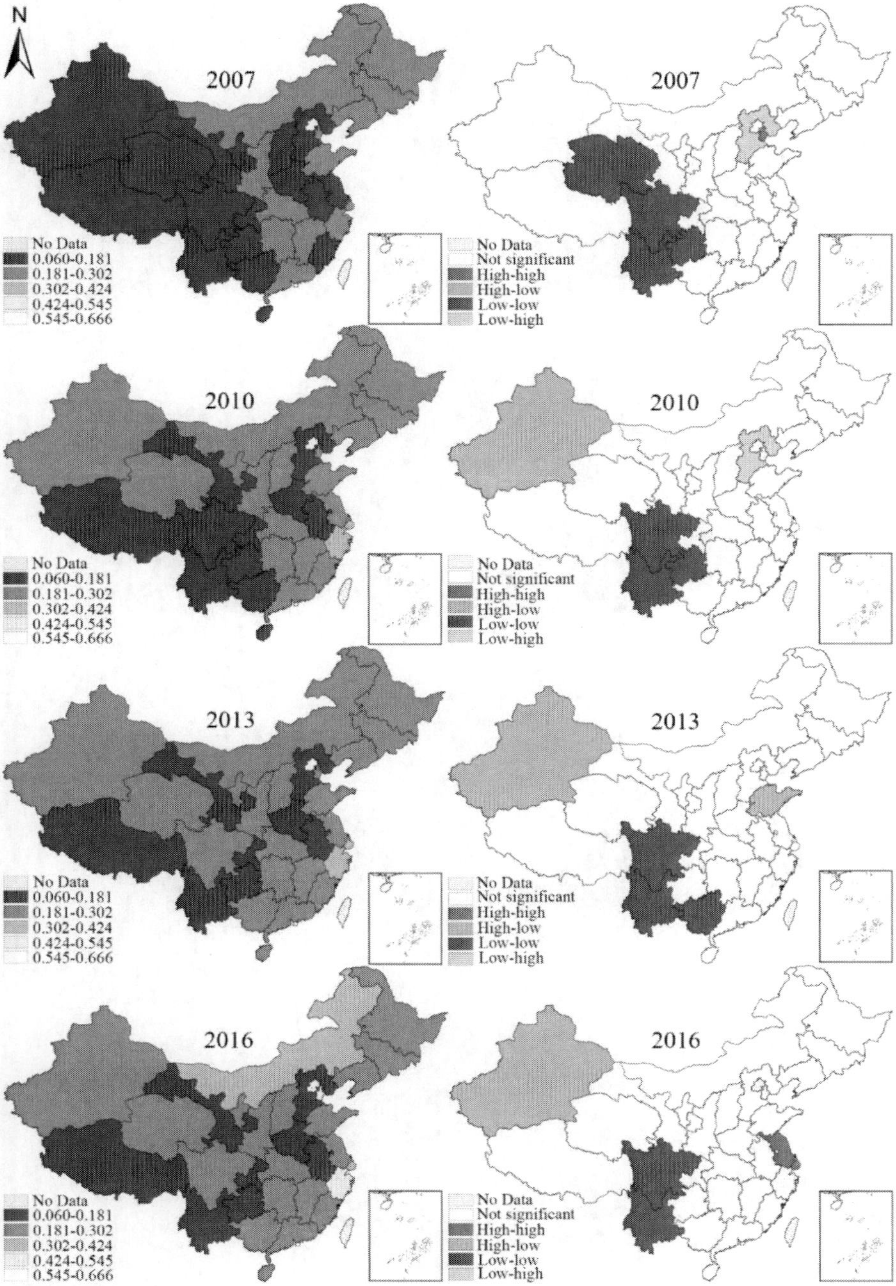

Figure B25. Hierarchical maps and univariate LISA cluster maps of the density of rural pharmacists in 2007, 2010, 2013, and 2016.

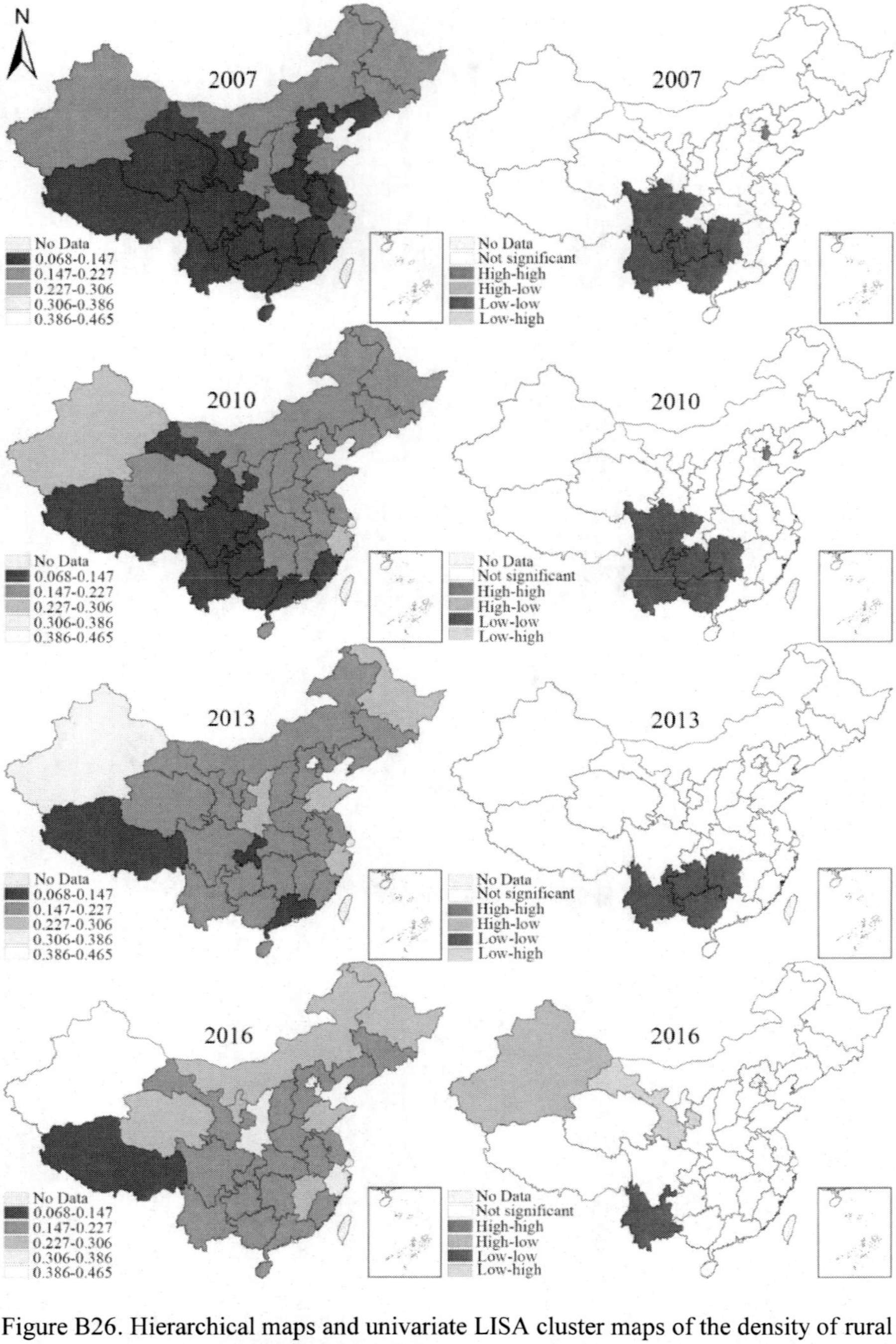

Figure B26. Hierarchical maps and univariate LISA cluster maps of the density of rural technologists in 2007, 2010, 2013, and 2016.

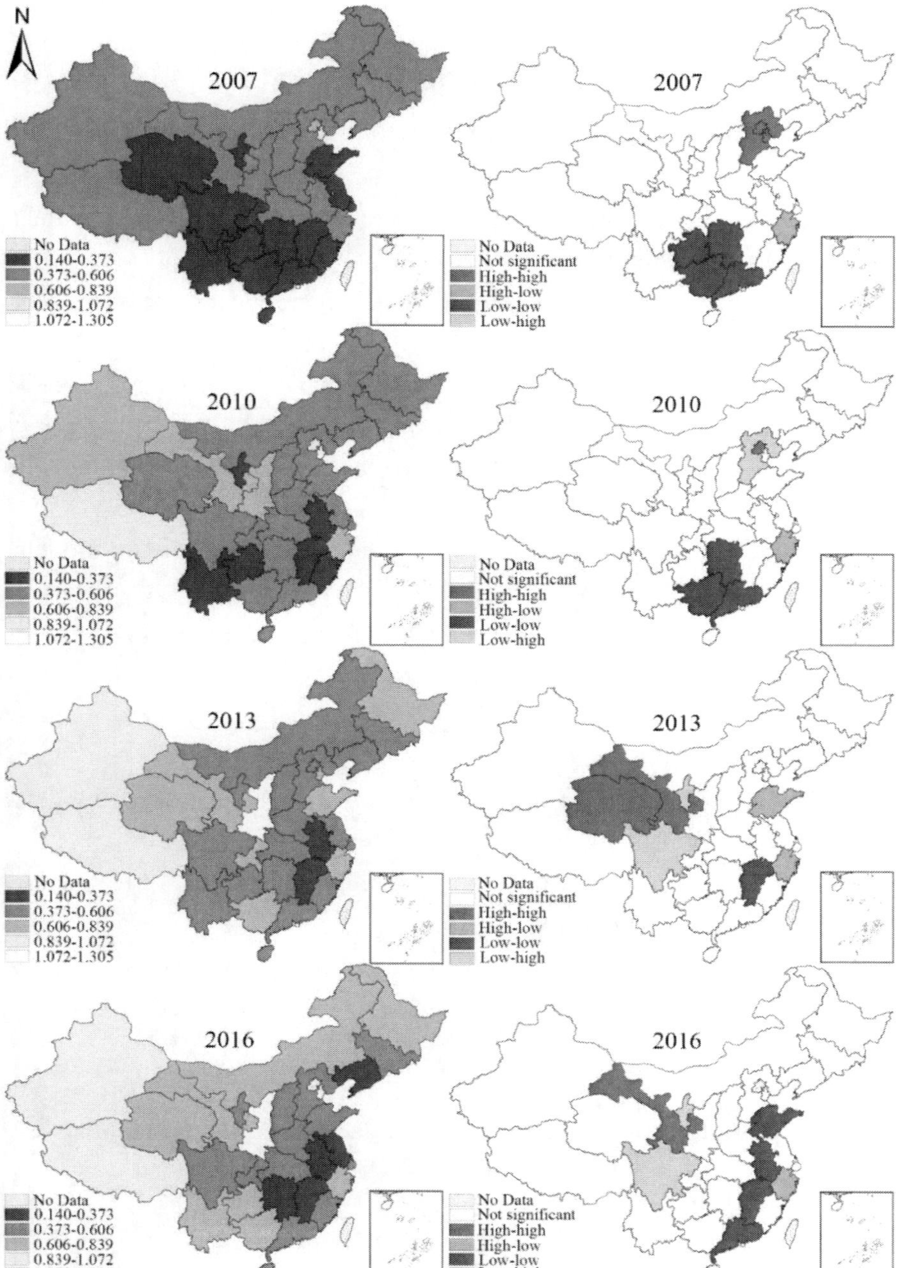

Figure B27. Hierarchical maps and univariate LISA cluster maps of the density of rural interns in 2007, 2010, 2013, and 2016.

APPENDIX C. EMPIRICAL RESULTS OF SPATIAL PANEL ECONOMETRIC MODELS

- Table C1 Estimation results of spatial panel econometric models for licensed doctor density
- Table C2 Estimation results of spatial panel econometric models for clinician density
- Table C3 Estimation results of spatial panel econometric models for traditional Chinese medicine doctor density
- Table C4 Estimation results of spatial panel econometric models for dentist density
- Table C5 Estimation results of spatial panel econometric models for public health doctor density
- Table C6 Estimation results of spatial panel econometric models for general practitioner density
- Table C7 Estimation results of spatial panel econometric models for registered nurse density
- Table C8 Estimation results of spatial panel econometric models for pharmacist density
- Table C9 Estimation results of spatial panel econometric models for technologist density
- Table C10 Estimation results of spatial panel econometric models for intern density

Table C1. Estimation results of spatial panel econometric models for licensed doctor density

Variable	SDPM with spatial fixed effects	SDPM with time fixed effects	SDPM with spatial and time fixed effects	SDPM with random effects	SEPM with spatial fixed effects	SLPM with spatial fixed effects
ln(OV)	**0.570***** **(0.080)**	−0.012 (0.040)	0.556*** (0.081)	0.402*** (0.073)	0.444*** (0.083)	0.370*** (0.080)

ln(IV)	**0.192*****	0.069	0.214***	0.207***	0.243***	0.206***
	(0.038)	(0.042)	(0.040)	(0.036)	(0.040)	(0.043)
ln(GHE)	**0.087****	0.078*	0.116***	0.098**	0.039	0.058
	(0.041)	(0.035)	(0.042)	(0.040)	(0.034)	(0.039)
ln(SHE)	**0.063****	0.225***	0.082***	0.085***	0.075***	0.083***
	(0.026)	(0.026)	(0.027)	(0.028)	(0.024)	(0.025)
ln(MGD)	**0.017**	−0.016	0.018	0.016	0.006	0.027
	(0.016)	(0.023)	(0.016)	(0.017)	(0.018)	(0.018)
W*	**−0.464*****	−0.269***	−0.283	−0.378***		
ln(OV)	**(0.136)**	(0.066)	(0.199)	(0.111)		
W*	**−0.236*****	−0.551***	−0.097	−0.256***		
ln(IV)	**(0.076)**	(0.074)	(0.100)	(0.067)		
W*	**−0.022**	−0.009	0.101	−0.009		
ln(GHE)	**(0.066)**	(0.073)	(0.086)	(0.063)		
W*	**0.036**	0.077	0.080	0.009		
ln(SHE)	**(0.050)**	(0.068)	(0.059)	(0.051)		
W*	**0.065****	0.221***	0.105***	0.068**		
ln(MGD)	**(0.031)**	(0.043)	(0.038)	(0.031)		
ρ	**0.319*****	−0.121	0.180	0.328***		−0.016
	(0.098)	(0.111)	(0.115)	(0.095)		(0.085)
λ					0.409***	
					(0.106)	
LL	**393.2808**	177.5314	397.9772	296.3392	379.0797	373.1585
R_w^2	**0.9119**	0.7198	0.8889	0.9081	0.8929	0.8966
R_b^2	**0.4538**	0.8277	0.4046	0.5305	0.2864	0.3177
R^2	**0.5011**	0.8124	0.4695	0.5787	0.3483	0.3841
Obs	**155**	155	155	155	155	155
Test	**Hausman test** **H_0: difference in coefficients not systematic**				**LR test**	**Wald test**
	$\chi^2(11) = 75.1$ $p = 0.000$				**$\chi^2 = 30.1$ $p = 0.000$**	**$\chi^2 = 44.6$ $p = 0.000$**

Note: Standard error in parentheses, ***p < 0.01, **p < 0.05,*p < 0.1

Table C2. Estimation results of spatial panel econometric models for clinician density

Variable	SDPM with spatial fixed effects (Best Model)	SDPM with time fixed effects	SDPM with spatial and time fixed effects	SDPM with random effects	SEPM with spatial fixed effects	SLPM with spatial fixed effects
ln(OV)	**0.660*****	−0.043	0.633***	0.410***	0.518***	0.426***
	(0.093)	(0.042)	(0.094)	(0.088)	(0.096)	(0.095)
ln(IV)	**0.275*****	0.151***	0.307***	0.302***	0.332***	0.279***
	(0.045)	(0.044)	(0.046)	(0.042)	(0.046)	(0.051)
ln(GHE)	**0.082***	0.022	0.125**	0.083*	0.006	0.035
	(0.048)	(0.038)	(0.049)	(0.046)	(0.039)	(0.045)
ln(SHE)	**0.038**	0.204***	0.062**	0.065**	0.041	0.048*
	(0.030)	(0.027)	(0.031)	(0.032)	(0.027)	(0.029)
ln(MGD)	**0.028**	−0.017	0.029	0.032	0.013	0.032
	(0.019)	(0.024)	(0.018)	(0.020)	(0.020)	(0.021)

Table C2. (Continued)

Variable	SDPM with spatial fixed effects (Best Model)	SDPM with time fixed effects	SDPM with spatial and time fixed effects	SDPM with random effects	SEPM with spatial fixed effects	SLPM with spatial fixed effects
W*	**−0.544*****	−0.150**	−0.364	−0.354***		
ln(OV)	**(0.158)**	(0.067)	(0.228)	(0.129)		
W*	**−0.309*****	−0.664***	−0.112	−0.345***		
ln(IV)	**(0.089)**	(0.079)	(0.120)	(0.078)		
W*	**−0.003**	−0.152**	0.164	0.009		
ln(GHE)	**(0.076)**	(0.076)	(0.101)	(0.073)		
W*	**0.029**	0.078	0.090	0.007		
ln(SHE)	**(0.058)**	(0.070)	(0.069)	(0.059)		
W*	**0.053**	0.178***	0.105**	0.053		
ln(MGD)	**(0.036)**	(0.045)	(0.045)	(0.036)		
ρ	**0.342*****	−0.134	0.191*	0.330***		−0.018
	(0.094)	(0.114)	(0.112)	(0.094)		(0.089)
λ					0.441***	
					(0.100)	
LL	**369.2911**	169.3556	374.6819	273.3824	354.9534	347.3901
R_w^2	**0.8740**	0.1464	0.8223	0.8676	0.8457	0.8508
R_b^2	**0.3642**	0.7997	0.3169	0.4467	0.2194	0.2436
R^2	**0.4095**	0.7078	0.3869	0.4977	0.2752	0.3062
Obs	**155**	155	155	155	155	155
Test	**Hausman test H₀: difference in coefficients not systematic**				**LR test**	**Wald test**
	$\chi^2(11) = 37.2$ $p = 0.000$				**$\chi^2 = 29.6$ $p = 0.000$**	**$\chi^2 = 45.3$ $p = 0.000$**

Note: Standard error in parentheses, ***p < 0.01, **p < 0.05,*p < 0.1

Table C3. Estimation results of spatial panel econometric models for traditional Chinese medicine doctor density

Variable	SDPM with spatial fixed effects	SDPM with time fixed effects	SDPM with spatial and time fixed effects	SDPM with random effects	SEPM with spatial random effects	SLPM with random effects (Best Model)
ln(OV)	0.302**	0.135	0.357***	0.320***	0.180*	**0.193****
	(0.121)	(0.105)	(0.122)	(0.110)	(0.101)	**(0.096)**
ln(IV)	−0.121**	−0.095	−0.139**	−0.130**	−0.079	**−0.092**
	(0.058)	(0.105)	(0.060)	(0.056)	(0.057)	**(0.056)**
ln(GHE)	0.070	0.237**	0.059	0.101	0.202***	**0.135****
	(0.062)	(0.098)	(0.063)	(0.063)	(0.050)	**(0.054)**
ln(SHE)	0.107***	0.174***	0.112***	0.100**	0.186***	**0.157*****
	(0.039)	(0.066)	(0.040)	(0.041)	(0.036)	**(0.036)**
ln(MGD)	−0.009	−0.015	−0.006	−0.018	0.006	**−0.006**
	(0.024)	(0.060)	(0.024)	(0.026)	(0.026)	**(0.025)**

Variable	SDPM with spatial fixed effects	SDPM with time fixed effects	SDPM with spatial and time fixed effects	SDPM with random effects	SEPM with spatial random effects	SLPM with random effects (Best Model)
W* ln(OV)	−0.218 (0.202)	-0.628^{***} (0.163)	0.206 (0.288)	-0.441^{**} (0.181)		
W* ln(IV)	0.013 (0.112)	0.339* (0.197)	−0.029 (0.139)	0.093 (0.105)		
W* ln(GHE)	0.009 (0.098)	0.911^{***} (0.203)	0.010 (0.122)	0.028 (0.100)		
W* ln(SHE)	0.138^{*} (0.078)	0.074 (0.137)	0.086 (0.090)	0.086 (0.081)		
W* ln(MGD)	0.064 (0.046)	0.640^{***} (0.111)	0.096^{*} (0.055)	0.091 (0.048)		
ρ	0.130 (0.113)	0.157 (0.125)	−0.007 (0.128)	0.207* (0.109)		**0.249^{***} (0.093)**
λ					0.109 (0.132)	
LL	337.9338	337.9338	337.9338	337.9338	218.9991	**222.0605**
R_w^2	0.8913	0.8801	0.8826	0.8891	0.8818	**0.8868**
R_b^2	0.2246	0.5406	0.1142	0.3515	0.2351	**0.2019**
R^2	0.2781	0.3401	0.1556	0.3909	0.2863	**0.2551**
Obs	155	155	155	155	155	**155**
Test	**Hausman test** **H_0: difference in coefficients not systematic**				**LR test**	**Wald test**
	$\chi^2(11) = 9.56$ $p = 0.5701$				**$\chi^2 = 12.0$ $p = 0.035$**	**$\chi^2 = 3.6$ $p = 0.462$**

Note: Standard error in parentheses, ***p < 0.01, **p < 0.05,*p < 0.1

Table C4. Estimation results of spatial panel econometric models for dentist density

Variable	SDPM with spatial fixed effects	SDPM with time fixed effects	SDPM with spatial and time fixed effects	SDPM with random effects	SEPM with spatial fixed effects	SLPM with spatial fixed effects
ln(OV)	**0.216 (0.135)**	0.405^{***} (0.086)	0.180 (0.136)	0.317^{***} (0.133)	0.177 (0.117)	0.184 (0.127)
ln(IV)	**−0.011 (0.064)**	-0.301^{***} (0.091)	−0.032 (0.067)	−0.035 (0.066)	0.044 (0.067)	0.040 (0.069)
ln(GHE)	**0.036 (0.069)**	0.046 (0.075)	−0.005 (0.071)	0.031 (0.074)	0.123^{**} (0.053)	0.118^{*} (0.063)
ln(SHE)	**0.223^{***} (0.044)**	0.644^{***} (0.053)	0.206^{***} (0.044)	0.260^{***} (0.049)	0.321^{***} (0.037)	0.301^{***} (0.042)
ln(MGD)	**0.042 (0.028)**	0.205^{***} (0.047)	0.051^{*} (0.028)	0.036 (0.030)	0.095^{***} (0.030)	0.057* (0.029)
W* ln(OV)	**−0.122 (0.226)**	-0.938^{***} (0.141)	−0.473 (0.298)	−0.206 (0.221)		
W* ln(IV)	**0.053 (0.125)**	-1.541^{***} (0.162)	−0.082 (0.154)	−0.082 (0.128)		

Table C4. (Continued)

Variable	SDPM with spatial fixed effects	SDPM with time fixed effects	SDPM with spatial and time fixed effects	SDPM with random effects	SEPM with spatial fixed effects	SLPM with spatial fixed effects
W*	**0.039**	−0.944***	−0.121	−0.040		
ln(GHE)	**(0.112)**	(0.155)	(0.136)	(0.117)		
W*	**0.237*** **	−0.158	0.263***	0.221**		
ln(SHE)	**(0.088)**	(0.160)	(0.101)	(0.097)		
W*	**0.253*** **	−0.180**	0.175***	0.208***		
ln(MGD)	**(0.053)**	(0.089)	(0.062)	(0.058)		
ρ	**−0.301** **	0.060	−0.377***	−0.093		0.063
	(0.125)	(0.110)	(0.127)	(0.125)		(0.089)
λ					−0.274*	
					(0.143)	
LL	**291.0669**	291.0669	291.0669	291.0669	300.4646	298.9125
R_w^2	**0.9263**	0.7547	0.9062	0.9254	0.9136	0.9156
R_b^2	**0.5394**	0.8886	0.6719	0.5896	0.5767	0.5481
R^2	**0.5336**	0.4860	0.6767	0.5978	0.5752	0.5518
Obs	**155**	155	155	155	155	155
Test	**Hausman test**				**LR test**	**Wald test**
	H_0: difference in coefficients not systematic					
	$\chi^2(11) = 25.4$ $p = 0.008$				**$\chi^2 = 26.7$**	**$\chi^2 = 10.6$**
					$p = 0.000$	**$p = 0.031$**

Note: Standard error in parentheses, ***$p < 0.01$,**$p < 0.05$,*$p < 0.1$

Table C5. Estimation results of spatial panel econometric models for public health doctor density

Variable	SDPM with spatial fixed effects (Best Model)	SDPM with time fixed effects	SDPM with spatial and time fixed effects	SDPM with random effects	SEPM with spatial fixed effects	SLPM with spatial fixed effects
ln(OV)	**0.975*** **	−0.127	0.913***	0.671***	0.636***	0.656***
	(0.183)	(0.098)	(0.183)	(0.170)	(0.184)	(0.186)
ln(IV)	**0.359*** **	−0.181*	0.395***	0.343***	0.432***	0.375***
	(0.089)	(0.100)	(0.091)	(0.085)	(0.101)	(0.100)
ln(GHE)	**0.263*** **	0.249***	0.305***	0.361***	−0.079	−0.065
	(0.094)	(0.094)	(0.095)	(0.098)	(0.079)	(0.079)
ln(SHE)	**−0.036**	0.292***	−0.014	−0.011	−0.152***	−0.157***
	(0.060)	(0.063)	(0.060)	(0.063)	(0.055)	(0.055)
ln(MGD)	**0.013**	−0.241***	0.016	−0.008	−0.012	0.003
	(0.036)	(0.055)	(0.036)	(0.039)	(0.041)	(0.039)
W*	**−0.442**	0.011	−0.538	−0.296		
ln(OV)	**(0.307)**	(0.160)	(0.406)	(0.262)		
W*	**−0.487*** **	−0.684***	−0.237	−0.470***		
ln(IV)	**(0.170)**	(0.185)	(0.218)	(0.154)		

Variable	SDPM with spatial fixed effects (Best Model)	SDPM with time fixed effects	SDPM with spatial and time fixed effects	SDPM with random effects	SEPM with spatial fixed effects	SLPM with spatial fixed effects
W*	**−0.178**	−0.724***	0.053	−0.185		
ln(GHE)	**(0.148)**	(0.180)	(0.195)	(0.149)		
W*	**−0.084**	−0.176	0.068	−0.139		
ln(SHE)	**(0.115)**	(0.148)	(0.134)	(0.118)		
W*	**0.085**	−0.272**	0.099	0.076		
ln(MGD)	**(0.070)**	(0.115)	(0.083)	(0.072)		
ρ	**0.167**	−0.105	−0.041	0.198*		−0.042
	(0.102)	(0.129)	(0.124)	(0.103)		(0.107)
λ					0.160	
					(0.116)	
LL	**285.3565**	285.3565	285.3565	285.3565	246.2362	245.3993
R_w^2	**0.4521**	0.0053	0.0868	0.4314	0.2926	0.2993
R_b^2	**0.0588**	0.6268	0.0708	0.1202	0.0486	0.0425
R^2	**0.0647**	0.4018	0.0691	0.1271	0.0369	0.0321
Obs	**155**	155	155	155	155	155
Test	**Hausman test** **H_0: difference in coefficients not systematic**				**LR test**	**Wald test**
	$\chi^2(11) = 42.9$ $p = 0.000$				**$\chi^2 = 36.9$ $p = 0.000$**	**$\chi^2 = 26.1$ $p = 0.000$**

Note: Standard error in parentheses, ***p < 0.01, **p < 0.05,*p < 0.1

Table C6. Estimation results of spatial panel econometric models for general practitioner density

Variable	SDPM with spatial fixed effects	SDPM with time fixed effects	SDPM with spatial and time fixed effects	SDPM with random effects	SEPM with random effects	SLPM with random effects	Non–spatial model with random effects (Best Model)
ln(OV)	0.715	0.326**	−0.213	0.515**	0.558***	0.565***	**0.756*****
	(0.499)	(0.138)	(0.441)	(0.253)	(0.154)	(0.153)	**(0.211)**
ln(IV)	0.525**	0.728***	0.738***	0.693***	0.303***	0.266***	**0.703*****
	(0.238)	(0.142)	(0.216)	(0.175)	(0.102)	(0.097)	**(0.161)**
ln(GHE)	1.001***	−0.347***	0.890***	0.260	0.010	0.015	**0.302****
	(0.257)	(0.127)	(0.226)	(0.208)	(0.083)	(0.082)	**(0.144)**
ln(SHE)	0.307*	0.529***	0.228	0.415***	−0.141**	−0.145**	**0.445*****
	(0.163)	(0.091)	(0.143)	(0.135)	(0.059)	(0.058)	**(0.117)**
ln(MGD)	−0.108	−0.308***	−0.101	−0.052	−0.058	−0.044	**0.013**
	(0.099)	(0.077)	(0.085)	(0.094)	(0.045)	(0.043)	**(0.086)**
W*	0.812	0.389*	−3.292***	0.610			
ln(OV)	(0.883)	(0.222)	(0.953)	(0.449)			
W*	0.787	−0.604**	1.340**	−0.274			
ln(IV)	(0.480)	(0.272)	(0.521)	(0.331)			
W*	0.487	0.167	0.483	0.363			
ln(GHE)	(0.429)	(0.259)	(0.453)	(0.313)			

Variable	SDPM with spatial fixed effects	SDPM with time fixed effects	SDPM with spatial and time fixed effects	SDPM with random effects	SEPM with random effects	SLPM with random effects	Non–spatial model with random effects (Best Model)
W*	−1.086***	0.645***	−0.380	−0.322			
ln(SHE)	(0.322)	(0.216)	(0.317)	(0.265)			
W*	0.528***	0.219	0.024	0.344**			
ln(MGD)	(0.197)	(0.154)	(0.196)	(0.167)			
ρ	−0.059	−0.295**	−0.523***	0.077		−0.003	
	(0.113)	(0.133)	(0.121)	(0.104)		(0.109)	
λ					0.139		
					(0.137)		
LL	227.938	227.938	227.938	37.152	146.344	145.839	
R_w^2	0.8220	0.7354	0.7204	0.8043	0.2739	0.2802	**0.7934**
R_b^2	0.2752	0.7602	0.0434	0.6558	0.0022	0.0021	**0.6463**
R^2	0.3682	0.7536	0.0073	0.6898	0.0006	0.0006	**0.6797**
Obs	155	155	155	155	155	155	**155**
Test	**Hausman test**				**LR test**	**Wald test**	**Hausman test**
	H₀: difference in coefficients not systematic						
	$\chi^2(11) = 12.0$ $p = 0.368$				**$\chi^2 = 5.9$ $p = 0.318$**	**$\chi^2 = 6.1$ $p = 0.196$**	**$\chi^2(5) = 1.5$ $p = 0.909$**

Note: Standard error in parentheses, ***p < 0.01,**p < 0.05, *p < 0.1

Table C7. Estimation results of spatial panel econometric models for registered nurse density

Variable	SDPM with spatial fixed effects (Best Model)	SDPM with time fixed effects	SDPM with spatial and time fixed effects	SDPM with random effects	SEPM with spatial fixed effects	SLPM with spatial fixed effects
ln(OV)	**0.442*****	0.041	0.379***	0.274***	0.381***	0.186*
	(0.116)	(0.054)	(0.118)	(0.102)	(0.114)	(0.110)
ln(IV)	**0.309*****	0.541***	0.371***	0.393***	0.338***	0.374***
	(0.055)	(0.057)	(0.059)	(0.056)	(0.054)	(0.059)
ln(GHE)	**0.172*****	0.128**	0.202***	0.124**	0.229***	0.106**
	(0.059)	(0.051)	(0.061)	(0.059)	(0.047)	(0.054)
ln(SHE)	**0.050**	0.288***	0.076**	0.125***	0.098***	0.082**
	(0.037)	(0.034)	(0.039)	(0.044)	(0.034)	(0.035)
ln(MGD)	**0.006**	0.042	0.004	0.030	0.010	0.022
	(0.023)	(0.030)	(0.023)	(0.025)	(0.024)	(0.024)
W*	**−0.593*****	0.179**	−0.697***	−0.225		
ln(OV)	**(0.190)**	(0.086)	(0.257)	(0.168)		
W*	**−0.146**	−0.904***	0.084	−0.262**		
ln(IV)	**(0.115)**	(0.119)	(0.149)	(0.107)		
W*	**−0.197****	−0.595***	−0.081	−0.109		
ln(GHE)	**(0.096)**	(0.100)	(0.122)	(0.095)		
W*	**0.103**	−0.246***	0.222**	0.040		
ln(SHE)	**(0.072)**	(0.092)	(0.086)	(0.077)		

Variable	SDPM with spatial fixed effects (Best Model)	SDPM with time fixed effects	SDPM with spatial and time fixed effects	SDPM with random effects	SEPM with spatial fixed effects	SLPM with spatial fixed effects
W*	**0.095****	−0.019	0.118**	0.058		
ln(MGD)	**(0.044)**	(0.058)	(0.053)	(0.046)		
ρ	**0.567*****	0.111	0.500***	0.447***		0.317***
	(0.087)	(0.121)	(0.094)	(0.098)		(0.072)
λ					0.569***	
					(0.094)	
LL	**331.9073**	128.5232	335.4882	234.3942	325.4707	320.6228
R_w^2	**0.9233**	0.6425	0.9164	0.9248	0.9247	0.9253
R_b^2	**0.4670**	0.8506	0.3157	0.6269	0.4174	0.4549
R^2	**0.5525**	0.3496	0.3797	0.6800	0.5104	0.5339
Obs	**155**	155	155	155	155	155
Test	**Hausman test**				**LR test**	**Wald test**
	H_0: difference in coefficients not systematic					
	$\chi^2(11) = 36.7$ $p = 0.000$				**$\chi^2 = 13.0$ $p = 0.024$**	**$\chi^2 = 25.1$ $p = 0.000$**

Note: Standard error in parentheses, ***p < 0.01, **p < 0.05, *p < 0.1

Table C8. Estimation results of spatial panel econometric models for pharmacist density

Variable	SDPM with spatial fixed effects	SDPM with time fixed effects	SDPM with spatial and time fixed effects	SDPM with random effects	SEPM with spatial fixed effects (Best Model)	SLPM with spatial fixed effects
ln(OV)	0.569***	0.128***	0.542***	0.506***	**0.536*****	0.412***
	(0.117)	(0.074)	(0.119)	(0.104)	**(0.113)**	(0.107)
ln(IV)	0.077	0.225***	0.138**	0.089	**0.105***	0.094*
	(0.056)	(0.077)	(0.060)	(0.054)	**(0.054)**	(0.057)
ln(GHE)	−0.082	0.144**	−0.037	−0.038	**0.015**	−0.050
	(0.060)	(0.069)	(0.062)	(0.062)	**(0.047)**	(0.048)
ln(SHE)	0.001	0.301***	0.033	0.048	**0.054**	0.045
	(0.038)	(0.048)	(0.039)	(0.042)	**(0.033)**	(0.032)
ln(MGD)	0.026	−0.023	0.021	0.024	**0.033**	0.022
	(0.023)	(0.041)	(0.023)	(0.025)	**(0.024)**	(0.023)
W*	−0.382*	−0.041	−0.220	−0.286*		
ln(OV)	(0.195)	(0.115)	(0.271)	(0.171)		
W*	−0.158	−0.691***	0.094	−0.181*		
ln(IV)	(0.110)	(0.141)	(0.144)	(0.101)		
W*	0.028	−0.467***	0.200*	0.023		
ln(GHE)	(0.094)	(0.141)	(0.121)	(0.095)		
W*	0.119	−0.222**	0.206**	0.060		
ln(SHE)	(0.073)	(0.111)	(0.087)	(0.077)		
W*	0.010	0.028	0.072	0.005		
ln(MGD)	(0.045)	(0.081)	(0.054)	(0.047)		
ρ	0.547***	0.250**	0.447***	0.469***		0.459***
	(0.087)	(0.110)	(0.100)	(0.094)		(0.086)

Table C8. (Continued)

Variable	SDPM with spatial fixed effects	SDPM with time fixed effects	SDPM with spatial and time fixed effects	SDPM with random effects	SEPM with spatial fixed effects (Best Model)	SLPM with spatial fixed effects
Λ					**0.519*****	
					(0.092)	
LL	329.5666	77.6135	334.6586	229.0749	**324.6614**	323.6405
R_w^2	0.7199	0.5596	0.6946	0.7220	**0.7224**	0.7090
R_b^2	0.3585	0.6920	0.3099	0.4149	**0.3704**	0.3083
R^2	0.3774	0.4257	0.2738	0.4317	**0.3890**	0.3291
Obs	155	155	155	155	**155**	155
Test	**Hausman test**				**LR test**	**Wald test**
	H_0: difference in coefficients not systematic					
	$\chi^2(11) = 24.0$ $p = 0.013$				**$\chi^2 = 9.5$**	**$\chi^2 = 12.6$**
					$p = 0.091$	**$p = 0.013$**

Note: Standard error in parentheses, ***p < 0.01, **p < 0.05, *p < 0.1

Table C9. Estimation results of spatial panel econometric models for technologist density

Variable	SDPM with spatial fixed effects (Best Model)	SDPM with time fixed effects	SDPM with spatial and time fixed effects	SDPM with random effects	SEPM with spatial fixed effects	SLPM with spatial fixed effects
ln(OV)	**0.438*****	−0.049	0.389***	0.279***	0.382***	0.234**
	(0.105)	(0.052)	(0.105)	(0.097)	(0.108)	(0.097)
ln(IV)	**0.048**	0.370***	0.114**	0.099**	0.091*	0.079
	(0.050)	(0.056)	(0.053)	(0.050)	(0.051)	(0.052)
ln(GHE)	**−0.074**	0.227***	−0.020	−0.035	0.058	−0.053
	(0.054)	(0.049)	(0.055)	(0.056)	(0.046)	(0.045)
ln(SHE)	**0.034**	0.201***	0.070**	0.084**	0.109***	0.089***
	(0.034)	(0.034)	(0.035)	(0.039)	(0.034)	(0.030)
ln(MGD)	**0.050****	0.024	0.048**	0.057**	0.060***	0.053**
	(0.021)	(0.029)	(0.020)	(0.023)	(0.023)	(0.021)
W*	**−0.465*****	−0.005	−0.390*	−0.268*		
ln(OV)	**(0.173)**	(0.088)	(0.234)	(0.154)		
W*	**−0.140**	−0.823**	0.122	−0.186**		
ln(IV)	**(0.099)**	(0.104)	(0.128)	(0.092)		
W*	**−0.035**	−0.405**	0.160	0.012		
ln(GHE)	**(0.084)**	(0.097)	(0.107)	(0.086)		
W*	**0.162****	−0.064	0.274***	0.082		
ln(SHE)	**(0.066)**	(0.083)	(0.078)	(0.072)		
W*	**0.037**	−0.009	0.102**	0.018		
ln(MGD)	**(0.040)**	(0.057)	(0.049)	(0.043)		
ρ	**0.617*****	0.071	0.512***	0.501***		0.546***
	(0.077)	(0.117)	(0.089)	(0.092)		(0.076)

Variable	SDPM with spatial fixed effects (Best Model)	SDPM with time fixed effects	SDPM with spatial and time fixed effects	SDPM with random effects	SEPM with spatial fixed effects	SLPM with spatial fixed effects
Λ					0.591***	
					(0.098)	
LL	**368.0546**	368.0546	368.0546	368.0546	331.9851	335.4246
R_w^2	**0.8312**	0.3832	0.8296	0.8404	0.8361	0.8328
R_b^2	**0.2543**	0.7656	0.2328	0.3705	0.3070	0.2112
R^2	**0.3157**	0.4898	0.2865	0.4357	0.3671	0.2823
Obs	**155**	155	155	155	155	155
Test	**Hausman test**				**LR test**	**Wald test**
	H$_0$: difference in coefficients not systematic					
	$\chi^2(11) = 24.0$ $p = 0.013$				**$\chi^2 = 22.7$**	**$\chi^2 = 20.0$**
					$p = 0.000$	**$p = 0.001$**

Note: Standard error in parentheses, ***p < 0.01, **p < 0.05, *p < 0.1

Table C10. Estimation results of spatial panel econometric models for intern density

Variable	SDPM with spatial fixed effects	SDPM with time fixed effects	SDPM with spatial and time fixed effects	SDPM with random effects (Best Model)	SEPM with random effects	SLPM with random effects
ln(OV)	0.639***	0.238**	0.497**	**0.450*** **	0.167**	0.153*
	(0.232)	(0.103)	(0.234)	**(0.156)**	(0.084)	(0.079)
ln(IV)	−0.100	−0.166	0.103	**−0.109**	0.141***	0.111**
	(0.111)	(0.106)	(0.121)	**(0.092)**	(0.046)	(0.049)
ln(GHE)	0.100	0.487***	0.146	**0.204* **	0.044	−0.034
	(0.119)	(0.096)	(0.120)	**(0.105)**	(0.043)	(0.046)
ln(SHE)	−0.027	0.085	0.036	**0.019**	0.150***	0.120***
	(0.075)	(0.067)	(0.076)	**(0.072)**	(0.035)	(0.034)
ln(MGD)	0.023	0.117**	0.005	**0.028**	0.065***	0.054**
	(0.046)	(0.057)	(0.045)	**(0.046)**	(0.023)	(0.023)
W*	−0.368	−0.605***	−0.550	**−0.374**		
ln(OV)	(0.385)	(0.163)	(0.507)	**(0.251)**		
W*	0.451**	0.089	1.092***	**0.351** **		
ln(IV)	(0.215)	(0.195)	(0.273)	**(0.167)**		
W*	0.034	0.414**	0.232	**0.115**		
ln(GHE)	(0.189)	(0.200)	(0.241)	**(0.168)**		
W*	−0.196	−0.292**	0.087	**−0.299** **		
ln(SHE)	(0.148)	(0.135)	(0.169)	**(0.135)**		
W*	−0.036	−0.049	0.034	**−0.064**		
ln(MGD)	(0.088)	(0.111)	(0.105)	**(0.084)**		
ρ	0.345***	−0.047	0.158	**0.340*** **		0.414***
	(0.097)	(0.119)	(0.114)	**(0.097)**		(0.089)
λ					0.542***	
					(0.105)	
LL	368.0546	368.0546	368.0546	**368.0546**	241.3807	**239.3328**
R_w^2	0.1733	0.0526	0.0604	**0.1572**	0.8371	0.8404

Table C10. (Continued)

Variable	SDPM with spatial fixed effects	SDPM with time fixed effects	SDPM with spatial and time fixed effects	SDPM with random effects (Best Model)	SEPM with random effects	SLPM with random effects
R_b^2	0.0739	0.4866	0.0972	**0.3199**	0.4389	0.3076
R^2	0.0765	0.4048	0.0523	**0.3116**	0.4963	0.3832
Obs	155	155	155	**155**	155	155
Test	**Hausman test** **H_0: difference in coefficients not systematic**				**LR test**	**Wald test**
	$\chi^2(11) = 10.8$ $p = 0.462$				**$\chi^2 = 13.7$ $p = 0.018$**	**$\chi^2 = 13.0$ $p = 0.011$**

Note: Standard error in parentheses, ***p < 0.01, ** p < 0.05, * p < 0.1

ABOUT THE AUTHORS

Dr. Bin Zhu

Post-doc Scholar

City University of Hong Kong; Xi'an Jiaotong University;

University of California, San Diego

Bin Zhu is a post-doctoral scholar of University of California, San Diego. He received the doctor degree of management sciences from Xi'an Jiaotong University and doctor degree of Philosophy from City University of Hong Kong. He does research with spatial statistics, spatial epidemiology and spatial econometrics. He has published articles on topics of health workforce distribution and notifiable infectious diseases in China. He received national scholarship from the Ministry of Education of the PRC twice. He was awarded the Peter Ho Conference Scholarship, Travel Fellowship Award of the China Health Policy and Management Society (CHPAMS), Best Paper Prize of China Health Insurance Research Association Annual Conference and Best Paper Prize of China Aging Industry and filial piety culture forum. This book was mainly adopted from his PhD thesis.

Dr. Ying Mao

Professor
Xi'an Jiaotong University

Prof. Ying Mao is a tenured professor of School of Public Policy and Administration, Xi'an Jiaotong University. She received her Bachelor and Master degree in Medical Science from Fudan University, and she obtained her PhD degree in Laws from Xi'an Jiaotong University. She has undertaken more than 100 international, national or provincial projects including one national project funded by the National Social Science Foundation. She has published 11 books and teaching materials and won 5 Ministerial and Provincial-Level Science and Technology Awards. She has supervised almost 80 PhD students and master students. Her research focuses on health security, including health policy and health technology assessment (HTA), health insurance policy and evaluation, regional health planning, healthy city, medical burden of the aging. She also took up several positions like the executive director of China Health Insurance Research Association; vice president of Shaanxi Health Insurance Research Association, China; deputy director of Economic and Social Committee in China Democratic League; and a consultant to Shaanxi Provincial Government, China.

Dr. Chih-Wei Hsieh

Assistant Professor
City University of Hong Kong

Dr. Chih-Wei Hsieh is an assistant professor of Department of Public Policy, City University of Hong Kong. He holds Ph.D in public administration from the Askew School of Public Administration and Policy, Florida State University. Before joining CityU in July 2014, he was Assistant Professor of Public Administration at the University of New Mexico in the United States. He has published articles on topics of emotional labor, public service motivation, and workplace diversity.

INDEX

A

access, 14, 15
accessibility, 32, 33, 115, 123
air pollutants, 21, 116
Albania, 18, 148
annual rate, 62, 68, 75

B

Bangladesh, 18, 137
Beijing, 52, 53, 54, 55, 56, 57, 62, 64, 65, 67, 69, 71, 72, 73, 74, 76, 114, 146, 151, 155, 156, 157, 158, 159, 160, 161, 162, 163, 164, 165, 166, 167, 168, 169, 170, 171, 172, 173, 174, 175, 180, 181, 182, 183, 184
benefits, 21, 118, 122
brain, 10, 114, 120, 131, 134
brain drain, 10, 114, 120, 131, 134

C

challenges, 4, 128
China, 1, 2, 3, 4, 5, 6, 7, 8, 9, 10, 11, 12, 13, 18, 20, 21, 25, 27, 28, 31, 32, 33, 35, 38, 39, 40, 45, 51, 53, 56, 57, 60, 61, 62, 66, 68, 71, 78, 81, 85, 89, 92, 93, 95, 112, 113, 114, 115, 116, 117, 118, 119, 121, 122, 124, 127, 128, 129, 130, 131, 132, 134, 136, 138, 139, 140, 141, 142, 143, 144, 145, 146, 147, 148, 149, 150, 151, 152, 154, 172, 221, 222
Chinese government, 3, 128
Chinese medicine, 3, 34, 210, 212
cities, 4, 136
classification, 2, 3, 118, 119
clustering, 11, 21, 31, 35, 39, 78, 81, 85, 88, 91, 92, 113, 115, 116, 118, 119, 128, 129, 133
clusters, 36, 38, 39, 60, 61, 62, 63, 64, 66, 67, 68, 69, 70, 71, 72, 73, 74, 75, 76, 81, 86, 88, 116, 118, 128, 131, 176, 180
collaboration, 125, 130
community, 5, 19
competition, 28, 123
composition, 116, 119, 127
culture, 22, 221

D

data availability, 120, 134, 136
defects, 6, 8

dentist, 62, 66, 105, 106, 120, 210, 213
dependent variable, 41, 42, 44, 45, 46, 95, 98
depth, 9, 12, 31, 134
developing countries, 1, 3
diseases, 21, 116, 123, 132, 133, 221
distribution, 4, 5, 6, 7, 8, 9, 10, 11, 12, 13, 14, 15, 16, 17, 18, 19, 20, 21, 22, 23, 24, 25, 28, 31, 33, 35, 37, 38, 39, 41, 51, 53, 56, 57, 60, 88, 93, 95, 103, 113, 114, 116, 118, 121, 124, 127, 128, 129, 130, 131, 132, 133, 134, 135, 136, 221
diversity, 135, 222
doctors, 2, 3, 4, 5, 10, 18, 33, 43, 53, 54, 57, 60, 61, 62, 66, 67, 68, 72, 74, 78, 79, 80, 81, 82, 83, 85, 86, 89, 90, 91, 98, 99, 100, 101, 102, 103, 104, 105, 106, 108, 111, 118, 119, 120, 123, 129, 130, 132, 153, 154, 156, 158, 164, 169, 176, 177, 180, 181, 182, 183, 193, 199, 205

E

economic indicator, 17, 18
education, 20, 27, 29, 42, 44, 103, 109, 115, 117, 122, 128, 129, 132, 134
empirical studies, 14, 18, 23
enrollment, 27, 121
epidemiology, 21, 133, 221
equity, 5, 6, 9, 13, 14, 15, 16, 17, 18, 19, 20, 93, 133
evidence, 9, 21, 128, 129

F

Fiji, 18, 150
financial, 24, 27, 123, 132, 133
formula, 16, 37, 46, 47
funds, 125

G

GDP, 5, 22
general practitioner, 18, 33, 43, 53, 63, 67, 82, 83, 98, 103, 104, 130, 210, 215
geography, 5, 119, 133, 134, 135
governments, 10, 42
gross domestic product, 5, 22
growth, 57, 60, 62, 68, 70, 71, 108, 113, 123
growth rate, 62, 70
Guangdong, 52, 54, 55, 56, 71, 72, 73, 76, 78, 81, 88, 89, 92, 155, 156, 157, 158, 159, 160, 161, 162, 163, 164, 165, 166, 167, 168, 169, 170, 171, 172, 173, 174, 175, 180, 181, 182, 183, 184

H

health care, 14, 22, 42, 117, 129, 131
health education, 3, 123
health expenditure, 10, 12, 22, 27, 42, 43, 100, 102, 104, 105, 106, 110, 111, 112, 122, 123, 124, 130, 136, 155, 173, 174
health insurance, 121, 222
health manpower distribution, 5, 6, 7, 8, 9, 10, 11, 12, 13, 14, 15, 16, 17, 18, 19, 20, 21, 22, 23, 24, 25, 28, 31, 33, 35, 38, 39, 40, 41, 51, 56, 57, 60, 68, 71, 77, 84, 88, 95, 103, 113, 114, 116, 121, 124, 127, 128, 129, 130, 132, 133, 134, 135, 136, 148
health services, 14, 15, 23, 26, 41, 100, 107, 108, 111, 120, 121, 123, 124, 129
health status, 14, 23, 26
health workforce, 1, 18, 24, 129, 137, 139, 140, 141, 142, 147, 148, 149, 150, 151, 152, 221
health workforce distribution, 18, 129, 152, 221
Hong Kong, 32, 221, 222
human, 1, 6, 44, 127, 131, 132

human resources, 1, 6, 127, 132
human resources for health, 1, 127
hypothesis, 28, 29

I

ideal, 15, 26
imbalances, 9, 22, 25, 41, 57, 114, 117, 118, 128, 132
income, 15, 16, 17, 19, 119
income inequality, 15, 19
independent variable, 12, 44, 45, 46, 48, 95, 98, 99, 101, 102, 103, 104, 105, 106, 109, 112, 136
indirect effect, 46, 47
industry, 42, 129
inequality, 5, 18
inequity, 5, 17, 19, 20
institutions, 26, 27, 41, 42, 115, 119, 120, 131, 132
investment, 23, 27, 28, 29, 42, 43, 100, 102, 111, 122, 123, 124, 130, 134
Iran, 18, 142
issues, 1, 134

J

Jamaica, 24, 145
job satisfaction, 23

L

labor force, 42
labor market, 9, 23, 24, 25, 112, 122, 124, 125, 130, 133
lead, 101, 102, 104, 105, 106, 119
location information, 17, 18
Lorenz curve, 5, 15, 17, 18
Luo, 19, 147, 150

M

management, 3, 119, 221
matrix, 37, 45, 47, 49
matter, 124, 135, 136
measurement, 14, 16, 43, 120
medical, 3, 10, 12, 19, 23, 26, 27, 42, 43, 101, 102, 105, 106, 109, 112, 117, 119, 120, 121, 122, 124, 129, 131, 132, 134, 136, 155, 175, 222
methodology, 31, 96, 98
Mexico, 18, 222
models, 10, 11, 12, 13, 23, 31, 44, 45, 46, 47, 48, 49, 95, 96, 97, 98, 99, 119, 124, 129, 210, 211, 212, 213, 214, 215, 216, 217, 218, 219
motivation, 23, 26, 222

N

neglect, 9, 19
null, 35, 98
null hypothesis, 35, 98
nurses, 2, 3, 4, 5, 10, 18, 19, 33, 43, 53, 57, 60, 61, 68, 74, 78, 79, 80, 85, 86, 90, 91, 98, 99, 100, 101, 102, 103, 108, 110, 111, 118, 119, 122, 129, 132, 153, 154, 160, 164, 169, 176, 177, 180, 182, 194, 200, 206

O

opportunities, 14, 120
outpatient, 12, 41, 43, 99, 101, 103, 105, 106, 107, 108, 112, 119, 120, 124, 129, 136
outpatients, 112, 129

P

physicians, 18, 22, 132
policy, 5, 10, 12, 13, 115, 116, 127, 129, 130, 131, 222
policy makers, 10, 13, 127, 130
population, 2, 5, 16, 17, 19, 20, 22, 23, 24, 26, 33, 41, 42, 43, 52, 53, 57, 96, 120, 121, 132, 133, 154, 162, 167, 172
population size, 5, 19, 24, 33, 42
positive correlation, 108, 110
positive relationship, 27, 100
PRC, 2, 3, 4, 33, 42, 122, 146, 221
principles, 14, 96
professionals, 2, 3, 118
profit, 27, 123
protection, 122, 132
public health, 3, 10, 21, 27, 33, 43, 53, 62, 67, 81, 82, 83, 98, 103, 104, 106, 108, 109, 111, 123, 130, 210, 214

Q

quotas, 10, 133

R

rate of change, 35, 36, 60
rationality, 10, 112, 115, 129
reality, 25, 26
reform, 19, 122
Reform, 5, 144, 151
regionalization, 117, 128
regression, 44, 45, 108, 110
requirements, 118, 119, 121, 128
researchers, 15, 47
resource management, 1, 131
resources, 1, 4, 14, 17, 20
rural areas, 56, 93, 114, 115, 118
rural population, 117

S

school, 3, 42
services, 1, 4, 12, 23, 26, 27, 41, 43, 107, 108, 119, 120, 121, 123, 129
shortage, 3, 4, 23, 93, 113, 114, 116, 117, 125, 128
significance level, 39, 98, 99, 102, 104, 105
social capital, 27, 123, 133
space-time, 11, 35, 36, 40, 60, 61, 62, 66, 68, 69, 71, 74, 133
spatial distribution, 6, 7, 9, 10, 11, 20, 21, 31, 33, 37, 38, 93, 127, 128
spatial econometrics, 7, 8, 138, 140, 144, 221
spatial location, 9, 19
spatial-temporal dynamics, 9, 11, 21, 31, 32, 127
spillover effects, 7, 8, 9, 12, 26, 28, 29, 44, 46, 101, 102, 105, 107, 108, 109, 110, 111, 112, 113, 120, 122, 124, 129, 130, 134, 136
spillovers, 9, 44, 136
state, 18, 29
statistics, 7, 8, 9, 10, 11, 20, 21, 31, 35, 36, 51, 60, 95, 96, 99, 101, 103, 104, 105, 106, 120, 121, 133, 149, 221
stock, 10, 25, 26, 27, 28, 29, 100, 113, 115, 128, 130, 131, 134, 153, 154, 155, 156, 157, 158, 159, 160, 161, 162, 163, 164, 165, 166, 168, 169, 170, 171, 172
structure, 13, 46
subgroups, 16, 17
Sun, 19, 120, 147, 148
supply chain, 23, 27
Sustainable Development, 1, 146, 148
Switzerland, 149, 150

T

target, 33, 46, 111, 114, 122

technician, 34, 43, 56, 62, 64, 68, 69, 71, 73, 75, 76, 77, 88, 97, 99, 100, 101, 102, 103, 110, 122, 176, 186, 187, 188, 189, 190, 191
technology, 20, 222
training, 27, 122, 128
treatment, 14, 41, 120

U

United Nations, 1, 22, 148
United States, 22, 141, 222
universities, 10, 133
urban, 5, 12, 18, 33, 41, 55, 56, 57, 59, 60, 68, 69, 70, 73, 74, 75, 84, 85, 86, 87, 88, 93, 114, 115, 117, 128, 131, 132, 175, 176, 177, 179, 188, 189, 198, 199, 200, 201, 202, 203
urban areas, 93, 114, 115
USA, 40, 49

V

variables, 11, 23, 42, 43, 45, 46, 48, 95, 96, 98, 99, 112, 129, 136
variations, 18, 35, 51, 60, 113, 115, 121, 133
vector, 45, 46
visualization, 17, 20

W

well-being, 14, 130
WHO, 1, 3, 13, 14, 15, 23, 33, 119, 121, 123, 142, 149, 150
workers, 1, 2, 3, 4, 5, 15, 22, 23, 24, 25, 26, 27, 28, 29, 32, 42, 113, 115, 121, 123, 124, 130, 131, 132, 133, 136
workforce, 1, 18, 19, 24, 27, 119, 129, 221
workload, 119, 120, 121
workplace, 122, 222
World Bank, 22, 25, 145
World Health Organization, 2, 139, 140, 146
worldwide, 1, 117